THE
TREMATODES

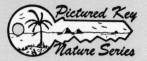

How To Know

THE
TREMATODES

Stewart C. Schell

University of Idaho

WM. C. BROWN COMPANY PUBLISHERS
Dubuque, Iowa

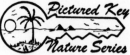

Copyright © 1970 by
Wm. C. Brown Company Publishers
Library of Congress Catalog Card Number 70-89537
SBN 697—04860—8 (Paper)
SBN 697—04861—6 (Cloth)

THE PICTURED-KEY NATURE SERIES

How To Know The—

AQUATIC PLANTS, Prescott, 1969
BEETLES, Jaques, 1951
BUTTERFLIES, Ehrlich, 1961
CACTI, Dawson, 1963
EASTERN LAND SNAILS, Burch, 1962
ECONOMIC PLANTS, Jaques, 1948, 1958
FALL FLOWERS, Cuthbert, 1948
FRESHWATER ALGAE, Prescott, 1954, 1970
FRESHWATER FISHES, Eddy, 1957, 1969
GRASSES, Pohl, 1953, 1968
GRASSHOPPERS, Helfer, 1963
IMMATURE INSECTS, Chu, 1949
INSECTS, Jaques, 1947
LAND BIRDS, Jaques, 1947
LICHENS, Hale, 1969
LIVING THINGS, Jaques, 1946
MAMMALS, Booth, 1949
MARINE ISOPOD CRUSTACEANS, Schultz, 1969
MOSSES AND LIVERWORTS, Conard, 1944, 1956
PLANT FAMILIES, Jaques, 1948
POLLEN AND SPORES, Kapp, 1969
PROTOZOA, Jahn, 1949
SEAWEEDS, Dawson, 1956
SPIDERS, Kaston, 1952
SPRING FLOWERS, Cuthbert, 1943, 1949
TAPEWORMS, Schmidt, 1970
TREMATODES, Schell, 1970
TREES, Jaques, 1946
WATER BIRDS, Jaques-Ollivier, 1960
WEEDS, Jaques, 1959
WESTERN TREES, Baerg, 1955

Printed in United States of America

PREFACE

"How to Know the Trematodes" is meant to serve as an identification manual for the undergraduate or graduate student in parasitology, the embryo parasitologist or any biologist who might find the study of trematodes interesting. It is hoped that the book will be informative and serve as a stimulus for collection and for research on the biology of trematodes. The work is restricted to the families and genera of trematodes known to occur in North America north of Mexico. Barring a few exceptions, the trematode parasites of deep-sea animals are excluded.

The classification followed for the higher categories of the Subclass Digenea is that outlined by La Rue (1957). For those of the Subclasses Monogenea and Aspidogastrea, the plan presented by Yamaguti (1963) is followed. This classification of the Monogenea is a combination of that set forth by E. W. Price (in numerous papers) and by S. Yamaguti (1963).

Sizeable gaps exist in our knowledge of the life cycles of trematodes. Less than 20 are known for the monogenetic trematodes. Several hundred are known for the digenetic trematodes but there are still a number of families in which no life cycles have been investigated. With increased knowledge of life cycles, a more satisfactory system of classification can be devised as phylogenetic relationship is based largely on similarity in anatomy of the larval stages. However, it is important to realize that an improved system of classification is not likely to simplify the identification of adult trematodes.

The keys are designed to facilitate identification and not to show phylogenetic relationship. A key for the identification of families is provided for each subclass of trematodes. Keys to the genera of adult trematodes follow under the individual family headings. In writing the keys, every effort was made to use the most easily-observed anatomical features. Host relations, habitat of the parasite and the abundant illustrations will also aid identification. Although the superfamilies of monogenetic trematodes are included in the keys, this plan is not followed for the digenetic trematodes because their diagnoses are based primarily on characteristics of the larval stages.

Some groups of digenetic trematodes, such as the Superfamilies Allocreadioidea and Plagiorchioidea are especially troublesome in that their classification is in an unsettled state. It is likely that additional knowledge of life cycles and more critical investigation of their anatomy will help to resolve this problem.

v

The author is responsible for the more than 1,000 separate illustrations included in the book. More than two-thirds of them were prepared from identified specimens, in many instances from type specimens. The type species is usually illustrated to represent the genus if this species is known to occur in North America. Whenever redrawn illustrations from the published papers of other authors are used, credit is given below each illustration.

I am especially indebted to W. W. Becklund of the Beltsville Parasitological Laboratory for the loan of numerous type specimens and to Harold W. Manter and Mary Hanson Pritchard, Dept. of Zoology, University of Nebraska for the loan of specimens and for their thorough review of the manuscript. I am also indebted to the following persons for the loan of identified specimens: Elon E. Byrd, Dept. of Biology, University of Georgia; J. Fred Denton, Dept. of Microbiology, Georgia School of Medicine; David J. Doran, Beltsville Parasitological Laboratory; Georges Dubois, Neuchâtel, Switzerland; Bernard Fried, Dept. of Biology, Lafayette College; William J. Hargis, Jr., Virginia Institute of Marine Science; Reinard Harkema, Dept. of Zoology, North Carolina State College; Ernest J. Hugghins, Dept. of Zoology, South Dakota State University; Wanda Hunter, Dept. of Zoology, Duke University; Ralph W. Macy, Dept. of Biology, Portland State College; Walter E. Martin, Dept. of Biology, University of Southern California; O. Wilford Olsen, Dept. of Zoology, Colorado State University; Ivan D. Pratt, Dept. of Zoology, Oregon State University; Robert B. Short, Dept. of Biological Sciences, Florida State University; Frank G. Wallace, Dept. of Zoology, University of Minnesota. In addition to the above acknowledgments, considerable credit is due the many parasitologists who have contributed to our knowledge of trematodes through their research on the taxonomy and life cycles of trematodes.

Moscow, Idaho   Stewart C. Schell

CONTENTS

Page

WHAT ARE TREMATODES?

The trematodes or flukes represent a class of animals in the Phylum Platyhelminthes. This phylum contains all of the so-called flatworms which are characterized as having a body that is flattened dorso-ventrally; an excretory or osmoregulatory system composed of flame cells, tubules and excretory vesicle; and internal organs embedded in a parenchyma tissue which develops from mesoderm and resembles the mesenchyme of the embryos of more advanced animals. Most species are hermaphroditic. The phylum contains three classes: The Class Turbellaria, or free-living flatworms; the Class Trematoda or flukes; and the Class Cestoidea or tapeworms. The animals in the two latter groups are all parasitic, living as external or internal parasites of invertebrates and vertebrates.

In the Class Turbellaria the epidermis is partially or wholly ciliated and pigmented eyespots are present in the adult. Almost all species are free-living in freshwater, marine or terrestrial habitats. Only a very few turbellarians are known to parasitize molluscs, crustaceans, echinoderms or other turbellarians. The class contains five orders of which the order Tricladida contains those

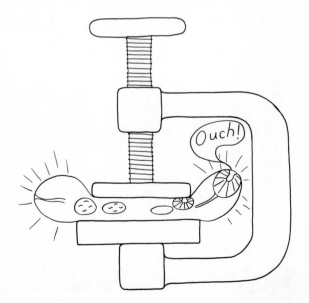

forms in which the digestive tract is composed of three main branches, one anterior and two posterior (Fig. 1a.). The common planarian is a representative of this order. The Orders Rhabdocoela (Fig. 1b.) and Alloeocoela have a digestive system in the form of a single sac or cecum, which in the latter order has lateral branches. Species in the Order Acoela are minute marine forms having a mouth but no digestive tract. Those of the Order Polycladida are marine animals having a broad leaflike body and a profusely-branched digestive system.

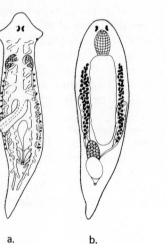
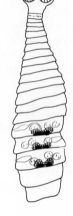

a.   b.   c.

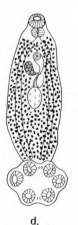
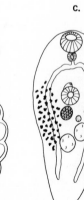

d.   e.   f.

Fig. 1.   Representatives of Classes in Phylum Platyhelminthes:
a. and b. Turbellaria (a. Tricladida, b. Rhabdocoela); c. Cestoidea
(Cestoda); d., e. and f. Trematoda (d. Monogenea, e. Aspidogastrea. f. Digenea)

The flatworms in the Class Cestoidea are without a digestive system; have a scolex for attachment to host tissues and a body composed of a linear series of proglottids, each of which functions as a separate reproductive unit (Fig. 1c.). Mature cestoids are parasites in the digestive tract of vertebrates. Fourteen orders are recognized but those of the Orders Proteocephala, Pseudophyllidea and Cyclophyllidea are encountered most frequently and contain most of the known species. Cestodes of the Order Proteocephala have a scolex with four suckers and in some cases a fifth apical sucker, the genital pores are marginal, vitelline follicles are restricted to narrow lateral bands in the medullary or inner zone of the proglottid and the uterus is saclike with lateral pouches and one or more median ventral pores. Eggs are nonoperculate and contain a six-hooked embryo (= onchosphere) at time of oviposition. Larval stages consist of a procercoid and plerocercoid. The adults parasitize fishes, amphibians and reptiles.

The Order Pseudophyllidea includes those forms in which the scolex contains a pair of dorso-ventral sucking grooves (bothria), vitelline follicles are located in the cortical or outer zone of the proglottid, the uterus is tubular and opens through a median uterine pore. The male and female reproductive pores are also median. Eggs are operculate and after an incubation period produce a ciliated six-hooked embryo known as a coracidium which hatches and is motile. Other larval stages are the procercoid and plerocercoid as in the proteocephalan cestodes. The adults parasitize the digestive tract of fishes, birds and mammals.

Cestodes of the Order Cyclophyllidea have a scolex with four suckers, with or without hooks; the proglottids have a genital pore that is usually marginal; vitelline glands are compact and are located in the posterior part of the proglottid, posterior to the ovary; the uterus is usually saclike, with or without lateral branches and without a uterine pore. Eggs are nonoperculate and contain an onchosphere when mature. The larva may be a cysticercus, cysticercoid, coenurus, strobilocercus or a hydatid cyst. The adults are parasites of reptiles, birds and mammals.

The trematodes or flukes are assigned to the Class Trematoda which contains those parasitic flatworms having a non-ciliated body in the adult stage; a well developed digestive tract which is usually in the shape of an inverted tuning fork and generally consists of a mouth, pharynx, esophagus and two blind intestinal ceca which have lateral branches in some species. The organs for attachment to the host vary greatly in the different groups. The class contains the Subclasses Monogenea (Fig. 1d.), Aspidogastrea (Fig. 1e.) and Digenea (Fig. 1f.). The Monogenea (monogenetic trematodes) and usually the Aspidogastrea utilize only one host in their life cycle. The monogenetic flukes are chiefly ectoparasites

on the skin and gills of fishes, although a few species occur in the
mouth and urinary bladder of amphibians and reptiles. Holdfast
organs are highly developed in this group and are located on a
prohaptor at the anterior end and on an opisthohaptor at the posterior end of the body. The intestinal ceca have lateral branches
in many species. The eggs usually have one or more polar filaments.

Trematodes of the Subclass Aspidogastrea are distinct in having
the body divided into a dorsal hump which contains the internal
organs and a ventral adhesive disc which is a powerful holdfast
organ. They are internal parasites of freshwater clams (mussels),
fishes and turtles.

The majority of the known species of trematodes are assigned
to the Subclass Digenea (digenetic trematodes) which are endoparasites of vertebrates. Although their anatomy varies greatly
from group to group, they can be characterized generally as trematodes having one or two muscular suckers, a digestive tract with
two blind and generally unbranched intestinal ceca and a complex life cycle involving the production of several different larval
stages which develop in one or more intermediate hosts. The larval
stages can also reproduce.

WHAT DO TREMATODES DO FOR A LIVING?

All trematodes lead a parasitic life. A parasite is an organism
that lives on or in another living organism called the host. The
host provides shelter and food for the parasite. A host that har-
bors the sexually mature parasite is known as the final or definitive host. Larval stages of the parasite may parasitize one or
more intermediate hosts.

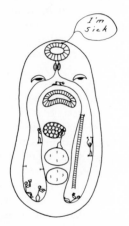

Some trematodes are thought to be
harmless, but they all require some
nutriment for survival and this can
be supplied only by the host. Trematodes can cause mechanical injury
to host tissues by the action of muscular suckers, hooks, spines, anchors
or clamps. Numerous tiny wounds
inflicted by these structures can become centers for invasion by bac-
teria. Trematodes that reside in the
blood vessels, kidneys or liver, where
they are in close contact with tissue
cells and body fluids, are capable of
injuring their host through the release of toxic excretory products.

Small ducts, such as the bile duct, pancreatic duct, the ureters, or even the small intestine of vertebrates, can become clogged when many trematodes are present. The attachment of numerous trematodes to the epithelial lining of the small intestine can interfere with absorption of digested food. An abundance of trematodes in the respiratory system can reduce the efficiency of gaseous exchange there and also result in excess secretions of mucus which can cause congestion in lungs and trachea. Injury to the host may be of an indirect nature, such as the transmission of the salmon-poisoning organism, *Neorickettsia helmintheca*, by the tiny fluke *Nanophyetus salmincola*, which is an intestinal parasite of dogs.

WHERE DO TREMATODES LIVE?

Adult monogenetic trematodes, which use only one host in their life cycles, are primarily ectoparasites on the gills or skin of fishes, however, a few occur in the mouth, nasal cavities, urinary bladder or urinary ducts of vertebrates. Mature aspidogastrid trematodes, which also usually use only one host, are endoparasites in the intestine of bony fishes and turtles, the bile duct and gall bladder of cartilaginous fishes or in the pericardial cavity, kidney or gill lamellae of freshwater clams (Family Unionidae). Digenetic trematodes, which utilize two or more hosts, are generally endoparasites

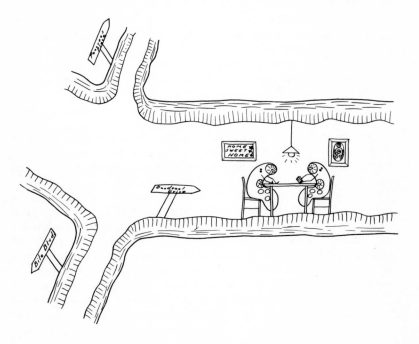

as adults in the digestive, respiratory, urinary, circulatory system, or in the gall bladder, bile duct or pancreatic duct of vertebrates. Some are known to inhabit the connective tissue and muscle of their host. Of these habitats, the digestive tract is most commonly involved. Some rather unusual habitats are the pharynx and Eustachian tubes of amphibians (*Halipegus* spp.), the naso-lacrimal duct, conjunctiva and nictitating membrane of birds (*Philophthalmus* spp.), the bursa Fabricii and oviducts of birds (*Prosthogonimus* and *Parorchis* spp.), encysted in the skin of birds (*Collyriculum* spp.), encysted in pairs on the duodenum of frogs (*Loxogenes* spp.), in the swim bladder of bony fishes (*Acetodextra* spp.) and in the coelom of cartilaginous fishes (*Nagmia* and *Probolitrema* spp.). A few digenetic trematodes are progenetic i.e., attain sexual maturity in invertebrates, for example, *Proterometra dickermani* can develop to maturity in the same snail that produces the larval stages. Mature specimens of *Allocreadium neotenicum* have been found in the larvae and adults of diving beetles.

THE LIFE CYCLES OF TREMATODES

The trematodes in the three subclasses differ in their life cycles. The life cycles of monogenetic and aspidogastrid trematodes are direct, there being only one host and no complicated series of larval stages. The few known life cycles in these groups are described in the taxonomic part of the text under the appropriate genus. Among the monogenetic trematodes, the embryo that hatches from the egg is usually a ciliated oncomiracidium which bears some resemblance to the adult. With subsequent development this larva slowly attains the size and appearance of the adult but usually retains some of the larva armature. Figure 2 provides an example of how this gradual transition from ciliated oncomiracidium to adult occurs.

The life cycles of digenetic trematodes involve a series of larval stages, such as miracidium, sporocyst, redia, cercaria and metacercaria, which develop in one or more intermediate hosts and precede the adult stage (Fig. 3). Upon entering a suitable mollusc, which serves as intermediate host, the miracidium undergoes a metamorphosis to the next larval stage which may be either a sporocyst or a redia. Sporocysts can produce embryos that develop into either a second generation of sporocysts or a generation of rediae. Sporocysts can produce rediae but the reverse procedure does not occur. If two consecutive generations of sporocysts develop, the first is designated the mother sporocyst and the second the daughter sporocyst generation. Two consecutive generations of rediae are likewise mother and daughter rediae. Both the redia

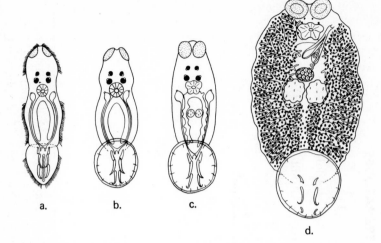

Fig. 2. Example of life cycle of a monogenetic trematode (a. onchomiracidium; b. and c. developmental stages; d. adult of *Neobenedenia melleni*) (Redrawn from Jahn & Kuhn, 1932)

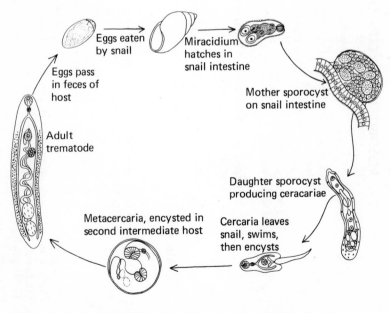

Eggs eaten by snail

Miracidium hatches in snail intestine

Eggs pass in feces of host

Mother sporocyst on snail intestine

Adult trematode

Daughter sporocyst producing ceracariae

Metacercaria, encysted in second intermediate host

Cercaria leaves snail, swims, then encysts

Fig. 3. Example of life cycle of digenetic trematode (*Telorchis* sp.).

POSSIBLE LIFE CYCLES OF DIGENETIC TREMATODES

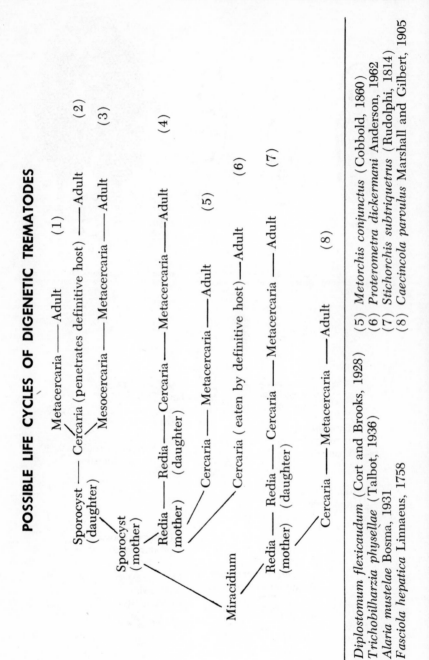

(1) *Diplostomum flexicaudum* (Cort and Brooks, 1928)
(2) *Trichobilharzia physellae* (Talbot, 1936)
(3) *Alaria mustelae* Bosma, 1931
(4) *Fasciola hepatica* Linnaeus, 1758
(5) *Metorchis conjunctus* (Cobbold, 1860)
(6) *Proterometra dickermani* Anderson, 1962
(7) *Stichorchis subtriquetrus* (Rudolphi, 1814)
(8) *Caecincola parvulus* Marshall and Gilbert, 1905

and the sporocyst are able to produce cercariae. The cercariae of most species of trematodes leave the mollusc and, after a brief free-living existence, encyst on or in a second intermediate host or on vegetation. The encysted stage undergoes some anatomical and possibly some physiological changes to become an infective metacercaria which, upon being ingested by the definitive host, develops to the sexually mature adult stage. This development of a series of larval stages involving multiplication of germinal cells which pass from one generation to the next is regarded as germinal lineage accompanied by polyembryony. Cercariae of trematodes of the families Schistosomatidae, Spirorchiidae, Azygiidae, Sanguinicolidae and Bivesiculidae infect the definitive host directly, without encystment in a second intermediate host. In contrast to this, a few strigeoid trematodes, such as species in the Genus *Alaria* (Family Diplostomatidae) produce an additional larval stage, the mesocercaria, which is interspersed between the cercaria and the metacercaria.

This variety of larval stages makes possible a considerable number of different kinds of life cycles. The table on page 8 illustrates the sequence of larval stages produced in the life cycles of several different species of trematodes. A knowledge of life cycles is of value in that it enables us to control a parasite by attacking the most vulnerable stage. It is also of use in devising a system of classification based on phylogenetic relationship. In some instances the adults of related forms do not resemble each other and their close relationship will be masked until the anatomy of the larval stages becomes known, as similarity in structure of larval stages indicates close relationship.

In undertaking investigations of life cycles, it is important to detect *all* larval stages that are produced in the life cycle. In the past, some earlier stages, such as miracidia, mother sporocysts and mother rediae, have been overlooked. Whenever possible, experimental infections should be established in laboratory-reared hosts and the development and anatomy of the larval stages should be observed.

THE ADULT TREMATODE
(= MARITA)

Sexually mature trematodes of the Subclasses Monogenea, Aspidogastrea and Digenea display considerable differences in their anatomy, as the illustrations in the following pages reveal. Those of the Subclass Monogenea are recognized most readily by the structure of the holdfast organs located at the ends of the body. The prohaptor at the anterior end (Fig. 4) may be in the form of a single oral sucker, a pair of buccal suckers which open into a buccal cavity, one or more pseudosuckers, a pair of bothria, a pair of head lappets, or it can be entirely glandular with the gland ducts distributed evenly along the margins or arranged in compact groups to form head organs. The opisthohaptor, at the posterior end of the body may be in the form of a muscular disc, with or without septa, anchors and hooks (Fig. 4), or it can be membranous with anchors and 14 to 16 marginal hooks. In some species the opisthohaptor contains muscular suckers, with or with-

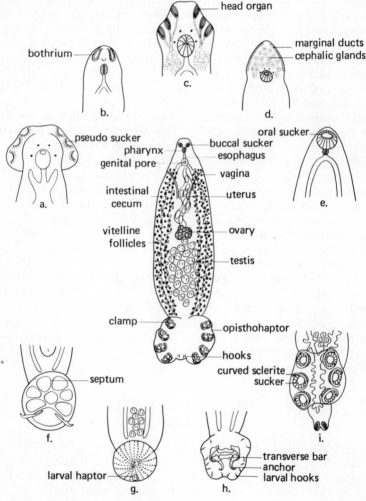

Fig. 4. Generalized monogenetic trematode (a. to e. prohaptors a. head lappets with pseudosuckers, b. bothria, c. head organs, d. marginal gland ducts, e. oral sucker; f. to i. opisthohaptors, f. muscular disc with septa, g. disc with larval haptor, h. membranes with anchors, i. suckers and sclerites).

out curved sclerites or it may contain jawlike clamps. In a few species the clamps are mounted directly on the posterior part of the body instead of on a separate opisthohaptor, thus converting part of the body into a holdfast organ. Clamps are bivalved structures, consisting of two membranous flaps which have a supporting framework of sclerites (Fig. 4). Size, number, shape and arrangement of the sclerites provide distinguishing features which are useful for the identification of the different families and genera. In some monogenetic trematodes the larval opisthohaptor persists, and after some increase in size, becomes the adult opisthohaptor on which the marginal hooks of the larva may be retained (Fig. 4h.). In a few species the opisthohaptor of the adult is a new one on which the small larval haptor is retained (Fig. 4g.).

The trematodes of the subclass Aspidogastrea have a ventral adhesive disc which contains numerous septa and alveoli (= loculi) or, as in the family Stichocotylidae, a longitudinal row of suckers on the ventral body surface. The dorsal part of the body, which contains the internal organs, is the hump (Fig. 5).

Among the Digenea, muscular oral and ventral suckers are the most typical holdfast organs (Fig. 6). The monostome trematodes have only an oral sucker and some trematodes in the Families Cyclocoelidae, Bivesiculidae, and some of the blood flukes are without suckers. The spiny retractile proboscides of trematodes in the Family Rhopaliasidae and the spiny collar of those in the Family Echinostomatidae might also serve as organs for attachment to host tissues. Trematodes of the Superfamily Strigeoidea have a bulbous or a lobed tribocytic organ in addition to the oral and ventral suckers.

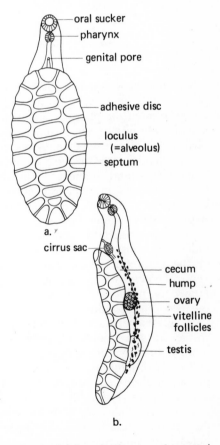

oral sucker
pharynx
genital pore
adhesive disc
loculus (=alveolus)
septum
a.
cirrus sac
cecum
hump
ovary
vitelline follicles
testis
b.

Fig. 5. Subclass Aspidogastrea (a. ventral view; b. lateral view).

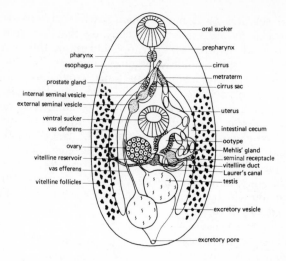

Fig. 6. Generalized digenetic trematode.

The digestive system usually consists of a mouth, prepharynx, pharynx, esophagus and one or two intestinal ceca. Depending upon the location of the pharynx, either the prepharynx or the esophagus may be absent. In some trematodes (e.g., Schistosomatidae) the pharynx is absent. The intestinal ceca may be short (e.g., some Lecithodendriidae) or long as in most species. The ceca have numerous lateral branches (diverticula) in many monogenetic trematodes and in some digenetic trematodes (e.g., Fasciolidae, Campulidae). A single cecum is present in species of the Subclass Aspidogastrea, some families of the Monogenea (e.g., Udonellidae, Tetraonchidae), and in some Digenea (e.g., Haplosplanchnidae). In most species the mouth is located at the anterior end of the body but in the Family Bucephalidae it is on the midventral body surface and leads to a muscular pharynx. In this family the intestine is also a single saclike cecum. In most species the ceca end blindly but in some they fuse to form a cyclocoel (e.g., Cyclocoelidae). A number of cecal variations occur among species of the Family Opecoelidae in which the ceca can end blindly, fuse to form a cyclocoel, open through separate ani, fuse and open through a single anus or fuse with the excretory vesicle to form a cloaca (= uroproct) which opens to the outside through a cloacal pore (see p. 120).

Most trematodes are hermaphroditic (monoecious) but those of the Family Schistosomatidae have separate sexes (dioecious). Female reproductive organs consist of an ovary, oviduct, ootype, Mehlis' gland, uterus, vitelline glands, Laurer's canal and seminal receptacle. The ovary can be sperical, ovoid, lobate, clubshaped, tubular or follicular. It produces the ovum which passes from the ovary to the ootype through an oviduct. The ootype seems to be an assembly area where ovum, vitelline cells and spermatozoa merge. Shell material is produced by the vitelline cells which surround the ovum. The function of the Mehlis' gland which surrounds the ootype, is unknown. From the ootype the eggs pass to the uterus where they are retained for a time. The terminal portion of the uterus is modified in many species to form a muscular metraterm or a spinous terminal organ as in the Family Monorchiidae. Laurer's canal of the Digenea and Aspidogastrea is comparable to the vaginae of the Monogenea. It may be present or abset. When present, it ends blindly, opens to the outside (many Digenea) or into the excretory vesicle (Aspidogastrea). The vagina of the monogenetic trematodes is either single, double or apparently absent. The vaginal pore or pores can be ventral, or dorsal; median or lateral.

The vitelline glands can be follicular, tubular or compact. They consist of clusters of vitelline cells which in many trematodes are known to secrete shell material and possibly yolk. The cells pass to a vitelline reservoir by way of a series of tubules and a transverse vitelline duct before they finally enter the ootype.

The male reproductive system is composed of one or more testes, vasa efferentia, vas deferens, seminal vesicle, prostate gland, cirrus and cirrus sac. There may be one testis or many, however, most species have two testes. The testes may be spherical, ovoid, lobate, dendritic or tubular. Spermatozoa are produced in the testes, pass through the vasa efferentia to the vas deferens and accumulate in the seminal vesicle where they are held temporarily. The seminal vesicle can be internal, inside the cirrus sac, or external, outside the cirrus sac. In some species both types are present or the cirrus sac may be absent and the seminal vesicle free in the parenchyma. The cirrus is a copulatory organ, spinous in some species, and usually enclosed in a cirrus sac. The prostate gland can also be contained in the cirrus sac or free in the parenchyma.

The reproductive system opens to the exterior through one or two (male and female) genital pores which can be located in almost any part of the body. If two pores are present they are usually close together but can be widely separated. If a single pore is present, it is usually ventral and median but can be lateral, sublateral or on the dorsal surface of the body.

Species in the Families Hemiuridae, Deropristiidae, Cryptogonimidae, Haploporidae and some others have the terminal portions of the male and female reproductive ducts fused to form a hermaphroditic duct. In trematodes of the Family Hemiuridae this duct

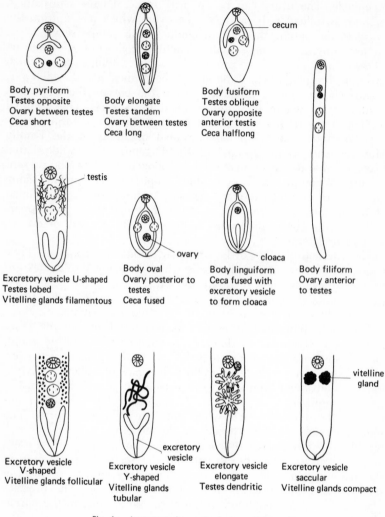

Body pyriform
Testes opposite
Ovary between testes
Ceca short

Body elongate
Testes tandem
Ovary between testes
Ceca long

Body fusiform
Testes oblique
Ovary opposite
anterior testis
Ceca halflong

Excretory vesicle U-shaped
Testes lobed
Vitelline glands filamentous

Body oval
Ovary posterior to
testes
Ceca fused

Body linguiform
Ceca fused with
excretory vesicle
to form cloaca

Body filiform
Ovary anterior
to testes

Excretory vesicle
V-shaped
Vitelline glands follicular

Excretory vesicle
Y-shaped
Vitelline glands
tubular

Excretory vesicle
elongate
Testes dendritic

Excretory vesicle
saccular
Vitelline glands compact

Fig. 6a. Important diagnostic features illustrated.

is enclosed in a sinus sac and in the Family Haploporidae it is in a hermaphroditic sac. Most species in the Superfamily Strigeoidea have a hermaphroditic duct that traverses a genital cone and opens into a copulatory bursa at the posterior end of the body.

In the Families Heterophyidae and Cryptogonimidae the ventral sucker and genital pore are withdrawn into a ventro-genital sac which might also contain one or more muscular gonotyls. Some families (e.g., Microphallidae, Bucephalidae) have a genital atrium, a chamber that receives the openings from the male and female reproductive ducts and opens on the body surface through a genital pore. In some species the genital atrium also contains male papillae, alveoli or spines.

The excretory system (osmoregulatory) is composed of a bilateral system of flame cells, tubules, collecting ducts and an excretory vesicle. The shape of the vesicle is of taxonomic value, especially for the identification of superfamilies and families. In the digenetic and aspidogastrid trematodes the excretory pore is almost always located at or near the posterior end of the body. In the monogenetic trematodes there are two pores and two vesicles near the anterior end of the body.

The nervous system consists of a transverse commissure which is located in the anterior part of the body and nerve fibers which extend anterior and posterior from the commissure. In a few species pigmented eyespots are also present as in the Families Deropristiidae, Cryptogonimidae and Lepocreadiidae as well as in numerous species of the Monogenea. All of the internal organs are embedded in the parenchyma tissue that is characteristically present in all animals of the Phylum Platyhelminthes.

THE EGGS OF TREMATODES

The trematode egg consists of an egg shell which encloses an ovum, one or more sperm and a cluster of vitelline cells. Shell material is secreted by the vitelline cells in most species. Following fertilization, an embryo or miracidium develops. The eggs of some species contain a miracidium at time of oviposition, whereas in other species some time is required for the development of the miracidium following oviposition, usually several weeks. Eggs that contain a miracidium are referred to as being embryonated. The miracidia of some species hatch when the eggs enter water. These hatched miracidia then penetrate the tissues of a mollusc. Embryonated eggs of certain species must be ingested by a suitable mollusc before hatching will occur. Secretions of the mollusc digestive tract seem to provide a stimulus for hatching.

Size, shape and color of the egg shell are of value for identification (Fig. 7). The egg shells of most species are ovoid or spindle-shaped and have a lid or operculum at one end. Operculate eggs are characteristic of most digenetic trematodes. Most monogenetic and a few digenetic trematodes produce non-operculate eggs.

The egg shell of some species is drawn out at one or both ends to form polar filaments. Filaments are present on the eggs of many monogenetic trematodes, as well as in some species of di-

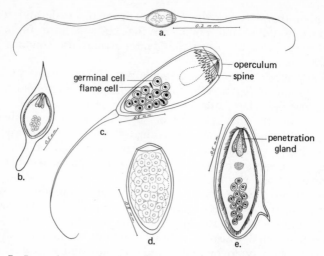

Fig. 7. Trematode eggs (a. *Notocotylus*; b. *Trichobilharzia*; c. *Halipegus*; d. *Paragonimus*; e. *Schistosoma*)

genetic trematodes (e.g., Notocotylidae, some Opecoelidae, Monoorchiidae, Hemiuridae). Trematodes in the Subclass Monogenea generally produce fewer eggs than those in the Subclasses Aspidogastrea and Digenea.

MIRACIDIUM

The miracidium is the embryo that develops in the egg. Those illustrated in Figure 8 represent different types. The miracidia of most species have the body covered by ciliated epidermal plates (Fig. 8a.). A few species differ from this in having ciliated plates covering only part of the body or have the cilia mounted on bars that protrude from the body (Fig. 8b). Cilia are absent in the miracidia of species, in the Families Didymozoidae, Hemiuridae, (Fig. 8c), Azygiidae. The cilia function as organs of locomotion.

Internal organs consist of germinal cells, penetration glands, apical gland, subepidermal cells, flame cells, excretory tubules, central nervous system and in some species pigmented eyespots. The germinal cells eventually multiply and produce embryos for succeeding generations of larvae which may be either sporocysts or rediae. The penetration glands and the apical gland are thought to secrete cytolytic substances which might aid hatching or enable the miracidium to penetrate the tissues of the molluscan host. The flame cells are connected with tubules that open to the outside through pores at the sides of the body.

It is generally assumed that closely related species of trematodes produce miracidia that are similar in their anatomy. Criteria for determining relationship are the number of flame cells, number of germinal cells and the number and arrangement of epidermal plates.

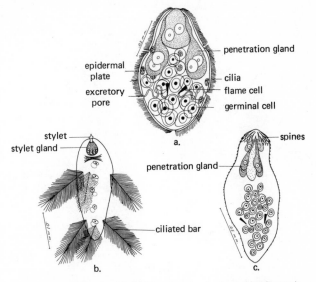

Fig. 8. Miracidia (a. *Phyllodistomum* sp.; b. *Leucochloridiomorpha constantiae*; c. *Halipegus* sp.). (Redrawn from Allison, 1943).

SPOROCYST

The miracidium of many species, upon entering a suitable mollusc, metamorphoses to the sporocyst stage through loss of ciliated epidermal plates, penetration glands and apical gland. The young sporocyst is barely more than a mass of proliferating germinal cells and flame cells enclosed in a delicate limiting membrane. The germinal cells eventually multiply and give rise to embryos of a second generation of larvae which might be either daughter sporocysts or rediae, depending upon the species involved. Daughter sporocysts (Fig. 9) can be branched or unbranched and produce embryos which develop into cercariae. The branched sporocysts of a few species of the Brachylaimidae produce one or more brightly pigmented brood sacs (Fig. 9b.) into which the cercariae migrate. Unbranched sporocysts may be elongate or ovoid, composed of a cellular body wall, a body cavity, germinal cells, excretory system and usually a terminal birth pore through which larvae of the succeeding generation escape. The term "parthenita," meaning parthenogenetic mother, is a somewhat obsolete term formerly used to denote the sporocyst and the redial stages.

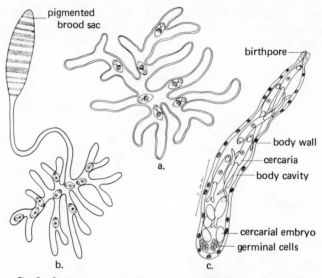

Fig. 9. Sporocysts (a. branched sporocyst of *Postharmostomum* sp.; b. branched with pigmented brood sac, *Leucochloridium* sp.; c. unbranched sporocyst of *Strigea* sp.

REDIA

A redia (plural-rediae) can be distinguished most readily by the muscular pharynx at the anterior end of the body. Attached to the posterior end of the pharynx of most rediae is a sac-like intestine. Like sporocysts, the rediae also have a cellular body wall enclosing a body cavity. Excretory tubules and flame cells are located in the body wall. Germinal cells in the body cavity produce embryos of the succeeding generations of larvae. In many rediae a birth pore is located near the pharynx. Procrusculi, lobe-like outgrowths of the body wall, might also be present as in the rediae of trematodes of the family Echinostomatidae.

One or two generations of rediae can be produced in the life cycle. If two generations appear, those of the first are designated as mother rediae (Fig. 10) and those of the second the daughter rediae (Fig. 11). The germinal cells in the latter eventually give rise to a generation of cercariae. The digenetic trematodes *Stichorchis subtriquetrus, Philophthalmus gralli, Tracheophilus cymbium* and *Parorchis avitus* are unique in that their miracidia contain a mother redia. In a few species three generations of rediae are known to be produced.

CERCARIA

Many different kinds of cercariae (singular-cercaria) are known and in some cases distinct types can be assigned to families or

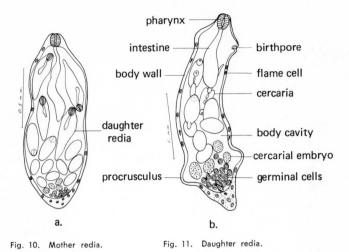

pharynx

intestine

body wall

daughter redia

procrusculus

birthpore

flame cell

cercaria

body cavity

cercarial embryo

germinal cells

a.

b.

Fig. 10. Mother redia.   Fig. 11. Daughter redia.

superfamilies. Cercariae are produced in either a daughter sporocyst or in a redia. They usually leave the host mollusc and lead a brief free-living existence until a suitable second intermediate host or place of encystment can be found. The cercariae of trematodes of several families of digenetic trematodes (e.g., Schistosomatidae, Spirorchiidae, Sanguinicolidae) penetrate the definitive host directly or the cercariae might be eaten by the definitive host (e.g., Azygiidae, Bivesiculidae), thus eliminating the need for a second intermediate host in the life cycle.

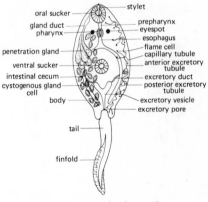

oral sucker

gland duct

pharynx

penetration gland

ventral sucker

intestinal cecum

cystogenous gland cell

body

tail

finfold

stylet

prepharynx

eyespot

esophagus

flame cell

capillary tubule

anterior excretory tubule

excretory duct

posterior excretory tubule

excretory vesicle

excretory pore

Fig. 12. Generalized cercaria.

Most cercariae have a long tail which is used for swimming, however, in some the tail is very short or absent. Locomotion in the latter is limited to creeping movements.

Many species of cercariae have been described and illustrated in published works on trematodes. When this is done, the generic name *Cercaria* is used for all species. The term cercaria can thus be regarded jointly as a generic name for described species of this larval stage and also as a group name for this type of larva. Considerable attention has been given to the anatomy of the excretory system of the cercarial stage, as similarity in anatomy

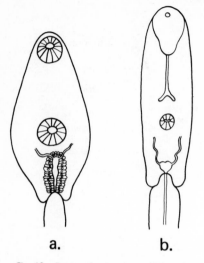

Fig. 13. Types of excretory vesicles (a. thick-walled, epithelial; b. thin-walled, non-epithelial).

of this system is thought atomy of this system is thought to denote phylogenetic relationship. The excretory vesicle is either thick-walled and cellular (epithelial) or thin-walled and noncellular (non-epithelial) (Fig. 13). The system is either *mesostomate*, with the main collecting ducts extending only to the midbody region where they receive the anterior and posterior tubules, or *stenostomate* with the main ducts extending into the anterior part of the body where they turn sharply posterior before joining the anterior and posterior tubules (Fig. 14).

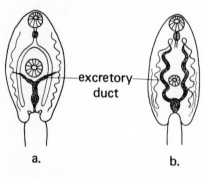

excretory duct

Fig. 14. Excretory systems of cercariae (a. mesostomate type; b. stenostomate type).

The number and arrangement of the flame cells is usually recorded as a flame cell formula which for plagiorchioid trematodes is written as $2[(3+3+3) + (3+3+3)] = 36$. In this formula the "2" represents the right and left sides of the body. In each side there are six groups of three flame cells. The parentheses indicate that half are attached to the anterior and half to the posterior collecting tubules.

The cercariae included in the following key are those most commonly encountered in life cycles of trematodes known to occur in North America.

KEY TO CERCARIAE

1a. Tail absent. ....Cercariaeum cercariae 2

This is an unnatural group with representatives in the Families Brachylaimidae, Monorchiidae, Zoogonidae and Cyclocoelidae.

1b. Tail present. 3

2a. Develop in branched sporocysts in terrestrial or amphibious snails; excretory vesicle small and thin-walled (Fig. 15). ....
....*Leucochloridium* cercaria

The sporocysts develop pigmented brood sacs into which the cercariae migrate for encystment. Produced by trematodes of the Genus *Leucochloridium* of the Family Brachylaimidae.

2b. Develop in rediae in aquatic snails; excretory vesicle has thick epithelial wall (Fig. 16). ....Mutabile cercaria

The cercariae leave the sporocysts and encyst in the same or a different snail. Produced by trematodes of the genus *Asymphylodora* of the Family Monorchiidae.

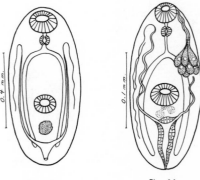

Fig. 15.   Fig. 16.

Fig. 15. Leucochloridium cercaria. Fig. 16. Mutabile cercaria.

3a. Tail short, knoblike or cupshaped. ....Microcercous cercariae 4

Several subgroups are recognized.

3b. Tail as long as or longer than body. 7

4a. Stylet absent; tail indistinctly set off from body; excretory vesicle thin-walled with two pronglike extensions in the tail (Fig. 17). ....Obscuromicrocercous cercaria

The main excretory ducts pass forward to the level of the pharynx then turn sharply posterior before they receive the collecting tubules. Develop in branched sporocysts in terrestrial snails. Produced by some trematodes of the Family Brachylaimidae.

4b. Stylet present; tail distinctly set off from body; excretory vesicle thick-walled, epithelial. 5

5a. Tail cup-shaped, contains unicellular glands; develop in sporocysts (Fig. 18). ....

........................Cotylomicrocercous (= Cotylocercous) cercaria

The tail apparently functions as an adhesive organ. These cercariae develop in snails and encyst in aquatic arthropods. This is thought to be the cercaria of trematodes of the Family Opecoelidae. Some species in the Family Dicrocoeliidae are known to produce similar cercariae.

5b. Tail knoblike or triangular with a ventral groove (sulcus), without unicellular glands; develop in a redia in freshwater operculate snails 6

6a. Tail knoblike; body and tail densely spinous (Fig. 19). ....

.... **Chaetomicrocercous cercaria**

Produced by trematodes of the Genera *Nanophyetus* and *Paragonimus* of the Family Troglotrematidae.

6b. Tail triangular with a ventral sulcus; body and tail nonspinous (Fig. 20). ....**Sulcatomicrocercous cercaria**

Produced by trematodes of the Genus *Sellacotyle* of the Family Troglotrematidae.

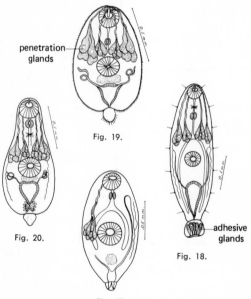

penetration glands

Fig. 19.

adhesive glands

Fig. 20.

Fig. 18.

Fig. 17.

Fig. 17. Obscuromicrocercous cercaria. Fig. 18. Cotylomicrocercous cercaria. Fig. 19. Chaetomicrocercous cercaria. Fig. 20. Sulcatomicrocercous cercaria.

7a. Tail unusually large, the base having a cavity which encloses the body of the cercaria. ....Macrocercous cercariae..........8
7b. Tail not greatly enlarged; body entirely anterior to tail. 10
8a. Tail bulbous and cystlike, having an excretory appendage (= handle), cellular streamers and containing body of cercaria and a long delivery tube (Fig. 21). ....
.... Cystophorous cercaria

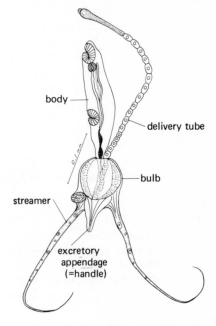

The body and the delivery tube can be ejected but remain attached to the bulb. These cercariae develop in rediae in freshwater and marine snails. When ingested by copepods, the body enters the hemocoel where it develops to a metacercaria. This type of cercaria is produced by trematodes of the Family Hemiuridae.

Fig. 21.   Cystophorous   cercaria.

8b. Tail not as described above. 9

9a. Tail very long and thick, tapering to a point; develop in sporocysts in bivalve molluscs of the Family Sphaeriidae (Fig. 22). .... Cystocercous ceraria

The body contains a stylet, penetration glands, well developed oral and ventral suckers, and an elongate epithelial excretory vesicle. This type of cercaria is produced by trematodes of the Family Gorgoderidae.

9b. Tail thick, with two broad paddlelike furcae; develop in rediae in freshwater operculate snails (Fig. 23). ....
.... **Furcocystocercous cercaria**

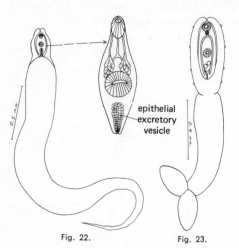

These cercariae are ingested by fishes which serve as definitive host, or some are known to develop to sexual maturity in the host snail. They are produced by trematodes of the Families Azygiidae and Bivesiculidae.

Fig. 22. Fig. 23.

Fig. 22. Cystocercous cercaria. Fig. 23. Furcocystocercous cercaria.

10a. Tail forked. ....Furcocercous cercariae..............**11**
10b. Tail not forked **17**
11a. Tail stem very short and broad; furcae very long; mouth on midventral surface of body and opening into a saclike intestine; head organ or sucker at anterior end of body (Fig. 24).
....**Bucephaloid or Gasterostome cercaria**

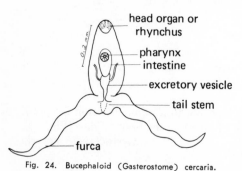

Fig. 24. Bucephaloid (Gasterostome) cercaria.

These cercariae develop in branched sporocysts in bivalve molluscs and encyst in fishes. Produced by trematodes of the Family Bucephalidae.

11b. Tail stem at least half as long as furcae; mouth at anterior end of body and surrounded by oral sucker; intestine composed of two ceca **12**

12a. Pharynx absent; cercariae penetrate definitive host directly, no second intermediate host. 13
12b. Pharynx present; cercariae encyst in a second intermediate host. 14
13a. Dorso-median finfold on body; penetration glands all of one kind; ventral sucker vestigial or absent (Fig. 25). ....
.... Lophocercous-apharyngeate cercaria
These cercariae are produced by trematodes of the Family Sanguinicolidae, the blood flukes of fishes.
13b. Body without dorso-median finfold; penetration glands of two kinds; ventral sucker well developed (Fig. 26). ....
.... Brevifurcate-apharyngeate cercaria.
These cercariae are produced by trematodes of the Families Schistosomatidae and Spirorchiidae, the blood flukes (schistosomes) of reptiles, birds and mammals.

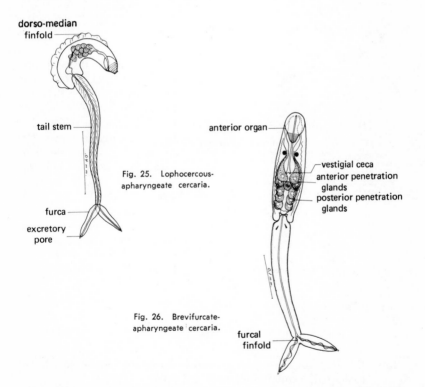

dorso-median
finfold

tail stem

Fig. 25. Lophocercous-apharyngeate cercaria.

furca

excretory
pore

anterior organ

vestigial ceca
anterior penetration glands
posterior penetration glands

Fig. 26. Brevifurcate-apharyngeate cercaria.

furcal
finfold

14a. Dorso-median finfold on body; ventral sucker vestigial; tail stem much longer than furcae; develop in rediae in aquatic snails (Fig. 27). ....Brevifurcate-pharyngeate-Clinostomatoid-cercaria.

These cercariae are produced by trematodes of the Family Clino-stomatidae. In having a pharynx and only one kind of penetration gland they resemble the longifurcate-pharyngeate cercariae of the Superfamily Strigeoidea (see couplet 16). The presence of ex-cretory pores at the tips of short furcae indicates relationship to the brevifurcate-apharyngeate cercaria of the Families Schisto-somatidae and Spirorchiidae (see couplet 13). The dorso-median finfold on the body shows resemblance to the lophocercous-apharyngeate cercaria of the trematodes of the Family Sanguini-colidae (see couplet 13).

14b. **Body without a dorso-median finfold; develop in sporo-cysts.** 15

15a. **Develop in sporocysts in marine bivalve molluscs; excretory vesicle large and U-shaped (Fig. 28).** ....Dichotoma cercaria

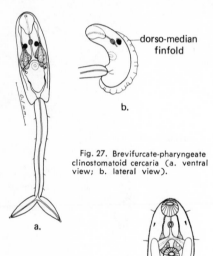

dorso-median finfold

b.

Fig. 27. Brevifurcate-pharyngeate clinostomatoid cercaria (a. ventral view; b. lateral view).

a.

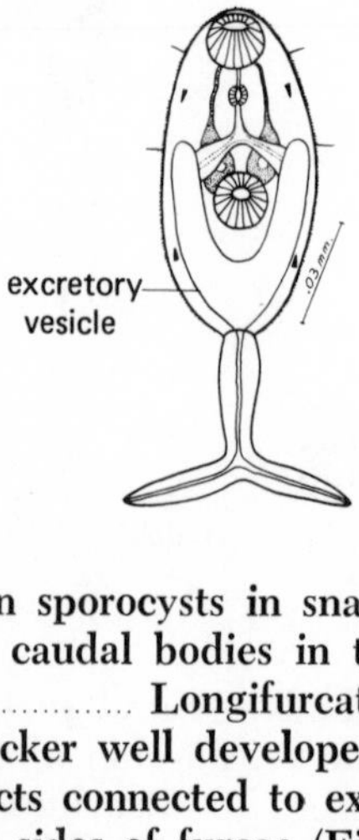

excretory vesicle

Fig. 28. Dichotoma cercaria.

The intestinal ceca are short and thick-walled. The tail stem is shorter than the furcae. In some species the tail is known to regress be-fore the cercaria leaves the sporocyst, causing the cer-caria to resemble a meta-cercaria. Produced by trem-atodes of the Family Gym-nophallidae. Resemblance to the cercaria of *Leucochlor-idiomorpha constantiae* sug-gests relationship to the Family Brachylaimidae.

15b. **Develop in sporocysts in snails; excretory vesicle small, not U-shaped; caudal bodies in tail stem** ....
.... **Longifurcate-pharyngeate cercariae**.........16

16a. **Ventral sucker well developed; one pair of longitudinal col-lecting ducts connected to excretory vesicle; excretory pores located on sides of furcae (Fig. 29).** ....Strigea cercaria

This is the type of cercaria produced by trematodes of the Families Strigeidae and Diplostomatidae. They develop in sporocysts in non-operculate snails.

16b. Ventral sucker vestigial or absent; two pairs of longitudinal collecting ducts connected to excretory vesicle, the median pair fused in the midline of the body; excretory pores located at tips of furcae; dorso-ventral finfolds on furcae (Fig. 30). ....Vivax cercaria

This type of cercaria is produced by trematodes of the Family Cyathocotylidae. The sporocysts develop in operculate snails. The posterior collecting tubules on each side of the body extend into the tail stem where they are connected with several flame cells.

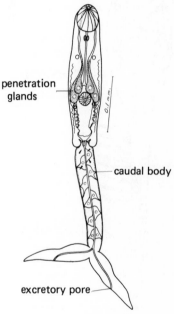

Fig. 29.   Strigea cercaria.

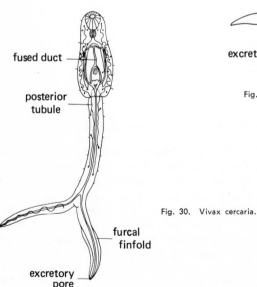

Fig. 30.   Vivax cercaria.

17a. Tail contains paired lateral fingerlike processes and one terminal process; one intestinal cecum present; body contains
many cytogenous glands; pigmented eyespots present (Fig.
31). ....Haplosplanchnid cercaria

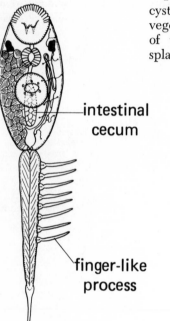

These cercariae are produced in sporocysts in marine snails and encyst on
vegetation. It is probably the cercaria
of trematodes of the Family Halplo-
splanchnidae.

intestinal
cecum

finger-like
process

Fig. 31. Haplosplanchnid cercaria.
(Redrawn from Cable, 1954 b.)

17b. Tail without finger-like processes; two intestinal ceca. 18

18a. Ventral sucker absent; two or three pigmented eyespots present; a pair of adhesive organs present at posterior end of
body; excretory system of the stenostomate type with the
main ducts united across the anterior part of the body; many
cystogenous glands in body (Fig. 32). ......Monostome cercaria
These cercariae develop in rediae and encyst in hemispherical
cyst membranes on aquatic vegetation. Produced by trematodes of
the Families Notocotylidae and Pronocephalidae.

18b. Oral and ventral suckers present. 19

19a. Ventral sucker large, located at posterior end of body; excretory system of stenostomate type; (Fig. 33). ....
.... **Amphistome cercaria**

These cercariae have an excretory system similar to that of the monostome cercariae. Adhesive glands are absent. Encyst on vegetation in hemispherical membranes. Produced by trematodes of the Families Paramphistomatidae.

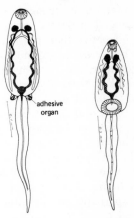

Fig. 32. Monostome cercaria. Fig. 33. Amphistome cercaria.

Fig. 32.   Fig. 33.

19b. Ventral sucker on midventral surface of body. 20
20a. Stylet in oral sucker (Fig. 34). 21
20b. Stylet absent. 25
21a. Excretory vesicle thick-walled, epithelial; pigmented eyespots present; develop in rediae in freshwater clams of the Family Sphaeriidae (Fig. 34). ....**Ophthalmoxiphidiocercaria**

These cercariae encyst in the larvae of aquatic insects. With increased knowledge of life cyles, this might prove to be the type of cercaria produced by trematodes of the Family Allocreadiidae.

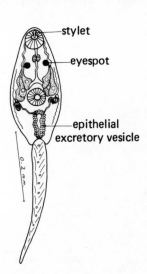

Fig. 34. Ophthalmoxiphidiocercaria.

21b. Excretory vesicle thin-walled; eyespots absent; produced in sporocysts in aquatic snails. ....Xiphidiocercariae........22

The cercariae encyst in a variety of aquatic invertebrates and vertebrates. At least six subgroups are known but only four are of common occurrence in North America.

22a. Tail provided with a dorso-ventral finfold; ventral sucker smaller than oral sucker (Fig. 35). ....Ornatae cercaria

The cercaria produced by trematodes of the Families Macroderoididae and Haplometridae.

22b. Tail without dorso-ventral finfold. 23

23a. Bilobed or pyriform virgula organ located in the region of the oral sucker; tail shorter than body; ventral sucker smaller than oral sucker (Fig. 36). ....Virgulate cercaria

The virgulate cercariae develop in sporocysts in operculate snails and are the cercariae of trematodes of the Family Lecithodendriidae. The virgula organ is used for the storage of mucoid secretions which are thought to provide some protection for the cercaria and perhaps aid in attachment to substrates. Hall (1960) published a key to species of virgulate cercariae.

23b. Virgula organ absent. 24

24a. Ventral sucker vestigial or absent (Fig. 37). ....
.... Ubiquita cercaria

Trematodes of the Family Microphallidae produce this type of cercaria.

24b. Suckers of equal size or ventral larger than oral sucker (Fig. 38). ....Armatae cercaria

Trematodes of the Families Plagiorchiidae and Telorchiidae produce this type of cercaria.

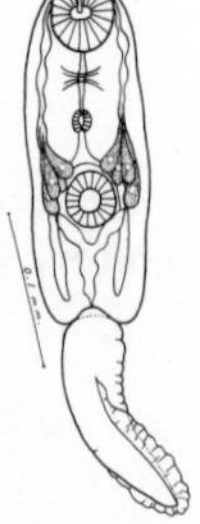

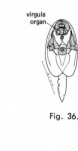

virgula
organ

Fig. 36.

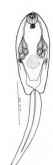

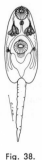

Fig. 38.

Fig. 35.

Fig. 37.

Fig. 35. Ornatae cercaria. Fig. 36. Virgulate cercaria. Fig. 37. Ubiquita cercaria. Fig. 38. Armatae cercaria.

25a. Oral sucker surrounded by a spiny collar (Fig. 39). ....
.... Echinostome cercaria

The excretory system is stenostomate as in the monostome and amphistome cercariae. They develop in rediae which have procrusculi and encyst in molluscs and other invertebrates. Produced by trematodes of the Family Echinostomatidae. The cercaria of the trematodes of the Family Psilostomatidae are similar but are without the spiny collar.

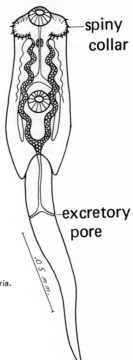

spiny collar

excretory pore

Fig. 39. Echinostome cercaria.

25b. Spiny collar absent. 26
26a. Tail provided with lateral setae or finlets. 27
26b. Tail without setae 29
27a. Cercariae develop in sporocysts in bivalve molluscs; pigmented eyespots absent; excretory vesicle large, U-shaped; tail has lateral finlets (Fig. 40). ....
....Non-oculate trichocercous cercaria
After more life cycles are known, this might turn out to be the type of cercaria produced by trematodes of the Family Fellodistomatidae. The large U-shaped excretory vesicle suggests relationship to the dichotoma type of furcocercous cercaria of the Family Gymnophallidae (see couplet 15). The finlets are clusters of long setae enclosed in a membrane.

27b. Cercariae develop in rediae in snails; pigmented eyespots present; excretory vesicle not large or U-shaped; tail has lateral setae singly or in clusters. 28

28a. Tail much longer than body; setae in clusters on tail only (Fig. 41). ....Oculate trichocercous cercaria
These cercariae develop in rediae in marine snails and encyst in marine polychaete worms. The adult flukes parasitize marine fishes. It is the cercarial type of some species in the Family Lepocreadiidae.

28b. Tail about as long as body; single setae on tail and body; excretory vesicle epithelial (Fig. 42). ....
.... Homalometronine cercaria (= Anallocreadine cercaria)
(Note: the Genus *Anallocreadium* is a synonym of *Homalometron*.)

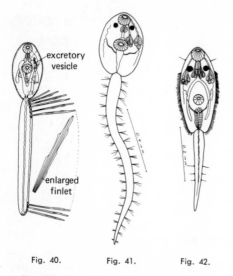

These cercariae encyst in clams of the Family Sphaeriidae. Some species in the Family Lepocreadiidae produce this kind of cercaria. A cercaria that resembles this type is produced by some species in the Family Deropristiidae.

Fig. 40.   Fig. 41.   Fig. 42.

Fig. 40. Non-oculate trichocercous cercaria. (Redrawn from Cable, 1954a.) Fig. 41. Oculate trichocercous cercaria. Fig. 42. Homalometronine cercaria.

29a. Tails provided with dorso-ventral and sometimes lateral finfolds; pigmented eyespots present; develop in rediae in gastropod molluscs 30

29b. Tail without finfolds; eyespots absent. 31

30a. Excretory vesicle bilobed, thick-walled, epithelial; ventral sucker vestigial or absent (Fig. 43). .... **Parapleurolophocercous cercaria**

If lateral finfolds are absent, the cercariae are designated as Pleurolophocercous. Both types develop in rediae in operculate snails and encyst in fishes. Both types of cercariae have been reported in the Family Heterophyidae. Pleurolophocercous cercariae are produced by species in the Families Opisthorchiidae and Cryptogonimidae.

30b. Excretory vesicle Y-shaped, thin-walled, non-epithelial; ventral finfold small, lateral finfolds large and supported by setaelike filaments; ventral sucker well developed (Fig. 44). .... **Megaperid cercaria**

These cercariae encyst on vegetation and are the cercariae of trematodes of the Family Megaperidae.

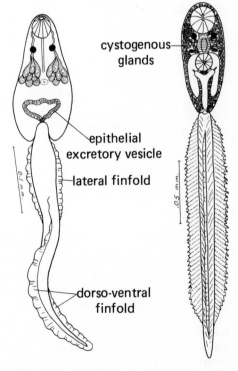

cystogenous glands

epithelial excretory vesicle

lateral finfold

dorso-ventral finfold

Fig. 43.   Fig. 44.

Fig. 43. Parapleurolophocercous cercaria. Fig. 44. Megaperid cercaria. (Redrawn from Cable 1954c.)

31a. Tip of tail contains adhesive gland cells; no excretory canal in base of tail (Fig. 45). ....**Megalurous cercaria**

Trematodes of the Family Philophthalmidae produce this type of cercaria.

31b. Tip of tail without adhesive gland cells; excretory canal in base of tail (Fig. 46). ....**Gymnocephalous cercaria**

This is the cercaria produced by trematodes of the Family Fasciolidae. The cercariae of both of the above groups encyst on vegetation.

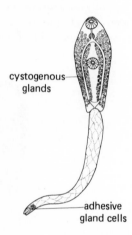

cystogenous glands

adhesive gland cells

Fig. 45. Megalurous cercaria.

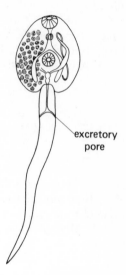

excretory pore

Fig. 46. Gymnocephalous cercaria.

MESOCERCARIA

Trematodes of the Genus *Alaria* of the Family Diplostomatidae produce an extra larval stage, the mesocercaria (Fig. 47), that is interspersed between the cercarial and metacercarial stages. They usually occur free in the coelom, lymph spaces or between the muscles of amphibians and reptiles. The body is pyriform, spinous, has two pairs of penetration glands and numerous flame cells. They develop from longifurcate-pharyngeate (strigea) cercariae from which they differ in being tailless, having more flame cells and a larger body. They differ from the metacercarial stage which follows in the life cycle in not being encysted and in having a much less extensive excretory system.

When ingested by a suitable definitive host, the mesocercaria transforms to a diplostomulum type of metacercaria, which after some migration, finally settles in the intestine where it develops to the adult stage. In some cases the mesocercariae might be eaten by a collector or paratenic host in which they accumulate but do not develop further until this host is eaten by a suitable definitive host.

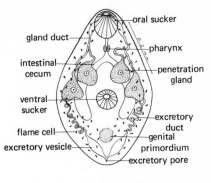

Fig. 47. Mesocercaria.

METACERCARIA
(= ADOLESCARIA)

With the exception of the few species of strigeoid trematodes in which a mesocercaria is produced, the metacercaria (Fig. 48) can be regarded as the larval stage interspersed between the cercaria and the adult trematode. Metacercariae of most species become encysted, however, some (e.g., Genera *Halipegus, Brachycoelium, Panopistus*) are not encysted. Most metacercariae occur in or on a second intermediate host. However, those of the Families Notocotylidae, Paramphistomatidae, Pronocephalidae and Fasciolidae generally occur on aquatic vegetation or on solid objects such as rocks, sticks or shells of molluscs.

Before encystment occurs, the cercaria loses its tail. The cyst membrane is secreted by cystogenous glands in the body of the cercaria. If the encysted metacercaria is located in the tissue of a second intermediate host, there is likely to be a host cellular response resulting in the production of a connective tissue capsule around the cyst membrane produced by the parasite. Most cyst membranes are spherical or ovoid (Fig. 48b), but a few notable exceptions are those of trematodes of the Families Notocotylidae and Paramphistomatidae which are hemispherical (Fig. 48c) and some of those in the Family Philophthalmidae which are flask-shaped (Fig. 48d).

Metacercariae of trematodes in the Families Strigeidae and Diplostomatidae have been studied intensively and a number of genera and species have been described. Their common and generic names are identical. Three of these are of common occurrence in North

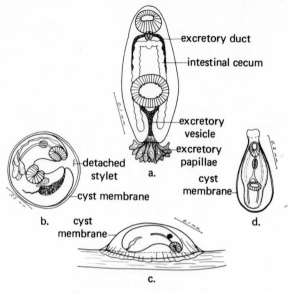

Fig. 48. Metacercariae (a. *Halipegus*; b. *Plagiorchis*; c. *Notocotylus*; d. *Philophthalmus*).

America. The tetracotyle (Genus *Tetracotyle*) (Fig. 49c) encysts in the tissues of snails, leeches and fishes. The cyst membrane is thick and transparent. Muscular pseudosuckers (cotylae) are located on the ventral body surface. The mature trematode is an intestinal parasite of birds, especially ducks. The diplostomulum

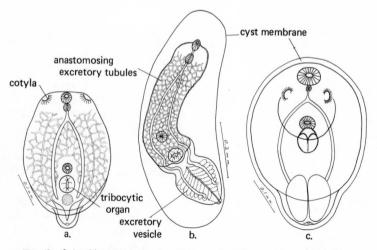

Fig. 49. Strigeoid metacercariae (a. Diplostomulum; b. Neascus; c. Tetracotyle).

(Genus *Diplostomulum*) (Fig. 49a) occurs in the eyes and central nervous system of fishes and amphibians. The host sometimes produces a connective tissue capsule around them. Cotylae are located on each side of the oral sucker. The adult trematodes occur in piscivorous birds and mammals. The neascus (Genus *Neascus*) (Fig. 49b) encysts on the viscera of fishes. The cyst membrane is thin and usually much larger than the enclosed larva. The body is divided into a distinct fore- and hindbody and contains an elaborate excretory system consisting of an extensive excretory vesicle and a network of anastomosing tubules. Cotylae are absent. The adult flukes develop in piscivorous birds.

HOW TO COLLECT AND PRESERVE TREMATODES

Since all trematodes are parasitic, collecting them involves the examination of a variety of host animals. Vertebrate animals harbor most of the adult trematodes whereas most larval stages occur in molluscs and arthropods. The techniques employed for the collection of some of the more delicate monogenetic trematodes differ from those used for collection of digenetic trematodes. Collection of Monogenetic Trematodes: Most species of monogenetic trematodes inhabit the skin and gills of fishes. A few species occur in the mesonephric ducts of fishes or in the mouth, nasal cavities or urinary bladder of amphibians and reptiles (turtles). The small and delicate specimens of the Families Dactylogyridae, Gyrodactylidae and Diplectanidae are best studied alive. To do this it is necessary to bring live fishes to the laboratory. First examine the skin with the aid of a dissecting microscope, then remove the gills and place them in fresh- or seawater, depending upon the habitat of the host. Separate and examine the gill filaments for live worms. Dislodge specimens with dissecting needles and transfer to a microscope slide in a drop of water and apply a coverslip. Slight flattening under a coverslip brings internal organs into clearer view.

If preserved specimens of these delicate monogenetic flukes are desired, freezing the gills or the entire fish for 6-24 hours will kill the worms in a relaxed condition and also loosens mucus that frequently clings to them. After freezing, place the gills or fish in a vial or jar of water for thawing, then shake the container vigorously for one or two minutes. Pour the liquid into a dish and remove extraneous particles by decanting the supernatant fluid after the specimens have settled. Decanting might have to be repeated several times. Remove specimens from the sediment with a medicine dropper and squirt them into formalin-acetic-alcohol solution (F.A.A.). After several rinses in water, mount the specimens in glycerine jelly. Usually these small delicate specimens are not stained.

The larger more muscular monogenetic trematodes from skin or gills of fishes or those from the urinary bladder or mouth of amphibians or reptiles can be removed with forceps. It is sometimes necessary to refrigerate this material overnight in water to relax and loosen the specimens. For preservation, place specimens on a microscope slide in a drop of water, apply a coverslip to flatten them slightly, then kill and preserve by adding several drops of F.A.A. solution at one edge of the coverslip. Place a piece of absorbent paper at the opposite edge to draw fluid across beneath the coverslip. After approximately 10 minutes, transfer the specimens to a dish containing some fixing fluid and leave them in this for at least one hour, then transfer them to 70% ethyl alcohol for storage.

Formalin-acetic-alcohol solution (F.A.A.):

Ethyl alcohol (95%)	50 pts.
Commercial formalin (37%)	10 pts.
Glacial acetic acid	2 pts.
Distilled water	40 pts.

If live fishes cannot be brought to the laboratory, the smaller specimens can be preserved with some success outdoors by first relaxing them in a 0.4% solution of chloretone (trichlor-tertiary-butyl alcohol). The solvent for the chloretone can be fresh- or seawater, depending upon the habitat of the host. To accomplish this, place gills, skin or fins in vials or jars containing the chloretone solution for 30-40 minutes with intermittent shaking. After relaxation, add two parts of F.A.A. solution to one part of the chloretone solution, shake container briefly to mix then set aside for at least 15 minutes. Specimens can remain in this mixture indefinitely. For examination, shake material again, pour it into a dish, remove large pieces of tissue, decant the supernatant fluid, then examine the sediment with the aid of a dissecting microscope. Pipette the worms into 70% ethyl alcohol for storage.

Collection of Digenetic Trematodes: Sexually mature digenetic trematodes are internal parasites of vertebrates. Almost any internal organ can be involved. First, remove the individual organs and place them in separate dishes of water. Slit open tubular organs such as the trachea, stomach, intestine, oviducts and ureters with scissors. Use dissecting needles to tear open small ducts such as the pancreatic duct, bile duct, Wolffian ducts or the intestine of very small vertebrates. After soaking for a few minutes, grasp the organs with forceps and shake vigorously to loosen parasites that might be attached. Examine the lining of organs to which parasites might cling, with the aid of a dissecting microscope. Gently use forceps to free specimens that are attached by their suckers or spines. Scrape inner surface of the intestine and stomach with scalpel or forceps to remove specimens. If mucus is abundant, loosen it by using saline solution in place of water. Finally, remove the organs from the dishes and clean the trematodes of debris by repeatedly decanting and refilling the dishes until the supernatant fluid is clear. Examine sediment with the aid of a dissecting microscope. Remove specimens with forceps or pipette.

The uterus of some trematodes contains so many eggs as to interfere with the observation of other internal organs. Place such specimens in water for 15 minutes or longer for release of excess eggs. This will also tend to relax contracted specimens. After specimens are isolated, they are ready for preservation, employing the same technique as for the larger monogenetic trematodes.

Keeping records: Host-parasite records can be kept on 3 x 5-inch cards. A card is used for each host examined and each host is given a number which is recorded on the card and also on the label that is placed in the vials with the specimens. In addition to the number, the card should contain the scientific name of the host, locality in which it was collected, list of parasitized organs and number of parasites in each organ. When the parasites are identified later, their genus and species names are recorded (Fig. 50). The label in each vial should contain the host number and name of the organ from which the parasites were obtained.

No. 157

Host : Ondatra zibethicus

Locality : Bonner Co. Idaho

Intestine : 16 Echinostoma coalitum
            13 Plagiorchis proximus

Cecum : 67 Quinqueserialis quinqueserialis
         21 Notocotylus spp.

Fur : mites

Fig. 50.

PREPARATION OF STAINED WHOLE MOUNTS OF TREMATODES

The primary reason for staining trematodes is to color internal organs so they can be observed more easily. Although many staining techniques have been devised, only a few need be considered.

Ehrlich's Hematoxylin Stain

Preparation of Staining Solution:

Powdered hematoxylin .... 2 gm.
Ethyl alcohol (100%) ....100 ml.
Glycerol ....100 ml.
Glacial acetic acid .... 10 ml.
Distilled water ....100 ml.
Aluminum potassium sulphate .... 10 gm.

Dissolve the hematoxylin in the alcohol, then add the glycerol and the acetic acid. Next dissolve the alum in warm distilled water, then slowly pour this solution into the hematoxylin solution with stirring. This is a stock solution that should ripen for three to four weeks. For use, dilute one part stock solution with three to four parts of 35% ethyl alcohol.

Procedure: Transfer stored specimens from 70% alcohol to 35% alcohol for 10 to 15 minutes, then to the diluted stain for 15 to 20 minutes. Remove excess stain by soaking specimens in 70% alcohol to which a few drops of strong hydrochloric acid have been added. Allow specimens to remain in this until the body cells are nearly free of stain, and internal organs, such as testes, ovary, vitelline glands and seminal vesicle become pink. Transfer the specimens to 70% alcohol to which a few crystals of sodium bicarbonate have been added. This alkaline solution will cause the internal organs to become blue. After 1/2 to 1 hour, transfer specimens to 95% alcohol (30 minutes) and then to 100% alcohol (30 minutes). Finally, clear in toluene or xylene (10 to 15 minutes), then place specimens on a microscope slide, add a drop or two of resinous mounting medium such as gum damar or synthetic resin and apply a coverslip.

Gower's Acetic Carmine Stain

Preparation of Powdered Stain: Add 10 gm. of powdered carmine to 100 ml. of 45% acetic acid. Dissolve the carmine by heating until it starts to boil. Allow solution to cool, then filter through coarse filter paper. Remove filter paper, containing residue, from funnel and spread out to dry. Store dried acidified carmine in vial until needed.

Preparation of Staining Solution:

Dried acidified carmine .... 1 gm.
Aluminum ammonium sulphate (alum) .... 10 gm.
Distilled water ....200 ml.

Dissolve the alum in warm distilled water, then add the powdered carmine. When cool, filter into a bottle and add a crystal of thymol for preservation. Store staining solution in a refrigerator.

Procedure: Transfer specimens from 70% ethyl alcohol to distilled water for 10 to 15 minutes, then place them in staining solution for 1 to 8 hours, the time depending upon the size of specimens. Pour off the staining solution and rinse specimens in distilled water. Dehydrate through 35% then 70% alcohol (15 minutes in each). Remove excess stain in 70% alcohol to which several drops of strong hydrochloric acid have been added. Continue destaining until the parenchyma cells are free of stain and internal organs are pink or red. Replace acid alcohol with alkaline 70% alcohol. After 30 to 60 minutes place specimens in 95% alcohol (30 minutes) then in 100% alcohol (30 minutes). Finally clear in toluene or xylene (10-15 minutes) then mount in resinous mounting medium.

Labeling the Microscope Slide: The microscope-slide label, placed at one end of the slide, should contain the genus and species name of the trematode, the name of the host, the organ or part of the body in which the parasite was found, the locality in which the host was collected, the date of collection and the host number as recorded on the record card. This information should be printed neatly, using a fine pen point and waterproof ink (Fig. 51).

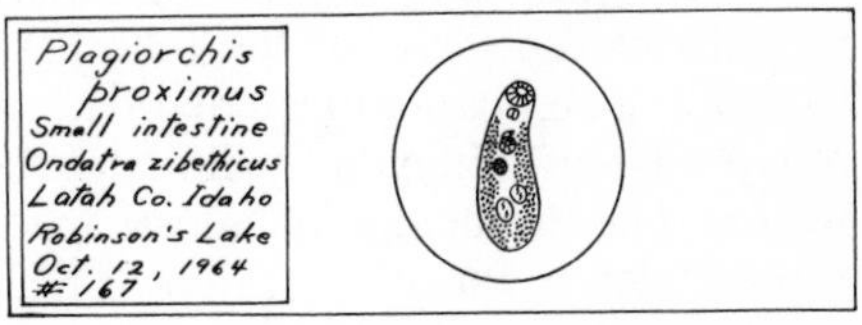

Fig. 51.

TECHNIQUES FOR THE STUDY OF LIVING LARVAL TREMATODES

As digenetic trematodes always use a mollusc as intermediate host, the latter serve as an excellent source of living larval stages such as sporocysts, rediae, cercariae and in some instances the metacercariae. Molluscs (snails and clams), collected in their natural habitat, can be kept alive indoors in dishes or pans containing aquarium or pond water. Snails survive longer if fed fresh green lettuce daily.

Extract the body of large snails (1/4 inch or more) by grasping the muscular foot with forceps and exerting a continuous but gentle pull. If smaller snails or fingernail clams (Sphaeriidae) are examined, first crush the shell and then remove the pieces with forceps. Place the body of the mollusc on a microscope slide in a drop of water or dilute sodium chloride solution (0.1%) and pull apart with dissecting needles to free the larvae. Rediae and cercariae usually float free of the other debris but sporocysts are frequently attached to each other and to the host tissues and must be dissected free.

The anatomy of larval stages is best observed in living specimens. Sporocysts and rediae are nearly non-motile and can be observed more clearly when slightly flattened under a coverslip. Vital dyes, such as neutral red or Nile blue sulphate, can be used as 0.1% aqueous solutions to stain germinal cells and the nuclei of the body wall. A drop of the dye is placed at the edge of the coverslip and allowed to run under slowly.

Obtain naturally-emerged cercariae by placing molluscs in small containers of water for several hours or overnight. Stain and anaesthetize living cercariae by placing them in very dilute solutions of neutral red or Nile blue sulphate, using just enough dye to color the water. The best procedure is to add one or two drops of a 0.1% solution of the dye to 50 to 75 ml. of water containing the larvae. After 10 to 15 minutes, the cercariae become relaxed and are stained sufficiently for observation. Slight flattening under a coverslip is helpful in bringing flame cells, excretory tubules and gland cells into view.

Living miracidia can be obtained from embryonated eggs of trematodes especially of the Families Echinostomatidae, Strigeidae, Gorgoderidae, Paramphistomatidae or Schistosomatidae and some others. Their miracidia will hatch when the eggs are placed in water. The miracidia of most species are motile and must be slowed down for observation. Fresh egg albumen is useful for this. Make a one-half inch ring of it on a microscope slide. Place a small drop of water containing one or more miracidia in the center of the ring, stir with a toothpick, apply a coverslip and examine. The viscid albumen will slow the movement of the cilia and keep the miracidia alive and in good condition for 15 minutes or longer. The first five minutes are ideal for observation of flame cells. If miracidia are observed in water, aqueous solutions of neutral red or Nile blue sulphate can be used to color the germinal cells and penetration glands. The technique is like that described above for cercariae.

It is sometimes necessary to demonstrate the number and arrangement of epidermal plates on miracidia. This can be accomplished with the Silver Impregnation Method of Lynch (1933). Greater success is achieved with the larger miracidia, especially if they can be obtained in quantity.

Procedure: Squirt live miracidia from a medicine dropper into hot (65-70° C.) 0.5% aqueous solution of silver nitrate. Allow specimens to settle to the bottom of the container then pour off the supernatant nitrate solution. Wash specimens in several changes of distilled water by alternate settling and decanting. Now place specimens in bright sunlight for 3-10 minutes. Wash in several more changes of distilled water, clear in glycerine and mount on microscope slides in glycerine jelly.

Results: The edges of the epidermal plates will be blackened and stand out sharply. Other parts of the miracidium will be almost colorless.

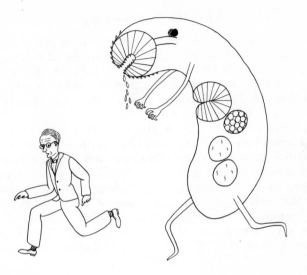

KEY TO SUBCLASSES

1a. Endoparasites; holdfast organs in the form of one or two suckers; life cycles indirect; reproduction by larval stages, involving two or more hosts (Fig. 6). ....Subclass Digenea p. 111
1b. Ectoparasites or rarely endoparasites; holdfast organs not in the form of oral and ventral suckers; life cycles usually direct; larvae do not reproduce. 2
2a. Posterior holdfast organ in the form of a large ventral disc. Excretory pore (rarely two) posterior; intestine a single cecum; internal parasites of lamellibranch and gastropod molluscs, fishes and turtles (Fig. 5). ....Subclass Aspidogastrea p. 106
2b. Posterior holdfast organ an opisthohaptor at the posterior end of the body, containing either one or more suckers, anchors or clamps; usually ectoparasites of fishes, more rarely endoparasites of frogs and turtles. Excretory pores (two) in anterior part of body (Fig. 4). ....Subclass Monogenea p.44

SUBCLASS MONOGENEA
Keys to Suborders, Superfamilies and Families

1a. Opisthohaptor a muscular disk, a muscular sucker or having one or two pairs of anchors; genito-intestinal canal absent (Fig. 52). ....Suborder Monopisthocotylea..........2
1b. Opisthohaptor bearing one or more pairs of muscular suckers or clamps; genito-intestinal canal present (Fig. 53). ....
.... Suborder Polyopisthocotylea........14

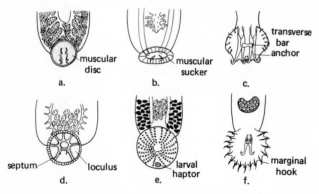

Fig. 52. Opisthohaptors of Monopisthocotylea.

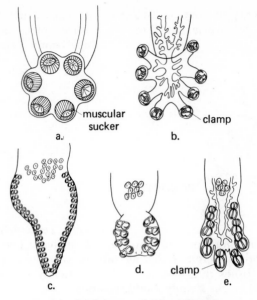

Fig. 53. Opisthohaptors of Polyopisthocotylea.

2a. Opisthohaptor membranous with one or two pairs of anchors and one or two transverse bars; (Fig. 52c, f.) prohaptor containing either head lappets or cephalic glands and head organs (Fig. 54). 3

2b. Opisthohaptor in the form of a muscular disk or sucker usually without anchors (Fig. 52a, b, d, e), but if anchors are present, they are not supported by transverse bars; prohaptor usually contains paired preoral suckers or numerous cephalic glands with marginal ducts (Figs. 54b-d). 8

3a. Intestine composed of a single cecum. 4

3b. Intestine composed of two ceca. 5

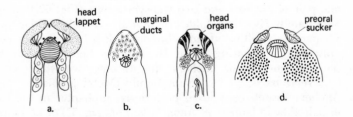

Fig. 54. Prohaptors (a. head lappets; b. marginal ducts; c. head organs; d. preoral suckers).

4a. Opisthohaptor contains two pairs of anchors and a butterfly-shaped transverse bar (Fig. 55); parasite of salmonid fishes. .... Superfamily Tetraonchoidea

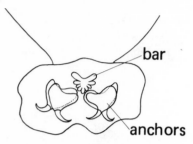

Fig. 55. *Tetraonchus alaskensis,* opisthohaptor.

....Family Tetraonchidae p. 66
4b. Opisthohaptor contains one pair of anchors, two transverse bars and numerous radiating tubular structures; parasites of marine fishes (Fig. 56). ....Superfamily Dactylogyroidea (in part) ....Family Bothitrematidae............................. p. 63

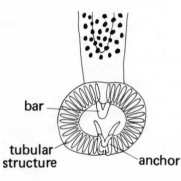

Fig. 56. *Bothitrema bothi,* opisthohaptor.

5a. Viviparous (embryo in uterus); vitelline follicles absent or weakly developed; opisthohaptor bearing 16 marginal hooks, one pair of anchors and two transverse bars (Fig. 52f). ....
Superfamily Gyrodactyloidea...... Family Gyrodactylidae p. 55
5b. Oviparous; vitelline glands abundant, distributed along ceca; opisthohaptor bearing 14 to 16 marginal hooks; one or two pairs of anchors or anchors absent; one, two, three or no transverse bars .... Superfamily Dactylogyroidea..........6
6a. Anchors absent; ceca fused posteriorly; prohaptor in the form of paired head lappets in *Anonchohaptor* (Fig. 57) or no lappets in *Acolpenteron* (Fig. 58); one testis; parasite of marine and freshwater fishes. ....Family Calceostomatidae p. 65

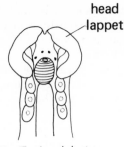

Fig. 57. Anonchohaptor.   Fig. 58. Acolpenteron.

6b. Anchors present. 7

7a. Posterior part of body covered with recurved spines; opistho-
     haptor contains two pairs of anchors and also squamodisks or
     plaques (Fig. 59). ....Family   Diplectanidae p. 63

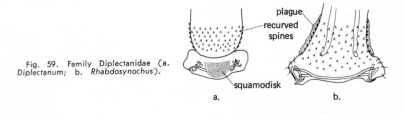

Fig. 59. Family Diplectanidae (a.
Diplectanum; b. Rhabdosynochus).

a.   b.

7b. Body without recurved spines, squamodisks or plaques; opis-
     thohaptor contains one or two pairs of anchors. ....
     ....Family Dactylogyridae p. 56

8a. Opisthohaptor contains numerous radiating rows of spines and
     a small larval haptor; on skin and gills of elasmobranchs
     (Fig. 60). ....Superfamily Acanthocotyloidea
     ....Family Acanthocotylidae p. 78

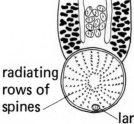

Fig. 60. Pseudacanthocotyla sp., opisthohaptor.

radiating
rows of
spines

larval haptor
with hooks

8b. Opisthohaptor without anchors or radiating rows of spines and
     without a separate larval haptor. 9

9a. Intestine composed of a single cecum; opisthohaptor a concave disk, without anchors or septa; parasite of marine parasitic copepods and perhaps marine fishes. ....Superfamily
Udonelloidea............Family Udonellidae.................... p. 66

9b. Intestine composed of two ceca; parasite of marine fishes.
....Superfamily Capsaloidea 10

10a. Opisthohaptor a septate or aseptate disk, bearing one or more
pairs of anchors. (Fig. 52a. & d.). 11

10b. Opisthohaptor unarmed; in the form of an oval suction
cup, a muscular sucker or two muscular flaps (Figs. 61,
62, 63). 13

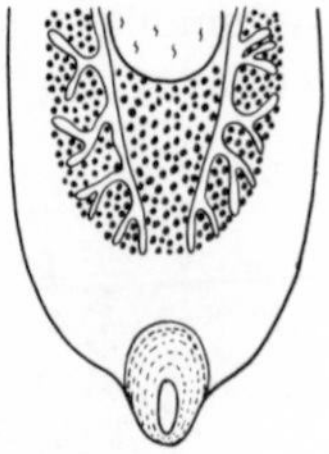

Muscular
flaps

anchor

Muscular
papillae

Fig. 61. *Microbothrium* sp. 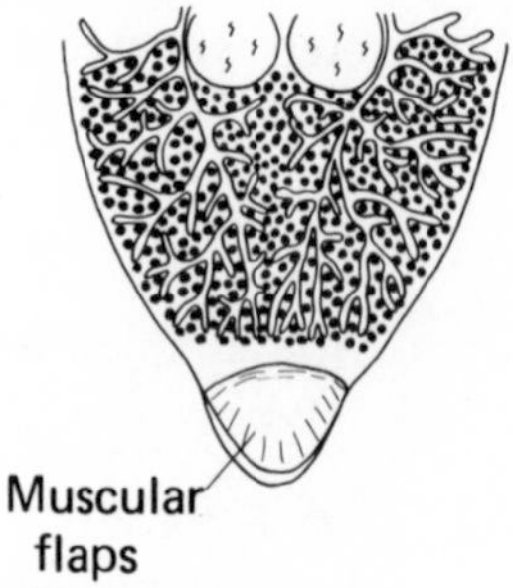   Fig. 62. *Loimopapillosum* sp. 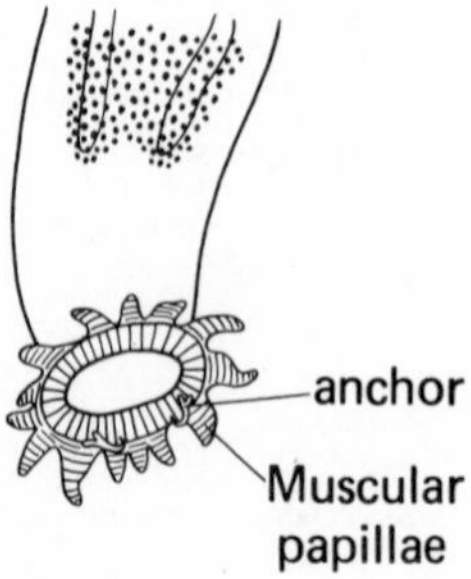   Fig. 63. *Dermophthirius* sp.

11a. Opisthohaptor septate with one pair of anchors (no anchors in
Empruthotrema); prohaptor contains a single sucker or numerous cephalic glands and marginal ducts or head organs;
one testis; parasite on skin, gills or in nasal cavities of marine
fishes (Fig. 64). ....Family Monocotylidae p. 72

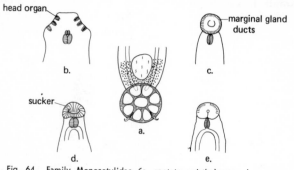

head organ

marginal gland
ducts

b.

c.

sucker

a.

d.   e.

Fig. 64. Family Monocotylidae (a. septate opisthohaptor; b. e. prohaptors).

11b. Opisthohaptor septate or aseptate with one, two or three
pairs of anchors; prohaptor containing either two preoral
suckers or numerous cephalic glands with marginal ducts;
two or more testes (Figs. 65, 66). 12

12a. Prohaptor contains cephalic glands with many marginal ducts; ceca unbranched; two testes, tandem; opisthohaptor septate, with one pair of anchors; on gills of sucking fishes (Fig. 65).
....Family **Dionchidae** p. 76

12b. Prohaptor contains a pair of preoral suckers; ceca branched; two opposite testes or testes numerous; opisthohaptor septate or aseptate with two or three pairs of anchors; parasite on gills, skin or in mouth or nasal cavities of marine fishes. (Fig. 66). ....Family **Capsalidae** p. 67

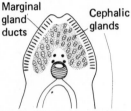

Fig. 65. *Dionchus* sp., prohaptor.

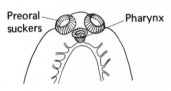

Fig. 66. *Capsala* sp.. prohaptor.

13a. Opisthohaptor a small oval suction cup or a bivalved muscular structure (Figs. 61 & 63); anchors absent; ceca branched; on the skin or in nostrils of elasmobranchs ....
....Family **Microbothriidae** p. 77

13b. Opisthohaptor a muscular sucker, with or without papillae (Fig. 62); one pair of anchors present; ceca unbranched; on the gills of elasmobranchs ....
....Family **Loimoidae** p. 76

14a. Opisthohaptor contains two or six muscular suckers; prohaptor either a single oral sucker or a pair of ventral bothria (Figs. 67-72). ....Superfamily **Polystomatoidea**........15

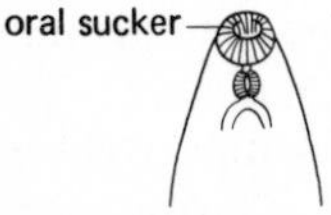

Fig. 67. Prohaptor, one sucker.

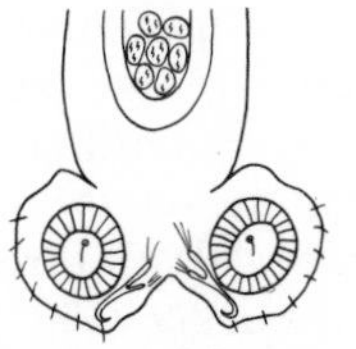

Fig. 68. Opisthohaptor, two suckers.

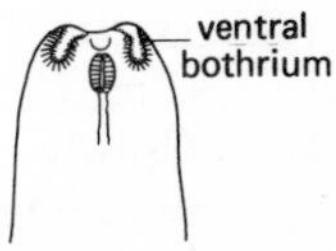

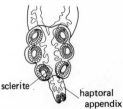

Fig. 69. Prohaptor, two bothria.

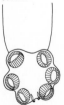

Fig. 70. Opisthohaptor, six muscular suckers.

haptoral appendix   sucker anchors

Fig. 71. Haptoral appendix without suckers.

sclerite   haptoral appendix

Fig. 72. Opisthohaptor, six suckers, haptoral appendix with suckers.

14b. Opisthohaptor contains eight or more clamps; prohaptor a
      pair of small suckers (Figs. 73-75). 18

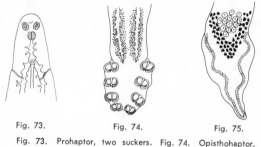

Fig. 73.   Fig. 74.   Fig. 75.

Fig. 73. Prohaptor, two suckers. Fig. 74. Opisthohaptor,
eight clamps. Fig. 75. Opisthohaptor, numerous clamps.

15a. Opisthohaptor contains an haptoral appendix; suckers have
      curved sclerites (Figs. 71, 72). 16
15b. Opisthohaptor without an haptoral appendix; suckers without
      sclerites (Figs. 68, 70). 17
16a. Prohaptor an oral sucker; haptoral appendix well developed,
      containing one pair of suckers and one pair of small anchors
      (Figs. 67, 72). ....Family Hexabothriidae p. 84
16b. Prohaptor contains a pair of ventral bothria; haptoral ap-
      pendix short, contains three pairs of large anchors but no
      suckers (Figs. 69, 71). ....Family Diclybothriidae p. 86
17a. Opisthohaptor contains six muscular suckers (Fig. 70). ....
      ....Family Polystomatidae p. 79
17b. Opisthohaptor contains two muscular suckers (Fig. 68). ....
      ....Family Sphyranuridae p. 83
18a. Opisthohaptor contains four pairs of clamps (Fig. 74). ....
      .... Superfamily Diclidophoroidea........19
18b. Opisthohaptor contains more than four pairs of clamps
      (Fig. 75). .... Superfamily Microcotyloidea........24
19a. Opisthohaptor indistinctly set off from body; clamps weakly
      developed, each composed of three X-shaped sclerites em-
      bedded in a muscular sucker (Fig. 76). ....
      .... Family Hexostomatidae p. 90

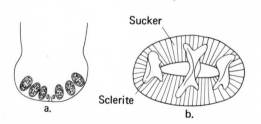

Sucker

Sclerite

a.   b.

Fig. 76. Family Hexostomatidae (a. opisthohaptor; b.
clamp).

19b. Opisthohaptor distinctly set off from body; clamps not as described above. 20

20a. Clamps oval, guitar or fire-tong shaped; prohaptor with a large terminal buccal cavity with two buccal suckers opening into the cavity (Fig. 77). ....
.... Family Macrovalvitrematidae p. 93

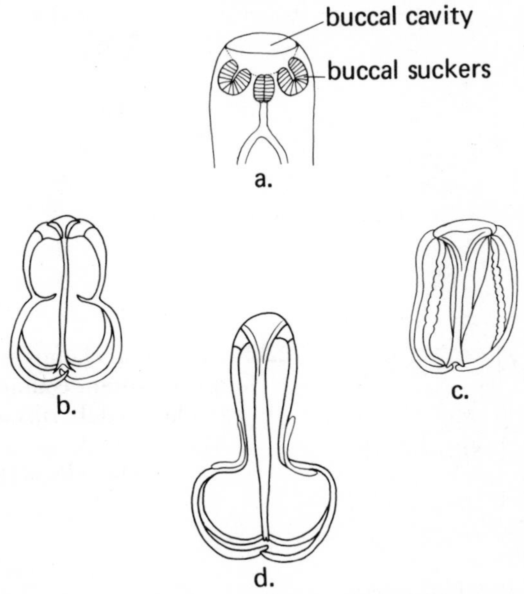

buccal cavity

buccal suckers

a.

b.

c.

d.

Fig. 77. Family Macrovalvitrematidae (a. prohaptor; b. guitar-shaped clamp; c. elongate clamp; d. fire-tong clamp).

20b. Clamps not as described above; prohaptor with a small, ventral oral opening 21

21a. Opisthohaptor contains four pairs of pedunculate clamps (Fig. 78). 22

21b. Opisthohaptor contains four pairs of sessile clamps (Fig. 79). 23

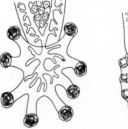
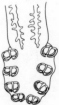

Fig. 78. Pedunculate clamps.
Fig. 79. Sessile clamps.

Fig. 78.   Fig. 79.

22a. Individual clamps asymmetrical, one quadrant containing a muscular sucker and/or a spinous or adhesive pad, wall of clamp contains ribs (Fig. 80). ....
....Family Diclidophoridae p. 87

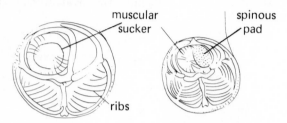

Fig. 80. Clamps of Diclidophoridae.

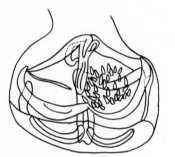

22b. Individual clamps symmetrical, one quadrant containing a denticulate patch, ribs absent (Fig. 81). .... Family
.... Dactylocotylidae p. 89

Fig. 81. Clamp of Dactylocotylidae.

23a. Clamps constructed of U-shaped sclerites (Fig. 82). ....
.... Family Mazocraeidae p. 95
23b. Clamps constructed of a median spring, slender lateral sclerites and spurs (Fig. 83). ....Family Discocotylidae p. 91

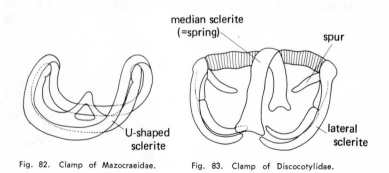

Fig. 82. Clamp of Mazocraeidae.   Fig. 83. Clamp of Discocotylidae.

24a. Opisthohaptor fish-tail shaped (Fig. 84). 25

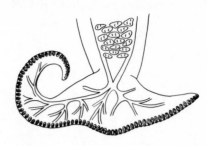

Fig. 84. *Allopyragraphorus* sp., opisthohaptor fish-tail shaped.

24b. Opisthohaptor not fish-tail shaped 26
25a. Clamps of two types, some fire-tong shaped and some microcotylid (Fig. 85); ceca branched, not anastomosing posteriorly.
.... Family Pyragraphoridae p. 104

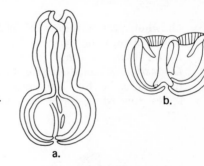

Fig. 85. Pyragraphorid clamps (a.
fire-tong; b. microcotylid).

25b. Clamps oval, longer than wide; ceca branched, anastomosing
posteriorly. ....
.... Family Allopyragraphoridae p. 105
26a. Clamps distributed along sides of body in some genera and
contain accessory pieces which join central sclerite, rib-like
thickenings in wall of clamps (Fig. 86). ....
.... Family Gastrocotylidae p. 105
26b. Clamps without accessory pieces and confined to a distinct
opisthohaptor. 27

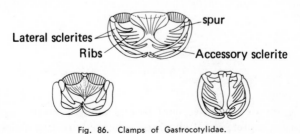

Fig. 86. Clamps of Gastrocotylidae.

27a. Opisthohaptor symmetrical; clamps of microcotylid type and evenly distributed on both sides of opisthohaptor (Fig. 87).
.... **Family Microcotylidae p. 97**

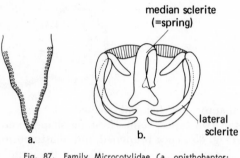

Fig. 87. Family Microcotylidae (a. opisthohaptor; b. clamp).

27b. Opisthohaptor asymmetrical, either triangular or truncate....28
28a. More clamps or larger clamps on one side of opisthohaptor than on other (clamps only on one side in genus *Leuresthicola*); median sclerite of clamps might be bifid or trifid at ends (Fig. 88); ovary U-shaped, the free ends directed toward posterior end of body. ....
.... **Family Heteraxinidae p. 102**

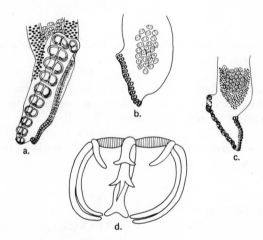

Fig. 88. Family Heteraxinidae (a., b., c. opisthohaptors; d. clamp).

28b. Clamps in two rows, end to end along posterior margin of opisthohaptor, the two rows separated by two pairs of an-

chors; median sclerite of clamp not bifid or trifid at ends;
ovary J- or U-shaped, the free ends directed anterior (Fig. 89).
.... Family Axinidae p. 99

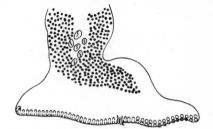

Fig. 89. Opisthohaptor of Axinidae.

SUBORDER MONOPISTHOCOTYLEA Odhner, 1912
SUPERFAMILY GYRODACTYLOIDEA Johnston
and Tiegs, 1922
FAMILY GYRODACTYLIDAE Cobbold, 1864

Viviparous; body minute (1 mm or less); opisthohaptor membranous with one pair of anchors, two transverse bars and 16 marginal hooks; prohaptor contains one pair of head organs; eyes
absent; ovary pre- or posttesticular; pharynx divided into two zones;
vitelline follicles absent or weakly developed and restricted to
area around ends of ceca; on gills and skin of freshwater and
marine fishes.

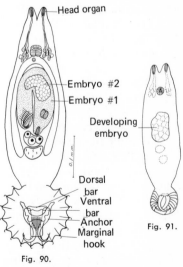

Gyrodactylus Nordmann,
1832 (Fig. 90) is the only
genus of the family known to
occur in North America.
Life cycle: *G. elegans*—
Species in this genus are viviparous, producing embryos
directly within the body of the
parent. This embryo (Fig. 91)
may in turn produce another
one within its body and still
another within this. This kind
of reproduction might be regarded as serial polyembryony.
After the embryo attains some
growth and produces an opisthohaptor with 16 hooks and
one pair of anchors, it is released by the parent. Newborn

Head organ
Embryo #2
Embryo #1
Developing
embryo
0.1 mm
Dorsal
bar
Ventral
bar
Anchor
Marginal
hook
Fig. 90.
Fig. 91.

Fig. 90. *Gyrodactylus rhinichthius*. Fig. 91.
Hatched embryo of *G. rhinichthius*.

larvae are without cilia and closely resemble the parent worm. They attach to the skin or gills of the same host. Mature specimens spread the infection by transferring to a different host when there is contact between hosts (Katheriner, 1904).

SUPERFAMILY DACTYLOGYROIDEA Yamaguti, 1963
FAMILY DACTYLOGYRIDAE Bychowsky, 1963

Oviparous; body small (1 mm or less); opisthohaptor membranous, containing one or two pairs of anchors, 14 to 16 marginal hooks and one, two, three or no transverse bars; prohaptor contains cephalic glands with their ducts grouped to form one or more pairs of head organs; one testis in most genera; ovary pretesticular; cirrus supported by an accessory piece; eyes usually present; vitelline follicles abundant, extending along ceca; primarily on gills of marine and freshwater fishes.

KEY TO GENERA

1a. Opisthohaptor has one pair of anchors. 2
1b. Opisthohaptor has two pairs of anchors. 4
2a. Opisthohaptor indistinctly set off from rest of body; transverse bars absent; parasites in nasal cavities of freshwater fishes (no illustration). ....
............................Genus *Aplodiscus* Rogers, 1967
2b. Opisthohaptor distinctly set off from rest of body; one transverse bar present; on gills of fishes. 3
3a. Tips of anchors doubly recurved; intestinal ceca end blindly (no illustration). ....
............................Genus *Pellucidhaptor* Price and Mizelle, 1964
3b. Tips of anchors not doubly recurved; intestinal ceca fused to form a cyclocoel (Fig. 92). ....
............................Genus *Dactylogyrus* Diesing, 1850

Life cycle: *D. vastator*—

The adult trematode is a parasite on the gills of carp, *Cyprinus carpio*, in Europe and the Near East. The eggs are nonoperculate and have a short polar filament. At temperatures of 24° to 28° C., the embryos develop and hatch in two to three days after oviposition. The host fish is believed to become infected when the ciliated larvae are swept into the mouth and pharynx with water currents. After attachment to the gills, the parasite attains sexual maturity in four to five days at 28° to 29° C. or in 20 days at 15° C. The parasites occupy the tips of the gill filaments, causing some injury there. Only very young carp, up to 60 mm, are infected. The rate of reproduction decreases in the fall and winter and increases again in the spring and summer. Over-wintering occurs as adults and as hibernating eggs. Many generations are produced annually. The entire life span requires 11 to 13 days at 24° to 28° C. (Wunder 1926, 1929; Kulwiec 1929; Iziumova, 1956; Paperna, 1963).

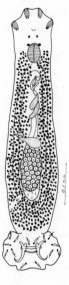

Fig. 92. *Dactylogyrus (Neodactylogyrus) banghami*

4a. Transverse bars absent; opistho-haptor lobed; on gills of elasmo-branchs (Fig. 93). ....
   Genus *Amphibdella* Chatin, 1874

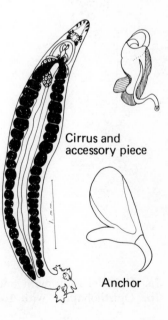

Cirrus and accessory piece

Fig. 93. *Amphibdella flavolineata*. (Redrawn from Price, 1937.)

Anchor

4b. Opisthohaptor contains one to three transverse bars. 5

5a. Opisthohaptor contains three transverse bars. 6
5b. Opisthohaptor contains one or two transverse bars. 7
6a. All three transverse bars separated; vas deferens forming a
loop, but not around the cecum; anchors nearly equal (Fig. 94).
.................................Genus *Pseudomurraytrema* Bychowsky, 1957
6b. Dorsal anchors supported by two articulated bars; ventral
anchors supported by one slender ventral bar; dorsal anchors
much larger than ventral; vas deferens loops around left cecum;
parasites of marine fishes (Fig. 95). ....
....Genus *Hargitrema* Tripathi, 1959

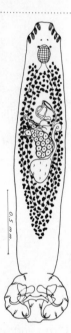

Fig. 94. *Pseudomurraytrema
copulata.*

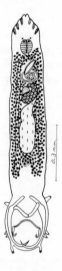

Fig. 95. *Hargitrema bagre.*

7a. Opisthohaptor with one transverse bar. 8
7b. Opisthohaptor with two transverse bars. 9

8a. Prohaptor contains one pair of head organs; ventral anchors much larger than dorsal (Fig. 96). ....Genus *Diplectanotrema*

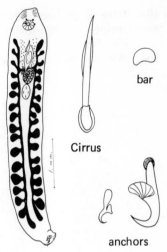

bar

Cirrus

Fig. 96. *Diplectanotrema balistes.* (Redrawn from Price, 1937.)

anchors

Johnston and Tiegs, 1922
8b. Prohaptor contains three pairs of head organs; anchors nearly equal in size (Fig. 97). ....
Genus *Amphibdelloides* Price, 1937

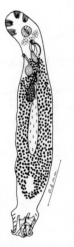

Transverse bar

Hook

Fig. 97. *Amphibdelloides narcine.*

Anchors

9a. Transverse bars articulating with each other. 10

9b. Transverse bars separated. 11

10a. Base of anchors greatly dilated, covering most of the ventral surface of opisthohaptor, tips of anchors directed lateral Fig. 98). ....Genus *Anchoradiscus* Mizelle, 1941

10b. Base of anchors not dilated (Fig. 99). ....
......................................Genus *Actinocleidus* Mueller, 1937

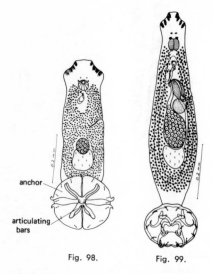

anchor

articulating bars

Fig. 98.   Fig. 99.

Fig. 98. Anchoradiscus anchoradiscus.
Fig. 99. Actinocleidus fusiformis.

11a. Ceca not fused posteriorly; vagina present (Fig. 100). ....
......................................Genus *Ancyrocephalus* Creplin, 1839

11b. Ceca fused posteriorly. 12

12a. Vagina absent (Fig. 101). ......Genus *Urocleidus* Mueller, 1934

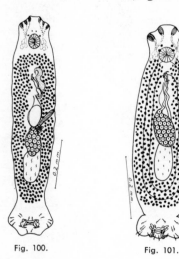

Fig. 100.   Fig. 101.

Fig. 100. Ancyrocephalus lactophrys.
Fig. 101. Urocleidus adspectus.

12b. **Vagina present, pore lateral.** 13

13a. **Parasites of marine fishes.** 14

13b. **Parasites of freshwater fishes.** 16

14a. **Ceca with lateral branches and fused posteriorly; vas deferens not looped around cecum (Fig. 102).** ....
Genus *Tetrancistrum* **Goto and Kikuchi, 1917**

14b. **Ceca without lateral branches but fused posteriorly.** 15

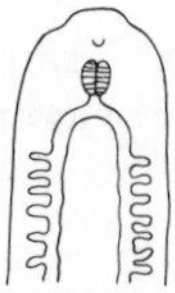

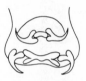

Branched ceca
(Diagrammatic)

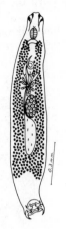

Fig. 102. *Tetrancistrum longiphallus.* (Redrawn from Price, 1937.)

15a. **Vas deferens passes medial to left cecum (Fig. 103).** ....
Genus *Pseudohaliotrema* **Yamaguti, 1953**

15b. **Vas deferens loops around left cecum (Fig. 104).** ....
Genus *Haliotrema* **Johnston and Tiegs, 1922**

Fig. 103. *Pseudohaliotrema mugilinus.*
Fig. 104. *Haliotrema* sp.

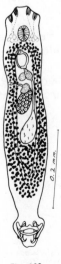

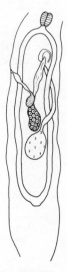

Fig. 103.   Fig. 104.

16a. Opisthohaptor wedge-shaped in lateral view, two anchors directed dorsal and two ventral. 17

16b. Opisthohaptor not wedge-shaped, usually rounded posteriorly. 18

17a. Transverse bars similar; marginal hooks large, heavy; vagina and vaginal pore on right side (Fig. 105). ....
....Genus *Onchocleidus* Mueller, 1936

17b. Transverse bars dissimilar; marginal hooks small, delicate; vagina and vaginal pore on left (Fig. 106). ....
....Genus *Cleidodiscus* Mueller, 1934

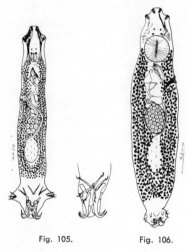

Fig. 105. *Onchocleidus ferox.*
Fig. 106. *Cleidodiscus capax.*

Fig. 105.   Fig. 106.

18a. Dorsal and ventral anchors of equal size; roots of dorsal anchors divided; tips of ventral anchors recurved (Fig. 107).
....Genus *Aristocleidus* Mueller, 1936

18b. Dorsal anchors twice as large as ventral; roots undivided; tips of dorsal and ventral anchors sharply recurved (Fig. 108).
....Genus *Haplocleidus* Mueller, 1937

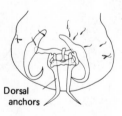

Dorsal anchors

Fig. 107. *Aristocleidus hastatus.* (Redrawn from Mueller, 1936.)

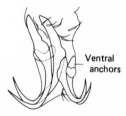

Ventral anchors

Fig. 108. *Haplocleidus dispar.* (Redrawn from Mueller, 1936.)

FAMILY BOTHITREMATIDAE Bychowsky, 1957

Opisthohaptor discoid with one pair of large anchors, two Y-shaped bars and a circle of radially-arranged tubular structures; prohaptor contains four pairs of cupshaped head organs; one intestinal cecum; one testis; ovary pretesticular; parasites on gills of marine teleosts.

The family contains a single genus and species, *Bothitrema bothi* (Fig. 109).

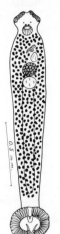

tubular structures

Fig. 109. *Bothitrema bothi.*

FAMILY DIPLECTANIDAE Bychowsky, 1957

Body small, posterior part usually covered with recurved spines; opisthohaptor contains two pairs of anchors, squamodisks or adhesive plaques and two to four transverse bars; prohaptor contains cephalic glands and head organs; one testis; ovary pretesticular, looped around intestinal cecum; parasites on gills of marine and freshwater fishes.

KEY TO GENERA

1a. Opisthohaptor pedunculate, the peduncle densely spinous and containing spinous dorsal and ventral plaques (Fig. 110). ....
.... Genus *Rhamnocercus* Monaco, Wood and Mizelle, 1954

The peduncle is formed by the narrowed posterior part of the body. The plaques contain chevron-like spines.

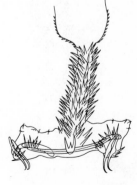

Fig. 110. *Rhamnocercus rhamnocercus*

1b. Opisthohaptor not pedunculate; either squamodisks or lateral adhesive plaques present. 2

2a. Lateral adhesive plaques present (Fig. 111). ....

.................**Genus *Rhabdosynochus* Mizelle and Blatz, 1941**

In this genus the posterior part of the body is widened; the opisthohaptor contains three transverse bars (two dorsal, one ventral); the ceca end blindly.

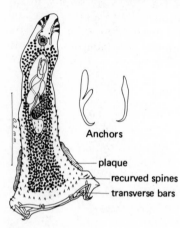

Anchors

plaque

recurved spines

transverse bars

Fig. 111. *Rhabdosynochus rhabdosynochus.* (Redrawn from Hargis, 1955a.)

2b. Dorsal and ventral squamodisks present. 3

3a. Two intestinal ceca present; opisthohaptor contains three separate transverse bars (Fig. 112). ....

.................**Genus *Diplectanum* Diesing, 1858**

Key to species in Tripathi (1957).

3b. One cecum present; opisthohaptor contains two fused transverse bars (Fig. 113). ....

.................**Genus *Neodiplectanum* Mizelle and Blatz, 1941**

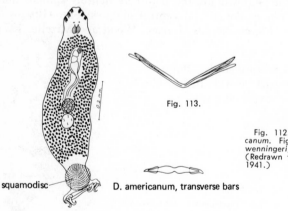

Fig. 113.

Fig. 112. *Diplectanum americanum.* Fig. 113. *Neodiplectanum wenningeri*, fused transverse bars. (Redrawn from Mizelle and Blatz, 1941.)

squamodisc

D. americanum, transverse bars

Fig. 112.

FAMILY CALCEOSTOMATIDAE
(Parona and Perugia, 1890)

Body small and delicate; opisthohaptor of North American forms without anchors but contains 14 marginal hooks; prohaptor in the form of two membranous head lappets or without lappets and containing head organs; one testis; ceca united posterior to testis; ovary pretesticular; North American forms are parasites of freshwater fishes. A taxonomic revision of the family was published by Fischthal and Allison (1941).

KEY TO GENERA

1a. Membranous head lappets present; head organs absent; no cephalic glands; on gills of freshwater fishes of the Family Catostomatidae (Fig. 114). ....
...............Genus *Anonchohaptor* Mueller, 1938

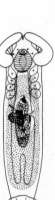

Fig. 114. *Anonchohaptor anomalus.*

1b. Head lappets absent; one pair of head organs present; cephalic glands in pre- and post-pharyngeal groups; in mesonephric ducts and urinary bladder of freshwater fishes (Fig. 115). ......
.... Genus *Acolpenteron* Fischthal and Allison,

Life cycle: *A. catostomi*—
The adult flukes occur in the urinary tract of smallmouth and largemouth bass. Eggs without polar filaments pass in the urine of the host. A ciliated larva develops and hatches in six to nine days (Fig. 115). Larvae have four tufts of cilia, two pairs of pigmented eyespots, a pharynx and 14 hooks (Fischthal and Allison, 1942).

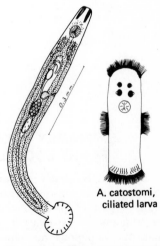

A. catostomi,
ciliated larva

Fig. 115. *Acolpenteron ureteroecetes.*

SUPERFAMILY TETRAONCHOIDEA Yamaguti, 1963
FAMILY TETRAONCHIDAE Bychowsky, 1957

Opisthohaptor membranous, sharply set off from body proper and contains two pairs of anchors and a winged or butterfly-shaped transverse bar; prohaptor contains one or more pairs of head organs; one testis; ovary pretesticular; intestine composed of a single cecum; cirrus and accessory piece present; parasites on gills of freshwater fishes.

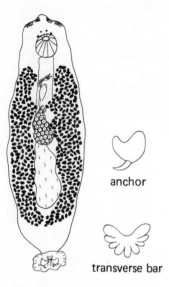

The family contains only the genus *Tetraonchus* Diesing, 1858 (Fig. 116) of which three species have been reported from North America, primarily as gill parasites of trout, grayling and pike.

anchor

transverse bar

Fig. 116. *Tetraonchus alaskensis.*

SUPERFAMILY UDONELLOIDEA Yamaguti, 1963
FAMILY UDONELLIDAE Taschenberg, 1879

Body small, nearly cylindrical; opisthohaptor in the form of a concave muscular disk without anchors or hooks; prohaptor contains a pair of pseudosuckers or head organs; intestine a single cecum; one testis; ovary pretesticular; vagina absent; parasites of parasitic copepods on marine fishes. Price (1938b) published a taxonomic revision of the family.

This family is represented in North America by only the genus *Udonella* Johnston, 1835 (Fig. 117). The disklike opisthohaptor without anchors or hooks and the single intestinal cecum are useful anatomical features for identification of the genus.

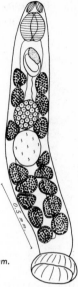

Fig. 117. *Udonella caligorum.*

SUPERFAMILY CAPSALOIDEA Price, 1936
FAMILY CAPSALIDAE Baird, 1853

Body large, broad and flat; opisthohaptor a muscular disk, with or without septa and containing two or three pairs of anchors; prohaptor in the form of two preoral suckers, bothria or glandular areas; testes two or many; ovary pretesticular; vitelline follicles abundant; parasites on skin and gills, or in mouth and nostrils of marine fishes. A taxonomic revision of the family was published by Price (1939a).

KEY TO GENERA

1a. More than two testes present. 2

1b. Two testes present. 5

2a. Opisthohaptor without septa; prohaptor contains two preoral bothria; on gills of sturgeon (Fig. 118). ....
....Genus *Nitzschia* Baer, 1826

2b. Opisthohaptor with septa; prohaptor contains two preoral suckers. 3

3a. **Pharynx constricted at middle; testes lateral and median to ceca; on skin and gills of marine fishes (Fig. 119).** ....
....**Genus** *Capsala* **Bosc, 1811**

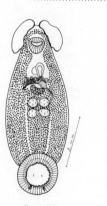

The posterior septa of the opisthohaptor are not bifid at the tips; anchors (if present) are without clawlike tips; the testes are usually distributed lateral and median to the intestinal ceca.

Fig. 118. *Nitzschia quadritestis.* Fig. 119. *Capsala martinieri.*

Fig. 118.   Fig. 119.

3b. **Pharynx globose, not constricted at middle; testes confined to intercecal area.** **4**

4a. **Posterior septa of opisthohaptor bifid at tip; anchors have clawlike tip; marginal body spines crownshaped (Fig. 120).**
....**Genus** *Capsaloides* **Price, 1938**

4b. **Posterior septa of opisthohaptor not bifid at tips; anchors not clawlike at tip; marginal body spines pointed, bifid or serrate at tip but not crown shaped (Fig. 121).** ....
....**Genus** *Tristoma* **Cuvier, 1817**

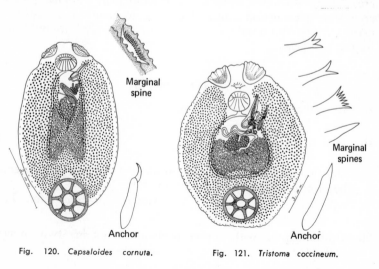

Marginal spine

Marginal spines

Anchor

Anchor

Fig. 120. *Capsaloides cornuta.*   Fig. 121. *Tristoma coccineum.*

5a. Opisthohaptor small, pedunculate; margins of body folded ventrally; preoral suckers surrounded by pleated membranes (Fig. 122). ....Genus *Encotyllabe* Diesing, 1850

The pedunculate opisthohaptor is attached to the ventral surface of the body and contains one pair of large anchors and 14 marginal hooks.

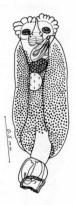

Fig. 122. *Encotyllabe lintoni.*

5b. Opisthohaptor discoid, sessile; body margins not folded; no preoral membranes. 6
6a. Opisthohaptor with septa, seven marginal loculi and three pairs of anchors (Fig. 123). ......Genus *Megalocotyle* Folda, 1929

All loculi on the opisthohaptor are marginal because of the fusion of the central and posterior loculi. The opisthohaptor has a scalloped margin.

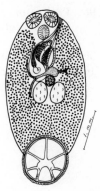

Fig. 123. *Megalocotyle trituba.*

6b. Opisthohaptor without septa. 7
7a. Prohaptor a single preoral lobe, containing glands, suckers or sucking grooves. 8
7b. Prohaptor not a single lobe, containing two preoral suckers or sucking grooves. 9

8a. Opisthohaptor with scalloped marginal membrane; ceca not fused posteriorly (Fig. 124). ....

................................Genus *Pseudobenedenia* Johnston, 1931

8b. Opisthohaptor without scalloped marginal membrane; ceca fused posteriorly (Fig. 125). ....

..........................Genus *Entobdella* Blainville in Lamarck, 1818

Life cycle: *E. soleae*—

The adult flukes inhabit the skin on the ventral surface of the common sole, *Solea solea*. The parasite releases eggs which are

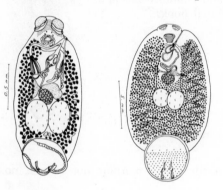

anchored to sand grains by a sticky egg stalk. Free-swimming oncomiracidia hatch and penetrate the skin on the dorsal surface of the fish. This is the only part of the fish that is exposed when they lie partially buried in the sand. After a brief developmental period, the parasite migrates to the ventral body surface where it matures (Kearn, 1963).

Fig. 124.   Fig. 125.

Fig. 124. *Pseudobenedenia noblei.* (Redrawn from Menzies, 1946.) Fig. 125. *Entobdella hippoglossi.*

9a. Prohaptor contains two sucking grooves or pseudosuckers; parasites of stingrays (Fig. 126). ....

................................Genus *Pseudentobdella* Yamaguti, 1963

9b. Prohaptor contains a pair of preoral suckers. 10

10a. Vagina long, opening on left margin of body; on skin of elasmobranchs (Fig. 127). ....

................................Genus *Benedeniella* (Johnston, 1929)

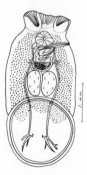

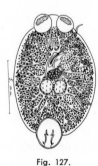

Fig. 126. *Pseudentobdella pacifica.* (Redrawn from Guberlet, 1936.) Fig. 127. *Benedeniella posterocolpa.* (Redrawn from Hargis, 1955b.)

Fig. 126.   Fig. 127.

10b. Vagina absent; on skin of marine teleost fishes (Fig. 128).
....Genus *Neobenedenia* Yamaguti, 1963

Life cycle: *N. melleni*—

Adults are parasites on the gills, cornea, conjunctiva and in the nasal cavities of several genera and species of marine fishes. Eggs are pyramidal and have one long filament. A ciliated larva develops and hatches in five to eight days. The newly-hatched larva (Fig. 129) has cilia on the sides of the body, two pairs of pigmented eyespots, pharynx, two ceca, excretory system and the primordia of two preoral suckers. The larval opisthohaptor remains folded lengthwise for a time, probably unfolding when the parasite attaches to the host. At this time the cilia are shed. The unfolded opisthohaptor is discoid and contains three pairs of anchors and 14 hooks (Jahn and Kuhn, 1932).

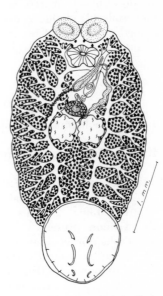

Fig. 128. *Neobenedenia melleni.* (Redrawn from Jahn and Kuhn, 1932.)

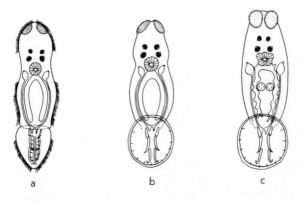

Fig. 129. *Neobenedenia melleni,* larval stages (a. hatched larva; b. cilia shed, opisthohaptor open; c. older larva). Redrawn from Jahn and Kuhn, 1932.)

FAMILY MONOCOTYLIDAE Taschenberg, 1879

Opisthohaptor discoid, containing septa and one pair of anchors (no anchors in *Empruthotrema*, and *Dendromonocotyle*); prohaptor an oral sucker, paired head organs or a single lobe containing numerous gland ducts; one testis; ovary pretesticular and usually looped around right cecum; parasites in nostrils or on skin or gills of marine fishes. Price (1938b) published a taxonomic revision of the family.

KEY TO GENERA

1a. Opisthohaptor contains more than nine loculi; two vaginae present. 2
1b. Opisthohaptor contains nine loculi or less; one vagina present. 5
2a. Anchors absent; opisthohaptor has one central, 14 marginal and five submarginal loculi; in the olfactory organs of rays (Fig. 130). ......Genus *Empruthotrema* Johnston and Tiegs, 1922
2b. Anchors present. 3
3a. Prohaptor contains many marginal gland ducts; many small loculi on ventral surface of opisthohaptor; in nasal cavities of elasmobranchs (Fig. 131). ....
..........................Genus *Cathariotrema* Johnston and Tiegs, 1922

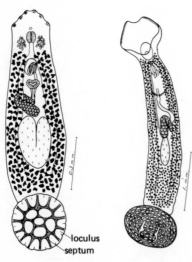

Fig. 130. *Empruthotrema raiae.* Fig. 131. *Cathariotrema selachii.*

loculus
septum

Fig. 130.   Fig. 131.

3b. Prohaptor contains three pairs of head organs; opisthohaptor
has marginal, submarginal and central loculi. 4

4a. Opisthohaptor contains one central, 13 marginal and four submarginal loculi; parasites of rays (Figs. 132, 133). ....
....Genus *Thaumatocotyle* Scott, 1904

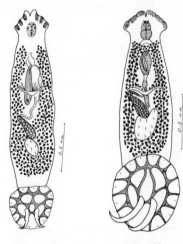

Fig. 132.   *Thaumatocotyle   dasybatis.*
Fig. 133.   *Thaumatocotyle pseudodasybatis.*

Fig. 132.   Fig. 133.

4b. Opisthohaptor contains one central, 18 marginal and seven
submarginal loculi; in nostrils of skate (Fig. 134). ....
....Genus *Merizocotyle Cerfontaine,* 1894

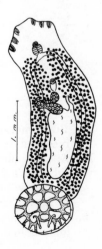

Fig. 134.   *Merizocotyle   pugetensis.*

5a. Opisthohaptor contains one central and seven marginal loculi; oral opening surrounded by a pseudosucker containing many gland ducts (Fig. 135); on gills of stingray. ....

....Genus *Dasybatotrema* Price, 1936

The posterior loculus is much larger than the others. The marginal membrane of the opisthohaptor is festooned.

5b. Opisthohaptor contains one central and eight marginal loculi. 6

6a. Lateral margins of posterior part of body with bilateral cuticular bars; opisthohaptor with transverse rows of recurved spines in addition to anchors; parasite of guitar fish (Fig. 136).

....Genus *Spinuris* Doran, 1953

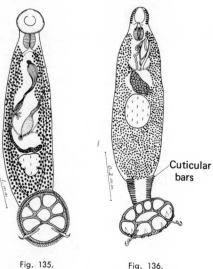

Cuticular bars

Fig. 135.   *Dasybatotrema dasybatis.*
Fig. 136.   *Spinuris lophosoma.*

Fig. 135.   Fig. 136.

6b. Body margins without cuticular bars; opisthohaptor without recurved spines. 7

7a. Anchors absent; opisthohaptor contains one central and eight submarginal loculi as well as numerous marginal ridges; ceca profusely branched; prohaptor contains preoral flap; on skin of rays (Fig. 137). ....Genus *Dendromonocotyle* Hargis, 1955

7b. Anchors present; opisthohaptor without marginal ridges; ceca unbranched. 8

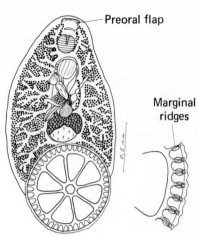

Fig. 137. *Dendromonocotyle octodiscus.*

8a. **Prohaptor an oral sucker; head organs or gland ducts absent; on gills of elasmobranchs (Fig. 138). .... Genus *Heterocotyle* Scott, 1904**

8b. **Prohaptor a single lobe containing numerous head organs or separate marginal gland ducts. 9**

9a. **Dorsal surface of opisthohaptor contains curved transverse row of muscular holdfast organs; vitelline follicles absent in posterior third of body; on gills of sawfish (Fig. 139). .... Genus *Neoheterocotyle* Hargis, 1955**

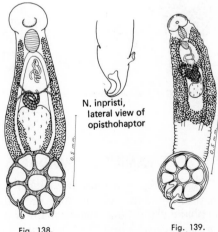

Fig. 138. *Heterocotyle papillata.*
Fig. 139. *Neoheterocotyle inpristi.*

Fig. 138. Fig. 139.

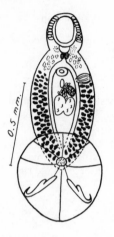

9b. **Dorsal surface of opisthohaptor without special holdfast organs; vitelline follicles fill posterior third of body; margin of opisthohaptor contains numerous ridges, each with a tetrapartite sclerite (Fig. 140).** ....
Genus *Heterocotyloides* **Yamaguti, 1963**

The opisthohaptor of this genus resembles that of *Dendromonocotyle* except that anchors are absent in the latter genus. The ceca of *Dendromonocotyle* are branched, whereas those of *Heterocotyloides* are unbranched. Their prohaptors differ greatly.

Fig. 140. *Heterocotyloides pricei.* (Redrawn from Pearse, 1949.)

FAMILY DIONCHIDAE Bychowsky, 1959

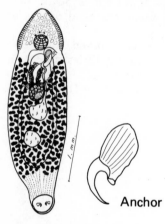

Opisthohaptor discoid with 10 marginal loculi, one pair of anchors and 14 marginal hooks; prohaptor has many cephalic glands and marginal gland ducts; ceca unbranched, united posteriorly; two tandem testes; ovary pretesticular; two pairs of eyespots; primarily parasites on gills of sucking fishes of the family Echeneidae.

The family contains only the genus *Dionchus* Goto, 1899 (Fig. 141). All three of the described species have been reported from North America as parasites of remoras (suckerfish).

Anchor

Fig. 141. *Dionchus agassizi.*

FAMILY LOIMOIDAE Bychowsky, 1957

Opisthohaptor a muscular sucker with one pair of anchors; prohaptor contains two or more preoral suckers or head organs and cephalic glands; one, two or many testes; ovary pretesticular; vagina present; ceca unbranched; parasites on the gills of elasmobranchs.

KEY TO GENERA

1a. Prohaptor contains head organs and cephalic glands; opisthohaptor with marginal papillae; ovary looped around right
cecum (Fig. 142). ....Genus *Loimopapillosum* Hargis, 1955
1b. Prohaptor contains one or more pairs of preoral suckers; opisthohaptor without marginal papillae; ovary not looped around
cecum. 2
2a. Testis large, deeply lobed; prohaptor contains three pairs of
preoral suckers (Fig. 143). ....Genus *Loimosina* Manter, 1944
2b. Testis small, ovoid; prohaptor contains one or two pairs of
preoral suckers (Fig. 144). ....Genus *Loimos* MacCallum, 1917

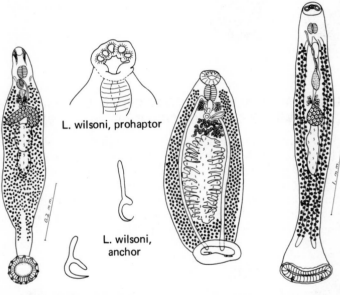

L. wilsoni, prohaptor

L. wilsoni,
anchor

Fig. 142.   Fig. 143.   Fig. 144.

Fig. 142. *Loimopapillosum dasybatis.* Fig. 143. *Loimosina wilsoni.* (Redrawn
from Manter, 1944.) Fig. 144. *Loimos salpinggoides.*

FAMILY MICROBOTHRIIDAE Price, 1936

Body small, flat; opisthohaptor, unarmed, either an oval muscular cup or two muscular flaps; prohaptor contains two small
suckers; one or two testes; ovary pretesticular; ceca branched;
parasites in nostrils and on skin of sharks. Price (1938b) published
a taxonomic revision of the family.

KEY TO GENERA

1a. One testis; opisthohaptor an oval muscular cup (Fig. 145). ....
....Genus *Microbothrium* Olsson, 1869

1b. Two testes; opisthohaptor in the form of two muscular flaps (?) (Fig. 146). ....Genus *Dermophthirius* MacCallum, 1926

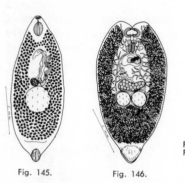

The structure of the opisthohaptor is not clearly evident, even on the type specimens. It was described formerly as a bell-shaped structure with cuticular thickenings. More critical examination of well-preserved specimens will be helpful.

Fig. 145. *Microbothrium apiculatum.*
Fig. 146. *Dermophthirius carcharini.*

Fig. 145.   Fig. 146.

SUPERFAMILY ACANTHOCOTYLOIDEA Sproston, 1948
FAMILY ACANTHOCOTYLIDAE Price, 1936

Opisthohaptor discoid with numerous radiating rows of spines and having a small larval haptor attached to the adult opisthohaptor; prohaptor contains cephalic glands and a pair of preoral suckers; testes numerous; ovary pretesticular; female genital pore marginal, male pore median; North American forms all obtained from the skin and gills of rays and skates. A taxonomic revision of the family was published by Price (1938b).

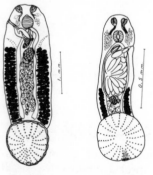

Fig. 147.   Fig. 148.

Fig. 147. *Pseudacanthocotyla williamsi.* (Redrawn from Price, 1938b.)
Fig. 148. *Allacanthocotyla pugetensis.* (Redrawn from Bonham and Guberlet, 1938.)

KEY TO GENERA

1a. Uterine pore on right margin of body; vitelline follicles distributed along more than half of body length (Fig. 147). ....
.... Genus *Pseudacanthocotyla* Yamaguti, 1963

1b. Uterine pore on left margin of body; vitelline follicles confined to posterior third of body (Fig. 148). .... Genus *Allacanthocotyla* Yamaguti, 1963

SUBORDER POLYOPISTHOCOTYLEA Odhner, 1912
SUPERFAMILY POLYSTOMATOIDEA Price, 1936
FAMILY POLYSTOMATIDAE Gamble, 1896

Opisthohaptor contains six cup-shaped suckers and usually one or more pairs of anchors and hooks; prohaptor an oral sucker; ceca branched or unbranched, ending blindly or anastomosing posteriorly; one, two or many testes; ovary pretesticular; parasites in the urinary bladder, nasal cavities, mouth, pharynx or esophagus of amphibians and reptiles. A taxonomic revision of the family was published by Price (1939b).

KEY TO GENERA

1a. **Testes numerous; uterus contains many eggs; opisthohaptor has one pair of anchors; in the urinary bladder of amphibians (Fig. 149).** ....Genus *Polystoma* Zeder, 1800

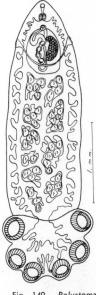

Fig. 149. *Polystoma integerrimum.*

Life cycle: *P. integerrimum*—

The mature trematode inhabits the urinary bladder of the frog, *Rana temporaria,* and the gills of its tadpole. Adult trematodes in the urinary bladder start to oviposit in the spring about the time that the frogs lay eggs. Eggs of the parasite leave the host in the urine. A ciliated larva (Fig. 150b) develops in the egg and hatches in 20 to 50 days, the time depending upon the temperature. The earliest ciliated larvae become attached to the external gills of very young tadpoles where they feed and develop within 20 to 25 days to mature adults. When the external gills are resorbed these flukes die, but while alive, they lay eggs which produce a ciliated larva that is identical to the first one. These larvae from eggs of the adults on the external gills attach to the internal gills of older tadpoles. Some of the later eggs of adults in the urinary bladder also produce ciliated larvae that attach to internal gills.

Little development occurs on the gills, but when the tadpoles metamorphose to frogs the larvae migrate by way of the digestive tract to the cloaca and then to the urinary bladder where they develop slowly to sexually mature trematodes. During development, the larvae lose their cilia (Fig. 150c) and at least some of their larval hooks (Fig. 150c). An opisthohaptor develops with six suckers and one pair of anchors. The adult trematodes of the gill generation differ in their anatomy from those of the bladder generation in having a rudimentary cirrus, no vaginae, no uterus, no genito-intestinal canal, small ovary, one testis, rudimentary vitellaria, sperm without heads and fewer ova. Like their host, the bladder parasites are reproductively dormant during the winter months. Complete development of this generation requires three years (Zeller, 1872, 1876; Gallien 1932, 1933; Bychowsky, 1957).

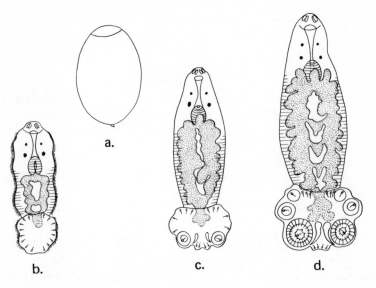

Fig. 150. *Polystoma integerrimum*, larvae (a. egg; b. hatched larva; c. larva, one pair suckers; d. larva, three pair suckers). (Redrawn from Zeller, 1872.)

Life cycle: *P. nearcticum*—

The adult is a parasite of the tree frogs, *Hyla versicolor* and *H. cinerea*. Oviposition occurs simultaneously by the host frog and by the mature trematodes in the urinary bladder in the springtime. Parasite eggs are released in masses and pass in the urine of the host. Ciliated larvae develop in the eggs and hatch in 12 to 13 days. Laboratory-reared tadpoles of *H. versicolor* were exposed to ciliated larvae which attached to their gills and developed to sexual maturity in 22 days. Some ciliated larvae that hatched later, entered the cloaca by way of the cloacal pore. They do not appear to migrate there by way of the digestive tract like *P. integerrimum*. The bladder forms develop slowly, maturing in the third year when the frogs become sexually mature. Eggs and larvae of the gill forms are identical to those of the bladder form but the adults of these two generations differ in their anatomy (Paul, 1938).

1b. One or two testes present. 2
2a. One testis; parasites in urinary bladder of turtles. 3
2b. Two opposite testes; in urinary bladder of amphibians. 5
3a. Opisthohaptor without anchors (Fig. 151). ....
....Genus *Neopolystoma* **Price, 1939**
3b. Opisthohaptor contains one or two pairs of anchors. 4
4a. Opisthohaptor contains one pair of anchors (Fig. 152). ....
....Genus *Polystomoidella* **Price, 1939**

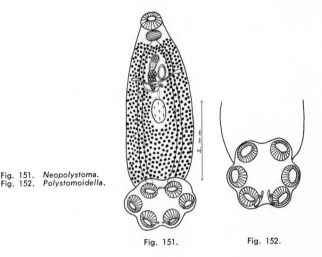

Fig. 151.   *Neopolystoma.*
Fig. 152.   *Polystomoidella.*

Fig. 151.   Fig. 152.

4b. **Opisthhaptor contains two pairs of anchors, one pair larger than the other (Fig. 153).** ....
Genus *Polystomoides* Ward, 1917...

Life cycle: *P. oris*—

Adults parasitize the oral cavity of the turtle, *Chrysemys picta*. Operculate eggs without polar filaments are produced throughout the year and are released singly at the rate of two or three every 24 hours. The development and hatching of a ciliated larva requires about 28 days. The rate of development is dependent upon temperature. At time of hatching the larva (Fig. 154) has two pairs of pigmented eyespots, an oral sucker, pharynx, two ceca, ciliated plates, excretory tubules

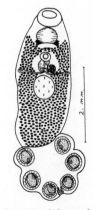

Fig. 153.   *Polystomoides coronatum.* (Redrawn from Price, 1939b.)

and an opisthohaptor containing numerous hooks. Muscular suckers develop gradually in pairs on the opisthohaptor. Mature specimens have six suckers. At least one year is required for development to sexual maturity in the turtle (Paul, 1938).

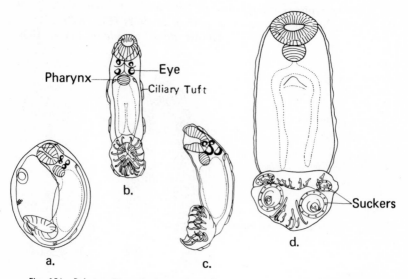

Fig. 154. *Polystomoides oris*, larvae (a. embryonated egg; b. and c. hatched larvae; d. four-sucker stage). (Redrawn from Paul, 1938.)

5a. Opisthohaptor contains one pair of anchors; testes near middle of body (Fig. 155). ....Genus *Neodiplorchis* Yamaguti, 1963
5b. Opisthohaptor without anchors; testes in anterior third of body (Fig. 156). ....Genus *Pseudodiplorchis* Yamaguti, 1963

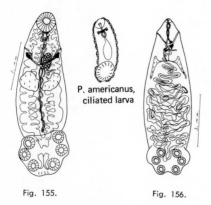

P. americanus, ciliated larva

Fig. 155. *Neodiplorchis scaphiopi.* (Redrawn from Rodgers, 1941.) Fig. 156. *Pseudodiplorchis americanus.* (Redrawn from Rodgers and Kuntz, 1940.)

Fig. 155.   Fig. 156.

FAMILY SPHYRANURIDAE Poche, 1926

Opisthohaptor bilobed, containing two cup-shaped suckers and one pair of anchors; prohaptor an oral sucker; ceca unbranched, united posteriorly; testes numerous; ovary pretesticular; two vaginae present; parasites on gills and skin of caudate amphibians.

The family contains only the genus *Sphyranura* Wright, 1879 (Fig. 157) of which four species have been reported from North America, primarily as parasites on the skin and gills of waterdog, *Necturus maculosus* and the Oklahoma salamander, *Eurycea tynerensis*.

Life cycle: *S. oligorchis—*

The adult trematode is a parasite on the gills and skin of *Necturus maculosus*. Eggs are non-embryonated when laid. Cleavage progresses for 15 to 18 days and by the 22nd day a U-shaped nonciliated larva is produced. Larvae hatch at 28 to 32 days following oviposition. The newly hatched larva (Fig. 158) has a bilobed opisthohaptor which contains 16 hooks, one pair of anchors and two small developing suckers. The larvae creep, inch-worm fashion, on the bottom in search of a host. They apparently attach to the gills first

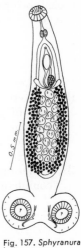

Fig. 157. *Sphyranura osleri.*

and move to the skin secondarily as young larvae are not found on the skin. Testes start to appear on the 12th to 15th days and the ovary on the 15th to 19th days following attachment. The entire cycle is completed in less than two months (Alvey, 1936).

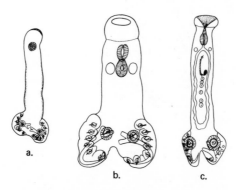

a.

b.

c.

Fig. 158. *Sphyranura oligorchis*, larvae (a. hatched larva; b. older larva; c. larva 16 days.) (Redrawn from Alvey, 1936.)

FAMILY HEXABOTHRIIDAE Price, 1942

Opisthohaptor contains six suckers with curved sclerites and an haptoral appendix with two terminal suckers; prohaptor contains an oral sucker; testes numerous; ovary pretesticular; two vaginae present; ceca branched, united posteriorly and extending into opisthohaptor; primarily parasites on the gills of elasmobranchs. A taxonomic revision of the family was published by Price (1942).

KEY TO GENERA

1a. Suckers and sclerites of opisthohaptor of different sizes. 2
1b. Suckers and sclerites of opisthohaptor of uniform size. 3
2a. Membranous collar surmounts oral sucker; cirrus large, spinous; vaginae fuse before joining other reproductive ducts; parasites of stingray (Fig. 159). ....
...................................Genus *Dasyonchocotyle* Hargis, 1955
2b. Membranous collar absent; cirrus small, unarmed; vaginae completely separate; parasite of sharks (Fig. 160). ....
...................................Genus *Heteronchocotyle* Brooks, 1934

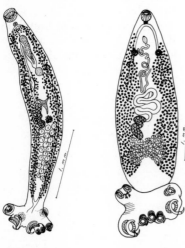

Fig. 159.   *Dasyonchocotyle spiniphallus.*
Fig. 160.   *Heteronchocotyle hypoprioni.*

Fig. 159.   Fig. 160

3a. Vaginae separate, opening individually into transverse vitelline duct (Fig. 162); eggs with one or two polar filaments......4

3b. Vaginae united before entering
vitelline reservoir; eggs without
polar filaments (Fig. 163, 164).
.......:.. 6

4a. Cirrus spinous; eggs have monopolar filaments; parasite of
smooth dogfish (Fig. 161). ....
.... **Genus** *Hexabothrium*
Nordmann, 1840

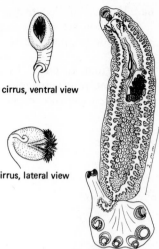

cirrus, ventral view

cirrus, lateral view

Fig. 161. *Hexabothrium canicula.* (Redrawn
from Sproston, 1946.)

4b. Cirrus non-spinous. 5
5a. Vitelline follicles not extending into haptoral appendix. ....
.... **Genus** *Erpocotyle van Beneden and Hesse,* 1863
5b. Vitelline follicles extending into haptoral appendix (Fig. 162).
.... **Genus** *Neoerpocotyle* Price, 1942

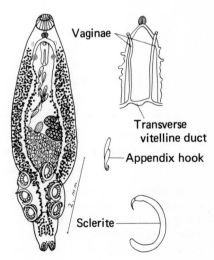

Vaginae

Transverse
vitelline duct

Appendix hook

Sclerite

Fig. 162. *Neoerpocotyle gingly-
mostomae.*

6a. Vaginae united to form a single median duct which joins the
vitelline reservoir; eggs have longitudinal ridges but no polar
filaments; parasite of skates (Fig. 163). ....
.... **Genus** *Rajonchocotyle* **Cerfontaine, 1899**
6b. Vaginae fused at two separate points before joining the vitelline reservoir; eggs without polar filaments and longitudinal
ridges; parasite of guitarfish (Fig. 164). ....
....**Genus** *Rhinobatonchocotyle* **Doran, 1953**

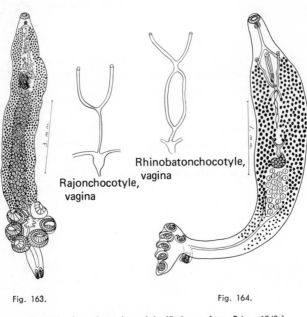

Rajonchocotyle,
vagina

Rhinobatonchocotyle,
vagina

Fig. 163.   Fig. 164.

Fig. 163.   *Rajonchocotyle wehri.* (Redrawn from Price, 1942.)
Fig. 164.   *Rhinobatonchocotyle cyclovaginatus.*

FAMILY DICLYBOTHRIIDAE Bychowsky
and Gussev, 1950

Opisthohaptor contains three pairs of suckers, each with a curved
sclerite; short haptoral appendix present, bearing three pairs of
anchors but no suckers; prohaptor contains a pair of ventral bothria;
testes numerous; ovary elongate, folded, pretesticular; vaginae
united; pores sublateral; parasites on gills of acipenserid fishes.

The family contains two genera of which only *Dicly-bothrium* Leuckart, 1835 occurs in North America (Fig. 165). This genus contains two species, both of which have been reported from North America as gill parasites of acipenserid fishes (*Acipenser* and *Polyodon*).

Fig. 165. *Diclybothrium hamulatum.*

SUPERFAMILY DICLIDOPHOROIDEA Price, 1936
FAMILY DICLIDOPHORIDAE Cerfontaine, 1895

Opisthohaptor contains eight pedunculate asymmetrical clamps, each of which has a muscular sucker and/or an adhesive pad in the inner quadrant; ventral wall of clamp has rib-like sclerites; prohaptor contains two small suckers which open into oral cavity; ceca branched; testes numerous; ovary pretesticular; parasites on the gills of marine fishes. Price (1943a) published a taxonomic revision of the family.

KEY TO GENERA

1a. Opisthohaptor has a large haptoral appendix; parasite of marine perch (Fig. 166). ....Genus *Pedocotyle* MacCallum, 1913

The haptoral appendix contains one pair of small, sessile clamps and the main part of the opisthohaptor has three pairs of pedunculate clamps. The vitelline follicles extend into the appendix.

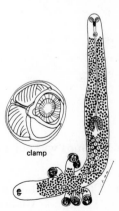

Fig. 166. *Pedocotyle morone.*

clamp

1b. Opisthohaptor without haptoral appendix. 2

2a. Posterior third of body narrow and without vitelline follicles; parasite of flounder and seatrout (Fig. 167). ....
....Genus *Neoheterobothrium* Price, 1943

2b. Posterior part of body as wide as the remainder of the body and contains vitelline follicles. 3

3a. Testes distributed all around ovary; clamps contain a muscular and a spinous pad (Fig. 168). ....
....Genus *Echinopelma* Raecke, 1945

3b. Testes all posterior to ovary. 4

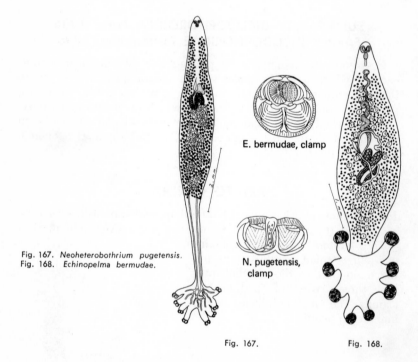

E. bermudae, clamp

Fig. 167. *Neoheterobothrium pugetensis.*
Fig. 168. *Echinopelma bermudae.*

N. pugetensis, clamp

Fig. 167.   Fig. 168.

4a. Clamps without a sucker or having a vestigial sucker (Fig. 169).
....Genus *Diclidophora* Kroyer, 1838

4b. Clamps contain a well-developed sucker (Fig. 170). ....
....................Genus *Choricotyle* van Beneden and Hesse, 1863

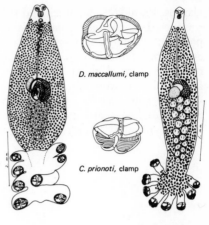

Fig. 169.   Diclidophora maccallumi.
Fig. 170.   Choricotyle prionoti.

D. maccallumi, clamp

C. prionoti, clamp

Fig. 169.   Fig. 170.

FAMILY DACTYLOCOTYLIDAE Brinkmann, 1942

Opisthohaptor with four pairs of pedunculate, asymmetrical clamps, each containing a denticulate patch; opisthohaptor without terminal lappets and anchors; prohaptor in the form of two small suckers; testes pre- and postovarian; ovary N-shaped; ceca branched; parasites on gills of marine fishes.

The family contains only the genus, *Dactylocotyle* van Beneden and Hesse, 1863 and one species, *D. denticulata* (Fig. 171).

Life cycle: *D. denticulata*—

The adult is a parasite on gills of the pollock (*Pollachius virens*). Eggs are laid in groups of 100 to 200 with their polar filaments entwined. Cleavage progresses to the morula stage within 48 hours and a ciliated larva (Fig. 172) is produced in 18 to 19 days at about 14° C. After hatching, the larvae swim for a time and attach to the gills of a host fish, lose the cilia and start to produce

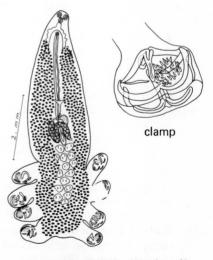

clamp

Fig. 171.   *Dactylocotyle denticulata*. (Redrawn from Price, 1943a.)

clamps. Frankland deparasitized fish in chloretone solution and then
reinfected them with ciliated larvae in the laboratory. These experimental infections were followed for 38 days, through the first
and second larval stages. Second stage larvae (Fig. 172) were produced five to thirteen days after hatching. Larval stages three,
four and five were obtained from natural infections. Clamps develop in pairs, starting with the posterior pair. As clamps develop,
the larval hooks are gradually replaced. The mature parasite develops within six months (Frankland, 1955).

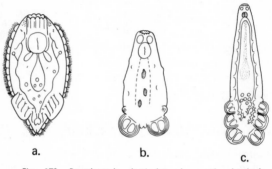

a.   b.   c.

Fig. 172. *Dactylocotyle denticulata,* larvae (a. hatched
larva; b. second-stage larva; c. fifth-stage larva.) (Redrawn
from Frankland, 1955.)

FAMILY HEXOSTOMATIDAE Price, 1936

Opisthohaptor indistinctly set off from the body and contains
four pairs of sessile clamps, each consisting of three X-shaped
sclerites embedded in a sucker; one or two pairs of anchors between posterior clamps; prohaptor contains a pair of small suckers;
testes numerous; ovary pretesticular, having the shape of an inverted U; eggs have polar filaments; vaginal pore dorso-median;
gill parasites of marine fishes. A taxonomic revision of the family
was published by Price (1961a).

KEY TO GENERA

1a. Body with a waist-like constriction anterior to opisthohaptor;
clamps arranged in two nearly longitudinal rows, clamps of
posterior pair only slightly smaller than the others (Fig. 173).
....Genus *Neohexostoma* Price, 1961

1b. Body without a waist-like constriction; clamps arranged in a
curved transverse row, clamps of posterior pair much smaller
than the others (Fig. 174). ....
....Genus *Hexostoma* Rafinesque, 1815

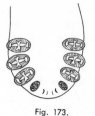

Fig. 173. Neohexostoma sp.
Fig. 174. Hexostoma sp.

Fig. 173. 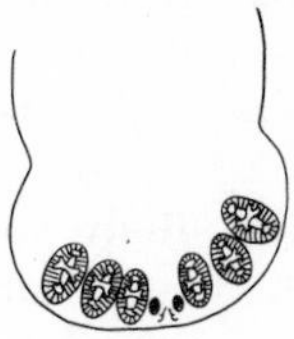   Fig. 174.

FAMILY DISCOCOTYLIDAE Price, 1936

Opisthohaptor contains eight sessile, symmetrical clamps without suckers or adhesive pads; prohaptor has two small suckers that open into buccal cavity; ceca branched; testes numerous (one large, lobed testis in *Octomacrum*); ovary pre- or posttesticular; parasites on gills of freshwater and marine fishes. Price (1943b) published a taxonomic revision of the family.

KEY TO GENERA

1a. One large, deeply lobed testis present; clamps of posterior pair smaller than the others; on gills of suckers (Fig. 175). ....
.................Genus *Octomacrum* Mueller, 1934

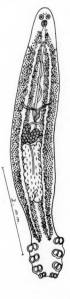

Fig. 175. Octomacrum lanceatum.

1b. Testes numerous. 2
2a. Ovary posttesticular; clamps have accessory sclerites. 3
2b. Ovary pretesticular; clamps without accessory sclerites. 4

3a. Anterior part of body narrow and oriented at right angles to wider posterior part; ceca fused in opisthohaptor; two vaginae with lateral pores; on gills of leatherjacket (Fig. 176). ....
................................Genus *Vallisia* Parona and Perugia, 1890

3b. Body straight, tapering gradually from anterior to posterior; ceca not fused in opisthohaptor; vagina single, pore lateral; on gills of lookdown (Fig. 177). ....
Genus *Pseudomazocraes* Caballero and Bravo-Hollis, 1955

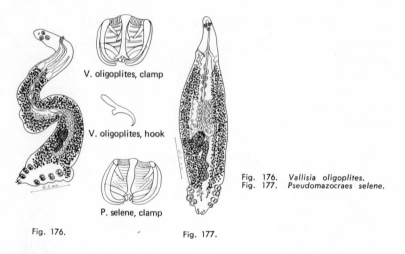

V. oligoplites, clamp

V. oligoplites, hook

P. selene, clamp

Fig. 176.

Fig. 177.

Fig. 176.   *Vallisia oligoplites.*
Fig. 177.   *Pseudomazocraes selene.*

4a. Clamps of anterior pair much larger than the others; terminus of opisthohaptor has three pairs of dissimilar anchors (Fig. 178).
...................Genus *Anthocotyle* van Beneden and Hesse, 1863

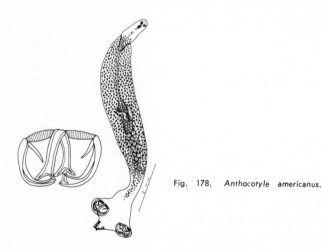

Fig. 178.   *Anthocotyle americanus.*

4b. Clamps all of equal size. 5
5a. Opisthohaptor deeply lobed with four clamps on each lobe; vagina single, pore dorso-median; parasite of marine fishes (Fig. 179). ....Genus *Bicotylophora* Price, 1936
5b. Opisthohaptor not lobed but somewhat rectangular; vagina Y-shaped, pores lateral; on gills of salmonid fishes (Fig. 180). ....Genus *Discocotyle* Diesing, 1850

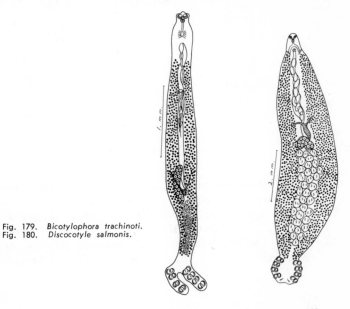

Fig. 179.   *Bicotylophora trachinoti.*
Fig. 180.   *Discocotyle salmonis.*

Fig. 179.   Fig. 180.

FAMILY MACROVALVITREMATIDAE Yamaguti, 1963

Body small, cylindrical; opisthohaptor contains eight guitar-shaped, fire-tong-shaped or oblong clamps; prohaptor has a large, terminal, cup-shaped buccal cavity with a pair of suckers opening into it; ceca branched, united posteriorly and extending into opisthohaptor; one testis or many; ovary pretesticular; vaginae present, pores lateral; parasites on gills of marine fishes.

KEY TO GENERA

1a. One testis; bilateral pleated placodes in anterior third of body; clamps of two different shapes; posterior pair of clamps oblong, others fire-tong-shaped; parasite of marine perch (Fig. 181). ....Genus *Hargisia* Yamaguti, 1963

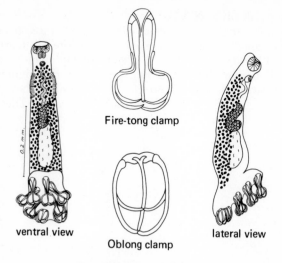

Fire-tong clamp

Oblong clamp

ventral view   lateral view

Fig. 181. *Hargisia bairdiella.*

1b. Testes numerous; body without pleated placodes; clamps similar in size and shape. 2

2a. Clamps guitar-shaped; parasite of croakers (Fig. 182). ....
..............................Genus *Macrovalvitrematoides* Yamaguti, 1963

2b. Clamps oblong with serrated margins; parasite of pigfish (Fig. 183). ....Genus *Pseudotagia* Yamaguti, 1963

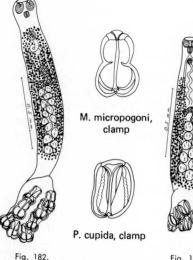

M. micropogoni, clamp

P. cupida, clamp

Fig. 182.   *Macrovalvitrematoides micropogoni.* Fig. 183. *Pseudotagia cupida.*

Fig. 182.   Fig. 183.

FAMILY MAZOCRAEIDAE Price, 1936

Opisthohaptor indistinctly set off from body or clamps mounted directly on sides of body, clamps pedunculate or sessile, clamp sclerites U-shaped; one or more pairs of anchors on terminal lappet; prohaptor contains two small suckers which open into buccal cavity; ceca branched; one testis or many; ovary folded on itself, anterior or opposite to testis; parasites on gills of herring and mackerel. A taxonomic revision of the family was published by Price (1961b).

KEY TO GENERA

1a. Clamps distributed along sides of body proper, extending at least as far forward as testis; parasite of herring. 2
1b. Clamps restricted to a distinct opisthohaptor some distance posterior to level of testis. 3
2a. Testis opposite ovary; clamps extending forward to level of ovary (Fig. 184). ....Genus *Mazocraeoides* Price, 1936
2b. Testis posterior to ovary; clamps very large, extending forward at least to level of testis (Fig. 185). ....
................................Genus *Pseudomazocraeoides* Price, 1961

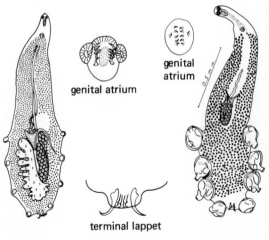

genital atrium

genital atrium

terminal lappet

Fig. 184.   Fig. 185.

Fig. 184. *Mazocraeoidies georgei.* (Redrawn from Price, 1961b.)
Fig. 185. *Pseudomazocraeoides megalocotyle.*

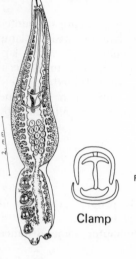

Clamp

3a. Opisthohaptor asymmetrical with four well-developed clamps on the right side and one very small one on the left; parasite of mackerel (Fig. 186). ....Genus *Grubea* Diesing, 1858

Fig. 186. *Grubea cochlear.* (Redrawn from Palombi, 1949.)

3b. Opisthohaptor symmetrical with four clamps on each side. 4

genital
atrium

4a. Terminal lappet a single lobe; clamps sessile or nearly so; testes numerous; clamps of anterior pair much larger than the others; parasite of gizzard shad (Fig. 187). ...... Genus *Pseudanthocotyloides* Price, 1958

4b. Terminal lappet bilobed, each lobe containing one anchor; clamps pedunculate; one testis; parasite of menhaden. 5

Fig. 187. *Pseudanthocotyloides banghami.*

5a. Clamps of anterior two pairs distinctly larger than the others (Fig. 188). ....Genus *Neoclupeocotyle* Price, 1961
5b. Clamps of uniform size (Fig. 189). ....
....Genus *Clupeocotyle* Hargis, 1955

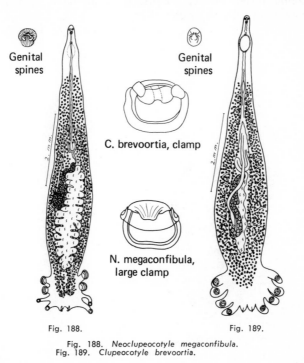

Genital spines

Genital spines

C. brevoortia, clamp

N. megaconfibula, large clamp

Fig. 188.   Fig. 189.

Fig. 188. *Neoclupeocotyle megaconfibula.*
Fig. 189. *Clupeocotyle brevoortia.*

SUPERFAMILY MICROCOTYLOIDEA Unnithan, 1957
FAMILY MICROCOTYLIDAE Taschenberg, 1879

Opisthohaptor symmetrical, clamps numerous and of microcotylid structure, without accessory sclerites; anchors absent; prohaptor contains paired suckers which open into buccal cavity; ceca branched, not united posteriorly; eyespots absent; testes numerous; ovary pretesticular, folded; vagina usually present, pore lateral or dorsal; on gills of marine fishes.

KEY TO GENERA

1a. Clamps distributed along lateral margins of body, extending forward to level of ovary; clamps slightly pedunculate, causing body margins to appear ruffled (Fig. 190). ....
....Genus *Prosomicrocotyla* Yamaguti, 1958

1b. Clamps confined to a distinct opisthohaptor at the posterior end of the body and confluent across the posterior end. 2

2a. Vitelline follicles absent in the posterior part of the body; vagina absent; suckers of prohaptor provided with prominent spines; on gills of mullet (Fig. 191). ....
................................Genus *Metamicrocotyla* Yamaguti, 1953

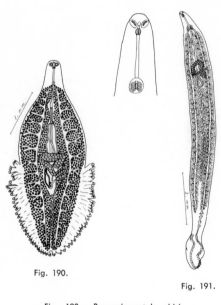

Fig. 190.

Fig. 191.

Fig. 190. *Prosomicrocotyla chiri.*
(Redrawn from Goto, 1895.)   Fig.
191. *Metamicrocotyla macracantha.*

2b. Vitelline follicles extending into posterior part of body; vagina present; suckers of prohaptor non-spinous or with very minute spines. 3

3a. Vaginal pore on right margin of body; parasite of gray snapper (Fig. 192). ....Genus *Microcotyloides* Fugii, 1944

3b. Vaginal pore on dorso-median surface of body. 4

4a. Genital atrium unarmed (Fig. 193). ....
....Genus *Aspinatrium* Yamaguti, 1963

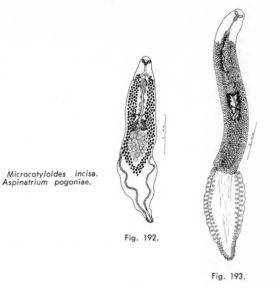

Fig. 192.   *Microcotyloides incisa.*
Fig. 193.   *Aspinatrium pogoniae.*

Fig. 192.

Fig. 193.

4b. Genital atrium armed (Fig. 194). ....
...................Genus *Microcotyle* van Beneden and Hesse, 1863

Life cycle: *M. spinicirrus*—
    The adult is a gill parasite of the freshwater drum, *Aplodinotus grunniens.* The eggs have bipolar filaments and an operculum. Larvae develop and hatch in five to eleven days following oviposition. The hatched larva (Fig. 195) has three bands of cilia, a pigmented eye, pharynx, six pairs of hooks, two pairs of anchors and three pairs of flame cells. The larva swims and upon contacting a suitable host fish, attaches to the gills. Following attachment, the cilia are shed and clamps start to form, new clamps developing throughout life from clamp primordia at the anterior end of the series. The larval haptor, containing hooks and anchors is eventually lost (Remley, 1942).

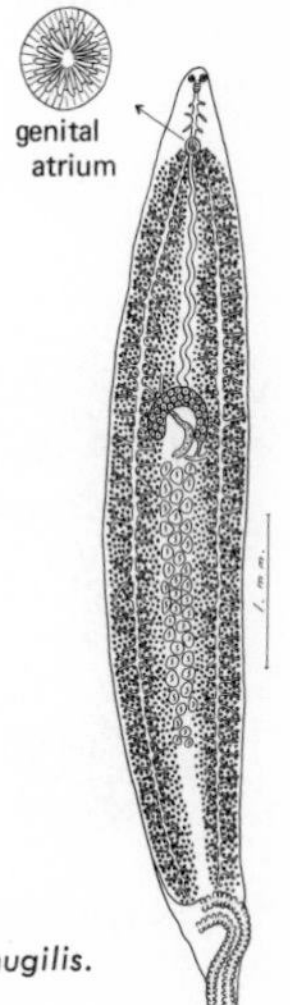

genital
atrium

Fig. 194.   *Microcotyle pseudomugilis.*

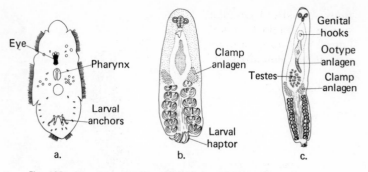

Fig. 195. *Microcotyle spinicirrus*, larval stages (a. hatched larva; b. attached stage; c. older attached stage.) (Redrawn from Remley, 1942.)

FAMILY AXINIDAE Unnithan, 1957

Opisthohaptor truncate, clamps arranged in two rows, end to end, the rows separated by anchors; prohaptor contains two small suckers which open into buccal cavity; testes numerous; ovary pretesticular, U- or J-shaped, the ends directed anteriad; parasites on gills of marine fishes. Price (1962a) published a taxonomic revision of the family.

KEY TO GENERA

1a. Genital atrium armed, spines arranged in two lateral and one median group (Fig. 196). ....Genus *Axine* Abildgaard, 1794

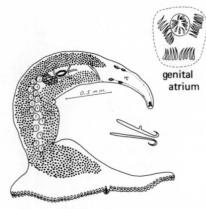

Fig. 196. *Axine hyporamphi.* (Redrawn from Price, 1962a.)

1b. Genital atrium unarmed. 2

2a. **Body broadly triangular; cirrus spinous; vaginal pore dorso-lateral and has hornlike spines; parasite of houndfish (Fig. 197).** .... **Genus** *Chlamydaxine* **Unnithan, 1957**

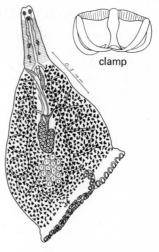

clamp

Fig. 197.   *Chlamydaxine truncata.*

2b. **Body elongate; parasite of houndfish or needlefish.** 3
3a. **Cirrus spinous; vaginal pore dorso-median, spinous (Fig. 198).** ....**Genus** *Axinoides* **Yamaguti, 1938**
3b. **Cirrus nonspinous; vaginal pore dorsal and sublateral, armed with horn-like spines (Fig. 199).** ....
....**Genus** *Nudaciraxine* **Price, 1962**

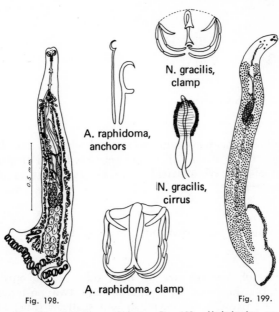

N. gracilis, clamp

A. raphidoma, anchors

N. gracilis, cirrus

A. raphidoma, clamp

Fig. 198.   Fig. 199.

Fig. 198.   *Axinoides raphidoma.*   Fig. 199.   *Nudaciraxine gracilis.* (Redrawn from Price, 1962a.)

FAMILY HETERAXINIDAE Price, 1962

Opisthohaptor triangular, asymmetrical, clamps more abundant or larger on one side than on the other (clamps only on one side in *Leuresthicola*); median sclerite (= spring) of clamp sometimes bifid or trifid at tip; prohaptor contains a pair of small suckers which open into buccal cavity; testes numerous; ovary pretesticular, in the shape of an inverted U; vagina present or absent; parasites on the gills of fishes. A systematic account of the family was published by Price (1962b).

KEY TO GENERA

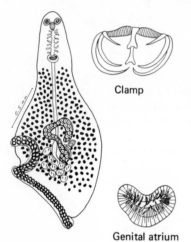

Clamp

Genital atrium

Fig. 200. *Leuresthicola olsoni*.

1a. Clamps present on only one side of opisthohaptor; vagina absent; on gills of grunion (Fig. 200). .... **Genus** *Leuresthicola* Price, 1962

1b. Clamps on both sides of opisthohaptor. 2

2a. Opisthohaptor has large and small clamps, the larger are asymmetrical, having the outer sclerites longer than the inner; small clamps symmetrical or nearly so; parasites of jackfish (Fig. 201). ....**Genus** *Cemocotyle* Sproston, 1946

2b. All clamps symmetrical but can be of two sizes. 3

3a. Clamps of uniform size on both sides of the opisthohaptor; genital atrium has two anterior and two posterior spinous pockets; parasites of weakfish and seatrout (Fig. 202). ....**Genus** *Cynoscionicola* Price, 1962

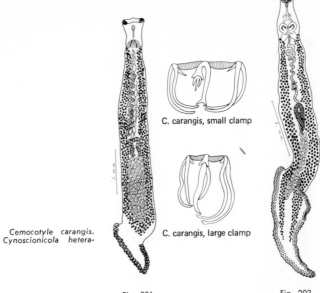

C. carangis, small clamp

C. carangis, large clamp

Fig. 201. *Cemocotyle carangis.*
Fig. 202. *Cynoscionicola hetera-cantha.*

Fig. 201.

Fig. 202.

3b. Clamps of one side of the opisthohaptor much larger than those of the other side. 4

4a. Sides of opisthohaptor of nearly equal length; clamps fewer and much larger on one side; genital atrium has two rows of spines attached to its anterior wall; parasites of freshwater drum (Fig. 203). ....Genus *Lintaxine* Sproston, 1946

4b. Sides of opisthohaptor of unequal length; clamps fewer and smaller on one side. 5

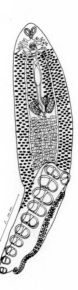

Fig. 203. *Lintaxine cokeri.*

5a. Vagina absent; eggs few; genital atrium has two antero-lateral spiny pockets; parasite of spot and margate (Fig. 204). ....
....Genus *Heteraxinoides* Yamaguti, 1963

5b. Vagina present; many eggs in uterus; on gills of amberjack (Fig. 205). ....Genus *Allencotyla* Price, 1962

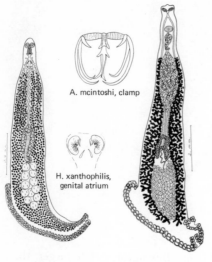

A. mcintoshi, clamp

H. xanthophilis, genital atrium

Fig. 204. *Heteraxinoides xantho-philis.* Fig. 205. *Allencotyla mcintoshi.*

Fig. 204.   Fig. 205.

FAMILY PYRAGRAPHORIDAE Yamaguti, 1963

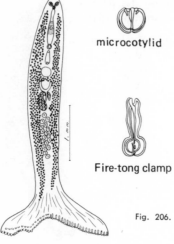

microcotylid

Fire-tong clamp

Opisthohaptor fish-tail-shaped; clamps of two types, microcotylid and fire-tong-shaped; prohaptor contains two small suckers; ceca branched but not anastomosing posteriorly; testes numerous; ovary pretesticular, elongate, sinuous; eggs with bipolar filaments; parasites on gills of marine fish.

The family contains a single genus and species, *Pyragraphorus pyragraphorus* (Fig. 206), a parasite of pompano, *Trachinotus carolinus*, on the Atlantic coast.

Fig. 206. *Pyragraphorus pyragraphorus.*

FAMILY ALLOPYRAGRAPHORIDAE Yamaguti, 1963

Opisthohaptor fish - tail - shaped, clamps all microcotylid, longer than wide; prohaptor contains two small suckers; ceca branched, anastomosing posteriorly and extending into opisthohaptor; testes numerous; ovary pretesticular, elongate, sinuous; eggs with bipolar filaments; parasites of marine fishes.

The family contains only the genus *Allopyragraphorus* Yamaguti, 1963 (Fig. 207).

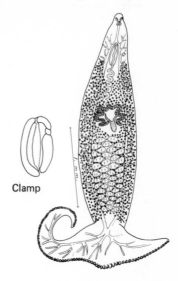

Clamp

Fig. 207. *Allopyragraphorus hippos.*

FAMILY GASTROCOTYLIDAE Price, 1943

Opisthohaptor symmetrical or asymmetrical; clamps distributed along margins of body proper or confined to a distinct opisthohaptor, contain accessory sclerites and sometimes ribs; small anchors present; prohaptor contains a pair of small suckers that open into buccal cavity; ceca branched; testes two to many; ovary pretesticular; elongate, folded; vagina present; eggs have bipolar filaments; parasites on gills of marine fishes.

KEY TO GENERA

1a. Rows of clamps of equal length on both sides of opisthohaptor. 2
1b. Rows of clamps of unequal length or having larger clamps on one side than on the other. 3
2a. Opisthohaptor extends far anteriad along ventral side of body; vitelline follicles confined to opisthohaptor; testes large, arranged in linear series; parasite of Spanish mackerel (Fig. 208).
..................................Genus *Thoracocotyle* MacCallum, 1913

2b. Opisthohaptor confined to posterior end of body; vitelline follicles restricted to body proper; testes small (Fig. 209). ....
....Genus *Gotocotyla* Ishii, 1936

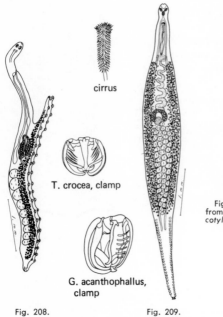

cirrus

T. crocea, clamp

G. acanthophallus,
clamp

Fig. 208. *Thoracocotyle crocea.* (Redrawn
from MacCallum, 1913.) Fig. 209. *Gotocotyla acanthophallus.*

Fig. 208.   Fig. 209.

3a. Clamps of longer row large and sessile, those of shorter row
small and pedunculate; testes two, tandem; terminal lappet
has three pairs of anchors; parasite of bumper (Fig. 210). ....
....Genus *Amphipolycotyle* Hargis, 1957
3b. All clamps sessile, similar in size and structure; testes numerous; end of opisthohaptor has one pair of anchors; parasite
of Spanish mackerel (Fig. 211). ....
....Genus *Scomberocotyle* Hargis, 1956

SUBCLASS ASPIDOGASTREA Faust and Tang, 1936
Key to Families

1a. Holdfast organ in the form of a large ventral adhesive disc
containing septa and alveoli (= loculi) and sometimes conical
papillae (Figs. 212-216). ....Family Aspidogasteridae p. 107
1b. Holdfast organ consisting of a longitudinal row of separate
suckers (Fig. 218). ....Family Stichocotylidae p. 111

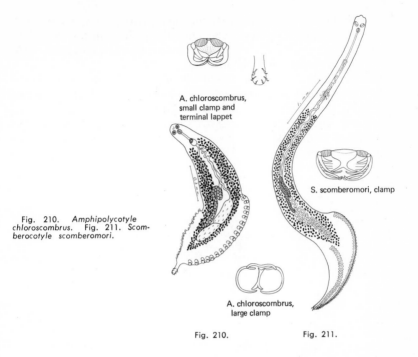

A. chloroscombrus, small clamp and terminal lappet

S. scomberomori, clamp

Fig. 210. *Amphipolycotyle chloroscombrus.* Fig. 211. *Scomberocotyle scomberomori.*

A. chloroscombrus, large clamp

Fig. 210.   Fig. 211.

FAMILY ASPIDOGASTERIDAE Poche, 1907

Body composed of a ventral adhesive disc and a dorsal hump. The adhesive disc contains one or more rows of alveoli separated by septa; the hump contains the internal organs; oral sucker usually absent; anterior end of body lobed; pharynx present; intestine a single cecum; one or two testes; cirrus sac present or absent; ovary anterior to testes; genital pore ventral, median or submedian, located anterior to the adhesive disc; vitelline glands follicular or tubular; uterus long, sometimes containing many eggs; excretory vesicle V-shaped, the arms extending anterior to level of pharynx; excretory pore near posterior end; endoparasites of poikilothermic vertebrates, gastropod and lamellibranch molluscs.

KEY TO GENERA

1a. Adhesive disc with three longitudinal rows of alveoli (one row median and transverse and two rows marginal) (Fig. 212). 2

1b. Adhesive disc with four longitudinal rows of alveoli (two rows median and transverse and two rows marginal) (Fig. 216). 3

2a.   One testis; vitelline glands follicular; cirrus sac present; parasites of turtles or freshwater lamellibranch molluscs. (Fig. 212).
....Genus *Cotylaspis* **Leidy, 1857**

Key to species in Skrjabin (1964).

Mature specimens were found adhering to the outer surface of the kidneys and the inner gill lamellae of unionid clams of the the genus *Anodonta*. Specimens survived for several weeks in dishes of water. Osborn (1903) regards them as scavengers which take up bits of debris. Mature specimens have also been found in the intestine of turtles.

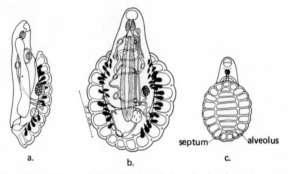

Fig. 212.   *Cotylaspis insignis* (a. lateral view, b. dorsal view, c. ventral view). (Redrawn from Osborn, 1903.)

2b.   Two testes; viteline glands tubular, asymmetrical; cirrus sac absent; parasites in the intestine of freshwater fishes and also in snails and freshwater clams (Fig. 213). ....
......................................Genus *Cotylogasteroides* **Yamaguti, 1963**

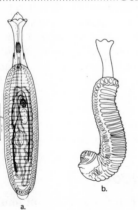

The genus contains a single species, *C. occidentalis* (= *Cotylogaster occidentalis*). Kelly (1926) found specimens in the freshwater clam *Lampsilis luteola*. Nickerson (1902) reported the species as a parasite of the sheepshead, *Aplodinotus grunnions*. Dickerman (1948) obtained mature specimens from the operculate snail, *Goniobasis* sp. from Lake Erie. The parasite is capable of undergoing its entire development in this host. He infected small sheepshead by feeding specimens from *Goniobasis*.

Fig. 213.   *Cotylogasteroides occidentalis* (a. ventral view, b. lateral view). (Redrawn from Nickerson, 1902.)

3a. **Median zone of adhesive disc with numerous conical papillae; cirrus sac absent; intestinal parasites of freshwater fishes and turtles and in the pericardial sac of lamellibranch molluscs (Fig. 214).** ....Genus *Lophotaspis* **Lo_oss, 1901**

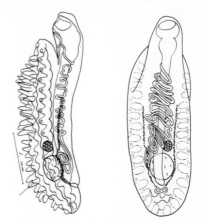

Fig. 214. *Lophotaspis interiora.* (Redrawn from Ward and Hopkins, 1931.)

3b. **Adhesive disc without conical papillae; cirrus sac present.** 4
4a. **Adhesive disc short, occupying about middle third of body; oral lobes around mouth; intestinal parasites of marine fishes (Fig. 215).** ....Genus *Lobatostoma* **Eckmann, 1932**

The median ridge, separating the two inner rows of alveoli, is weakly developed. Most specimens appear to have only three rows of alveoli. The oral lobes provide the best distinguishing feature.

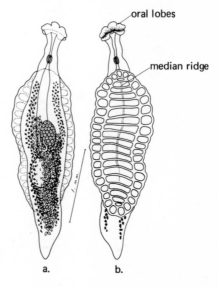

Fig. 215. *Lobatostoma ringens* (a. dorsal view, b. ventral view).

4b. **Adhesive disc long, extending nearly to posterior end of body; no oral lobes around mouth; intestinal parasites of freshwater fishes and lamellibranch and gastropod molluscs (Fig. 216).** ....Genus *Aspidogaster* **Baer, 1827**

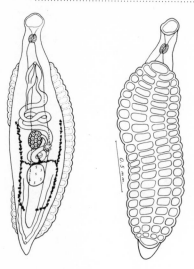

Fig. 216. *Aspidogaster conchicola* (a. dorsal view, b. ventral view).

Life cycle: *A. conchicola*—

The operculate eggs in the uterus of mature worms contain miracidia which hatch when eggs are placed in water. The hatched larvae (Fig. 217) resemble amphistome trematodes of the subclass Digenea in having a large ventral sucker near the posterior end of the body. As development progresses, the ventral sucker enlarges gradually, and slowly transforms to the ventral adhesive disc of the adult fluke. The larvae are thought to be transferred from host to host by water currents. Mature specimens inhabit the pericardial cavity and kidneys of freshwater clams of the family Unionidae (Williams, 1942).

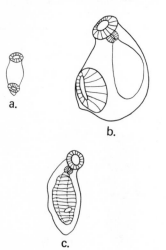

Fig. 217. Larvae of *Aspidogaster conchicola* (a. hatched larva; b. older larva; c. larva with developing disc). (Redrawn from Williams, 1942.)

FAMILY STICHOCOTYLIDAE Faust and Tang, 1936

Body very long and slender (up to 115 mm.); oral sucker absent, mouth at base of a depression; one intestinal cecum; pharynx present; holdfast organ consisting of a longitudinal series of 20-30 ventral suckers, distributed along most of length of the body, the more posterior ones smaller than the others; two testes, oblique; cirrus sac small; ovary anterior to testes; genital pore anterior to first sucker; vitelline glands partly tubular and partly follicular, unpaired; uterus very long, having many transverse folds; excretory system consisting of two longitudinal, sinuous canals, extending from posterior end of body to level of pharynx; parasites in bile ducts and gall bladder of elasmobranchs (rays).

The family contains a single genus and species, *Stichocotyle nephropis* (Fig. 218). Larval stages have been found encysted in the wall of the rectum of lobsters in Europe and North America.

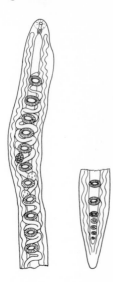

Fig. 218. *Stichocotyle nephropis*.

SUBCLASS DIGENEA
Key to Families

1a. Mouth on midventral surface of body, opening into saclike intestine (Fig. 219); a sucker or a rhynchus at anterior end of body (Fig. 221); genital pore near posterior end of body; parasites of fishes. ....Family Bucephalidae p. 176

1b. Mouth at anterior end of body, usually surrounded by a muscular sucker (Fig. 220); intestine usually composed of two ceca; genital pore usually in anterior half of body. 2

2a. Parasites in blood vessels of host; pharynx absent. 3

2b. Not in blood vessels of host; pharynx usually present. 5

3a. Sexes separate (dioecious); in blood vessels of birds and mammals; genital pore in anterior third of body. ....
....Family Schistosomatidae p. 141

3b. Hermaphroditic (monoecious); in blood vessels of fishes or reptiles (turtles); genital pore usually in posterior third of of body. 4

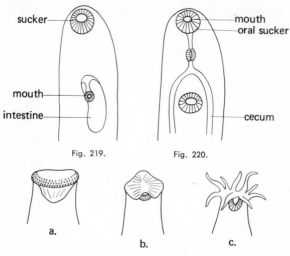

Fig. 219.   Fig. 220.

Fig. 221.

Fig. 219. Fig. 220. Fig. 221. Family Bucephalidae (a. rynchus, b. and c. suckers).

4a. Parasites in blood vessels of fishes; body without suckers; intestine X- or H-shaped due to presence of anterior intestinal ceca (Fig. 222). ....Family Sanguinicolidae p. 153

4b. Parasites in heart and arteries of turtles; muscular suckers usually present; intestine in shape of an inverted tuning fork with ceca sometimes fused in posterior part of body to form a common cecum (Fig. 223). ....Family Spirorchiidae p. 149

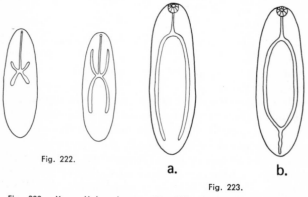

Fig. 222.

a.   b.

Fig. 223.

Fig. 222. X- or H-shaped ceca. Fig. 223. Intestinal ceca (a. blind ceca, b. common cecum).

5a. Embedded in muscles, connective tissue or visceral organs of fishes; body very long and threadlike or the anterior part narrow and posterior part thick; hermaphroditic or sexes sep-

arate; testes, ovary and vitelline glands tubular; ovary and
vitelline glands posterior to testes; genital pore close to mouth.
....Family Didymozoidae p. 330

5b. Body not as described above; usually in lumen of some in-
ternal organ of host. 6

6a. Ventral sucker or both suckers absent. 7
6b. Oral and ventral suckers usually present. 14

7a. Triangular unarmed head collar present
(Fig. 224). 8
7b. Head collar absent or armed with large
spines if present; ends of body rounded.
....9

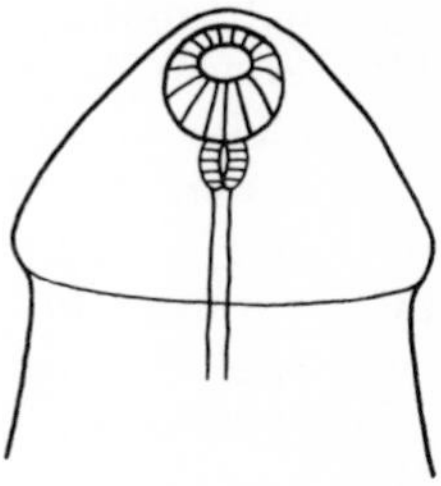

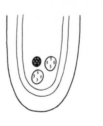

Fig. 224.   Triangular head collar.

8a. Parasites in urinary tract of birds; testes opposite, in middle
third of body. ....(Genus *Eucotyle*) Family Eucotylidae p. 241
8b. Parasites in intestine or urinary tract of turtles; testes opposite, near posterior end of body. ....
....Family Pronocephalidae p. 212

9a. Intestinal ceca fused posteriorly to form a cyclocoel
(Fig. 225). 10
9b. Intestinal ceca end blindly
(Fig. 226). 11

Fig. 225.   Cyclocoel.
Fig. 226.   Ceca blind.

Fig. 225. 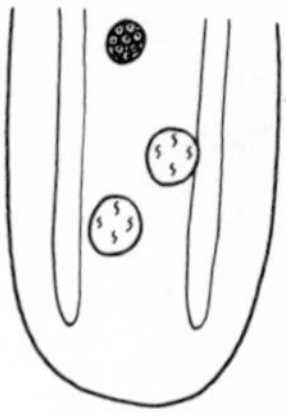   Fig. 226.

10a. Parasites in urinary tract of birds; testes tandem or oblique,
in middle third of body; ovary pretesticular; oral sucker
present. ....(Genus *Tanaisia*) Family Eucotylidae p. 241
10b. Parasites in respiratory tract of birds; testes near posterior
end of body; ovary between testes or opposite anterior testis;
oral sucker absent or rudimentary. ....
....Family Cyclocoelidae p. 161

11a. One testis; both suckers absent; pharynx present; excretory
system V-shaped, two excretory vesicles, the arm of each
extending anterior to level of esophagus; pigmented eyespots
usually present; in digestive tract of marine fishes. ....
....Family Bivesiculidae p. 160

11b. Two testes; oral sucker present; one excretory vesicle; parasites of reptiles, birds or mammals. 12

12a. Parasites in respiratory tract of turtles; testes and vitelline glands tubular; testes extend through 2/3 of body length; excretory pore dorsal to pharynx. ....
....Family Heronimidae p. 207

12b. Not in respiratory tract of turtles; testes and vitelline glands not tubular; excretory pore at posterior end of body. 13

13a. Intestinal parasites of turtles; testes tandem, in middle of body; ovary posterior to testes; oral sucker large with two muscular projections. ....
........................Family Microscaphidiidae (= Angiodictyidae) p. 214

13b. Parasites in cecum and colon of birds and mammals; testes opposite, near posterior end of body; ovary between testes; eggs have bipolar filaments. ....Family Notocotylidae p. 208

14a. Ventral sucker at or near posterior end of body. 15

14b. Ventral sucker on ventral body surface, usually in anterior half of body. 16

15a. Body nearly round; ventral sucker subterminal; ovary pretesticular; testes opposite; muscular ring between oral sucker and pharynx; parasites of marine fishes. ....
....Family Opistholebetidae p. 284

15b. Body oval, conical or elongate; ventral sucker terminal; ovary posttesticular; testes tandem or oblique; muscular ring absent; parasites of all classes of vertebrates. ....
....Family Paramphistomatidae p. 201

16a. Bulbous or foliaceous tribocytic organ arising posterior to ventral sucker (Figs. 227, 228); body usually divided into distinct fore- and hindbody regions; copulatory bursa and genital pore at posterior end of body. 17

16b. Tribocytic organ absent; body not as described above. 20

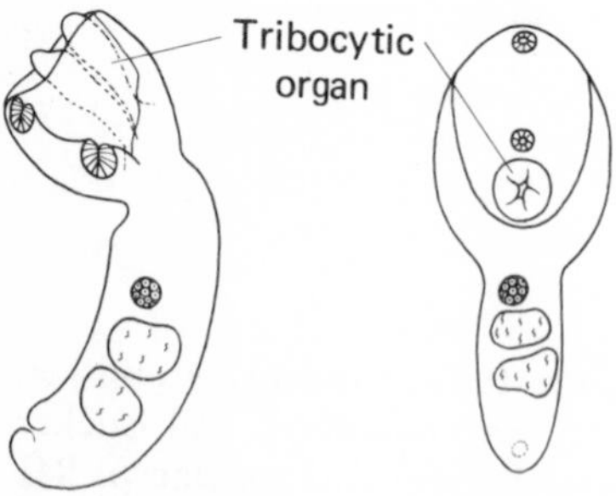

Fig. 227.   Fig. 228.

Fig. 227.   Foliaceous tribocytic organ.
Fig. 228.   Bulbous tribocytic organ.

17a. Cirrus sac present, located near posterior end of body; **body** small, not divided into distinct fore- and hindbody regions.
.... Family Cyathocotylidae p. 139

17b. Cirrus sac absent; body usually divided into distinct fore-
and hindbody regions. 18

18a. Forebody cup-shaped; tribocytic organ foliaceous (Fig. 227);
intestinal parasites of birds or mammals. ....
.... Family Strigeidae p. 124

18b. Forebody flat or spoon-shaped; tribocytic organ bulbous
(Fig. 228); intestinal parasites of reptiles, birds or mammals. 19

19a. Hindbody contains thick-walled paraprostate organ surrounded by gland cells (Fig. 229); intestinal parasites of
reptiles (alligators). ......Family Proterodiplostomatidae p. 136

19b. Paraprostate organ absent (Fig. 230); intestinal parasites of
birds and mammals. ....Family Diplostomatidae p. 128

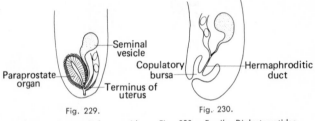

Fig. 229.   Fig. 230.

Fig. 229. Proterodiplostomatidae.   Fig. 230. Family Diplostomatidae.

20a. Genital pore in posterior third of body, some distance posterior to ventral sucker. 21

20b. Genital pore in anterior part of body, usuallly close to ventral
sucker. 23

21a. Ovary pretesticular, separated from testes by some folds of
uterus; intestinal parasites of bats. ....
.... Family Urotrematidae p. 249

21b. Ovary between testes or opposite anterior testis; parasites
of birds or of mammals other than bats. 22

22a. Parasites in the mouth and esophagus
of aquatic birds; anterior end retractile, the retraction producing a
collar-like fold around oral sucker
(Fig. 231); metacercariae precocial
(5-8 mm long), commonly encysted
in the tissues of fishes and frogs. ......
.... Family Clinostomatidae p. 156

22b. Intestinal parasites of birds and mammals or in bursa Fabricii of birds;
anterior end of body not retractile.
.... Family Brachylaimidae p. 164

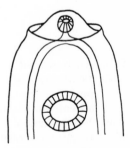

Fig. 231. Family Clino-
stomatidae.

23a. Body fusiform or elongate; telescoping ecsoma (= tail) sometimes present at posterior end of body (Fig. 232); cuticle annulated in some genera; terminus of male and female ducts (Fig. 233) fused to form genital sinus (= hermaphroditic duct) which is enclosed in a sinus sac (= false cirrus sac); vitelline glands compact follicular or tubular (Fig. 232); parasites in stomach and esophagus of marine fishes (rarely in pharynx or Eustachian tubes of amphibians). ....
.... Family Hemiuridae p. 319

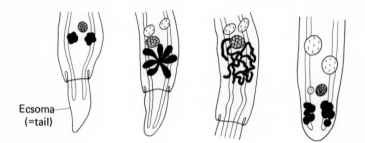

Fig. 232. Family Hemiuridae, vitelline glands and ecsoma.

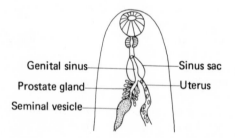

Fig. 233. Family Hemiuridae, Terminal reproductive organs.

23b. Anatomy not as described above. 24
24a. Ventro-genital sac present, containing ventral sucker, genital pore and usually a muscular gonotyl (Fig. 234); cirrus sac absent; hermaphroditic duct usually present. 25
24b. Ventro-genital sac absent; cirrus sac present or absent. 26
25a. Intestinal parasites of fishes; uterus extends posterior to testes; arms of excretory vesicle extend forward to pharynx; intestinal ceca usually long; pigmented eyespots some times present. .... Family Cryptogonimidae p. 315

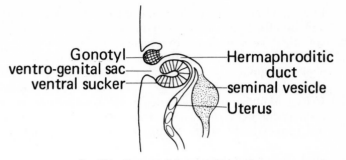

Fig. 234. Ventro-genital sac, sagittal section.

25b. Intestinal parasites of birds and mammals; uterus usually not extending posterior to testes; arms of excretory vesicle not extending far forward; intestinal ceca sometimes short. .... Family Heterophyidae p. 306

26a. Hermaphroditic sac present (Fig. 235), enclosing hermaphroditic duct, metraterm, internal seminal vesicle and prostate cells; external seminal vesicle also present; eggs usually large; usually one testis; parasites of marine fishes. .... Family Haploporidae p. 198

26b. Anatomy not as described above. 27

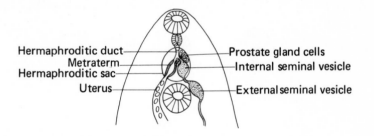

Fig. 235. Family Haploporidae, terminal reproductive organs.

27a. Uterus entirely anterior to ovary. 28
27b. Uterus extending posterior to ovary, frequently to posterior end of body. 45
28a. Testes follicular (15 or more), filling intercecal space. 29
28b. One or two testes present (rarely 9-11). 30
29a. More than 20 testes, arranged in longitudinal rows in hindbody; intestinal ceca have one pair of anterior diverticula; cirrus sac present; intestinal parasites of marine fishes. .... Family Pleorchiidae p. 285
29b. Testes filling intercecal space but not in longitudinal rows; cecal diverticula absent; cirrus sac absent; in trachea, nasal cavities or esophagus of birds. ....Family Orchipedidae p. 284

30a. Intestinal ceca have at least one pair of anterior diverticula and usually numerous lateral diverticula. 31

30b. Intestinal ceca without diverticula. 32

31a. Intestinal ceca have anterior and usually lateral diverticula; eggs triangular in cross section; in liver and bile passages of marine mammals. .... Family Campulidae p. 191

31b. Ceca without anterior diverticula but have numerous lateral diverticula; eggs rounds in cross section; in liver and bile passages of herbivorous mammals and in human beings. .... Family Fasciolidae p. 192

32a. Oral sucker has two ventro-lateral muscular papillae and a muscular dorsal transverse ridge; (Fig. 236); excretory vesicle Y-shaped, the arms extending far anterior and having many lateral diverticula; in intestine of turtles. .... Family Rhytidodidae p. 189

32b. Anatomy not as described above. 33

33a. One testis; one intestinal cecum; cirrus sac absent; parasites of marine fishes. .... Family Haplosplanchnidae p. 197

33b. Two testes (rarely 9-11); two intestinal ceca; cirrus sac present or absent. 34

34a. Retractile spiny proboscis on each side of oral sucker; intestinal parasites of opossum (Fig. 237). .... Family Rhopaliasidae p. 200

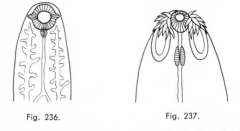

Fig. 236.   Fig. 237.

Fig. 236. Family Rhytidodidae. Fig. 237. Family Rhopaliasidae.

34b. Spiny proboscides absent. 35

35a. Vitelline follicles few, arranged in a U-shaped pattern along ends of ceca; some genera have spiny collar around oral sucker (*Parorchis*); parasites in cloaca (*Cloacitrema*), bursa Fabricii, beneath the conjunctiva or nictitating membrane (*Philophthalmus*) of birds. ...... Family Philophthalmidae p. 194

35b. Vitelline follicles not arranged as described above; primarily parasites in digestive tract of vertebrates. 36

36a. Spiny collar or one or two circles of large spines around oral sucker, or anterior part of body densely spinous. 37

36b. Large spines absent at anterior end of body or body not densely spinous. 38

37a. Spiny collar present (Fig. 238); testes tandem; vitelline follicles abundant; hermaphroditic duct absent; intestinal parasites of birds and mammals. ....
.... Family Echinostomatidae p. 179

37b. One or two circles of large spines around oral sucker (Fig.
239) or body very densely spinous; hermaphroditic duct present; intestinal parasites of fishes. ....
.... Family Acanthocolpidae p. 281

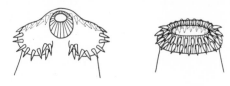

Fig. 238.   Fig. 239.

Fig. 238. Family Echinostomatidae, spiny collar.
Fig. 239. Family Acanthocolpidae, circumoral spines.

38a. Testes opposite, anterior to ventral sucker; anterior margin
of pharynx scalloped; oral sucker larger than ventral sucker;
intestinal parasites of marine fishes. ....
.... Family Megaperidae p. 283

38b. Testes posterior to ventral sucker; pharynx not scalloped. 39

39a. Parasites in kidneys of aquatic birds; body rounded anteriorly
and tapered posteriorly; testes opposite; ventral sucker weakly
developed, difficult to observe. ....
.... Family Renicolidae p. 251

39b. Parasites in intestine, gall bladder or bile duct of vertebrates;
body oval or elongate. 40

40a. Cirrus sac absent; seminal vesicle free in parenchyma; body
translucent, musculature weakly developed; ovary and testes
near posterior end of body; parasites in bile duct or gall
bladder of vertebrates. .... Family Opisthorchiidae p. 302

40b. Cirrus sac usually present; intestinal parasites of vertebrates;
testes and ovary some distance from posterior end of body.
....41

41a. Intestinal parasites of reptiles, birds or mammals. 42
41b. Intestinal parasites of fishes. 43

42a. Body elongate or oval with subcutaneous network of excretory canals; testes round or oval; parasites of reptiles,
birds or mammals; anatomy resembling that of echinostomes,
but without the spiny collar. ..... Family Psilostomatidae p. 186

42b. Body elongate, without subcutaneous canals; testes lobed;
parasites of birds. .... Family Cathaemasiidae p. 190

43a. Body spinous; pigmented eyespots present in younger specimens; primarily parasites of marine fishes. ....
.... Family Lepocreadiidae p. 271

43b. Body non-spinous; eyespots absent. 44
44a. Body muscular; suckers large; excretory vesicle Y-shaped; ceca long, end blindly; primarily parasites of freshwater fishes. .... Family Azygiidae p. 157
44b. Body not muscular; ventral sucker frequently provided with marginal papillae; intestinal ceca end blindly, open through one or two ani, fuse to form a cyclocoel or fuse with excretory vesicle to form a cloaca (Fig. 240); excretory vesicle I-shaped; primarily parasites of marine fishes. ....
.... Family Opecoelidae p. 262

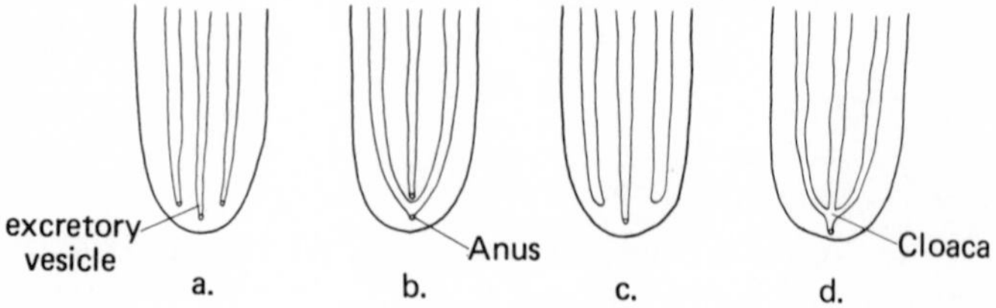

Fig. 240. Family Opecoelidae (a. two ani; b. one anus; c. ceca blind; d. cloaca).

45a. Body long, cylindrical; ventral sucker pedunculate; ovary posterior to testes; parasites of marine fishes. 46
45b. Body not as described above; ventral sucker sessile. 47
46a. Two testes, tandem; vitelline glands tubular; intestinal ceca with one pair of anterior diverticula in region of pharynx; ceca fused to excretory vesicle to form cloaca. ....
.... Family Accacoeliidae p. 329
46b. Sixteen to 20 testes; five to seven vitelline follicles posterior to ovary; ceca without anterior diverticula; ceca fused posteriorly to form cyclocoel. .... Family Syncoeliidae p. 330
47a. Genital pore immediately posterior to ventral sucker; testes opposite; parasites in lungs or intestine of mammals, or encysted in skin of birds (Collyriclum has no ventral sucker).
.... Family Troglotrematidae p. 290
47b. Genital pore not posterior to ventral sucker. 48
48a. Metraterm in the form of a spiny terminal organ enclosed in a metraterm sac (Fig. 241); usually one testis (infrequently two testes); intestinal parasites of fishes. ....
.... Family Monorchiidae p. 297
48b. Spiny terminal organ and metraterm sac absent; two testes.
....49
49a. Primarily parasites of bats (a few in amphibians or birds); intestinal ceca usually short; testes opposite; vitelline follicles

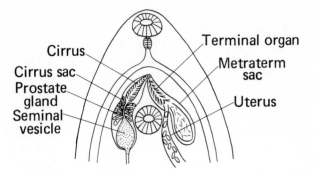

Fig. 241.   Family Monorchiidae, terminal reproductive organs.

in anterior half of body; body broadly oval or pyriform; genital pore sometimes marginal or submarginal. ....
.... Family Lecithodendriidae p. 242

49b. Parasites of vertebrates other than bats. 50

50a. Genital atrium present in ventral surface of body, receiving openings from male and female reproductive ducts (Fig. 242); body small, oval, pyriform or elongate. 51

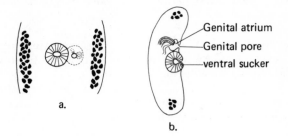

Fig. 242.   Genital atrium (a. ventral view, b. cross section).

50b. Genital atrium absent. 52

51a. Genital atrium and genital pore anterior to ventral sucker; excretory vesicle U-shaped, the arms extending forward as far as oral sucker; in intestine, bursa Fabricii or gall bladder of shore birds. ....Family Gymnophallidae p. 174

51b. Genital atrium and genital pore lateral to ventral sucker, atrium frequently containing a muscular papilla; excretory vesicle V-shaped, the arms not extending far forward; primarily intestinal parasites of birds, a few in fishes and mammals. .... Family Microphallidae p. 252

52a. Intestinal ceca and arms of excretory vesicle have diverticula anteriorly; testes opposite; intestinal parasites of turtles. .... Family Pachypsolidae p. 225

52b. Intestinal ceca and arms of excretory vesicle not as described above. 53

53a. Genital pore marginal or submarginal. 54
53b. Genital pore usually median. 56
54a. Testes tandem; body elongate; parasites of freshwater fishes.
.... Family Lissorchiidae p. 233
54b. Testes opposite; body oval or fusiform. 55
55a. Parasites of birds; body non-spinous; vitelline glands follicular. .... Family Stomylotrematidae p. 252
55b. Parasites of fishes; body spinous; vitelline glands usually
compact, rarely follicular. .... Family Zoogonidae p. 293
56a. Ovary posterior to testes; body weakly muscular; parasites
in liver, gall bladder, bile or pancreatic ducts of reptiles,
birds or mammals. .... Family Dicrocoeliidae p. 236
56b. Ovary between or anterior to testes; not in liver or bile
passages. 57
57a. Parasites in urinary bladder of fishes and amphibians or in
coelom of elasmobranchs; cirrus sac absent; body non-spinous;
pharynx sometimes absent; body translucent, muscles weakly
developed; vitelline glands compact or dendritic. ....
.... Family Gorgoderidae p. 286
57b. Parasites not in urinary bladder or coelom of host. 58
58a. Body non-spinous; parasites of fishes, rarely in amphibians.
....59
58b. Body spinous. 60
59a. Excretory vesicle Y- or V-shaped, the arms extending forward
to level of pharynx; seminal vesicle bipartite; body muscular, thick; parasites of marine fishes. ....
.... Family Fellodistomatidae p. 170
59b. Excretory vesicle I-shaped; parasites of freshwater fishes or
amphibians; oral sucker has muscular papillae in some genera.
.... Family Allocreadiidae p. 257
60a. Oral sucker with lateral muscular papillae and a dorsal transverse ridge; intestinal parasites of turtles. ....
.... Family Auridistomatidae p. 232
60b. Oral sucker without muscular papillae. 61
61a. One or two circles of large spines around oral sucker or
anterior part of body densely covered with large spines;
hermaphroditic duct present; seminal vesicle bipartite; vitelline follicles confined to hindbody; intestinal parasites of
fishes. .... Family Deropristiidae p. 279
61b. Body spines small throughout; hermaphroditic duct absent;
seminal vesicle not bipartite. 62
62a. Cirrus sac near anterior end of body; genital pore opening
antero-dorsal to oral sucker; excretory vesicle with lateral
diverticula; intestinal parasites of amphibians and reptiles.
.... Family Cephalogonimidae p. 232

62b. Genital pore on ventral surface of body. 63
63a. Genital pore at lateral margin of oral sucker or ventral to pharynx; body translucent, muscles weakly developed. 64
63b. Genital pore posterior to pharynx. 65
64a. Testes opposite; parasites in bursa Fabricii, cloaca or oviducts of birds, or in liver of mammals. ....
.... Family Prosthogonimidae p. 250
64b. Testes oblique, rarely opposite; parasites in lungs of amphibians. .... Family Haplometridae p. 231
65a. Intestinal ceca short, usually not extending more than halfway through body; testes opposite or nearly so; vitelline follicles confined to anterior half of body; intestinal parasites of amphibians and reptiles. .... Family Brachycoeliidae p. 234
65b. Intestinal ceca long; vitelline follicles not confined to anterior half of body. 66
66a. Excretory vesicle I-shaped (Fig. 243a); intestinal parasites of fishes, amphibians or reptiles; testes tandem or oblique, in middle third of body. .... Family Macroderoididae p. 227
66b. Excretory vesicle Y-shaped. 67
67a. Testes tandem, one or both testes near posterior end of body; excretory vesicle with long stem, arms of Y embrace ventral sucker (Fig. 243b); cirrus sac elongate; body slender; intestinal parasites of amphibians and reptiles. ....
.... Family Telorchiidae p. 225
67b. Testes opposite or oblique, some distance from posterior end of body; stem and arms of excretory vesicle short. 68
68a. Parasites in lungs, mouth or esophagus of snakes; testes opposite or slightly oblique; seminal receptacle absent; genital pore usually submedian; main collecting ducts attached behind tips of arms of excretory vesicle (Fig. 243 c). ....
.... Family Ochetosomatidae p. 221
68b. Intestinal parasites of all classes of vertebrates; testes opposite or oblique; seminal receptacle present; main collecting ducts attached to tips of arms of excretory vesicle (Fig. 243 d).
.... Family Plagiorchiidae p. 215

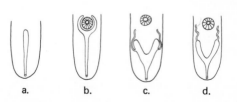

a.   b.   c.   d.

Fig. 243. Excretory vesicles (a. I-shaped; b., c., d. y-shaped).

ORDER STRIGEATIDA Larue, 1926*

*(This order name provides for uniformity in order-name endings and is used in place of Strigeatoidea LaRue, 1926 which is too suggestive of a superfamily name).

SUPERFAMILY STRIGEOIDEA Railliet, 1919

Miracidia have two pairs of flame cells; cercariae of the longifurcate-pharyngeate type, develop in sporocysts in aquatic snails; adult body usually divided into distinct fore- and hindbody, genital pore at posterior end of body; at least three hosts involved in life cycle; intestinal parasites of vertebrates.

Dubois (1938 and 1968) published taxonomic monographs on this group.

FAMILY STRIGEIDAE Railliet, 1919

Body divided into a cup-shaped forebody, containing the suckers, pharynx and tribocytic organ, and a cylindrical hindbody containing the reproductive organs; tribocytic organ foliaceous; testes usually tandem; cirrus sac absent; copulatory bursa well developed; genital pore dorso-terminal; ovary pretesticular; vitelline follicles numerous, restricted to either fore- or hindbody or present in both areas; uterus short; eggs large, few; intestinal parasites of birds and mammals.

KEY TO GENERA

1a. Vitelline follicles in fore- and hindbody. 2
1b. Vitelline follicles restricted to hindbody. 5
2a. Only a few vitelline follicles in forebody; hindbody 6 to 17 times longer than forebody; parasites of birds (Fig. 244). ....
....Genus *Ophiosoma* Szidat, 1928

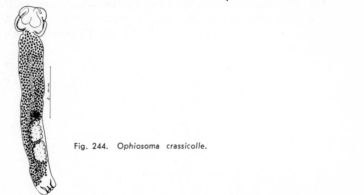

Fig. 244. *Ophiosoma crassicolle.*

2b. Vitelline follicles evenly distributed in fore- and hindbody; hindbody less than five times longer than forebody. 3

3a. Pharynx absent (Fig. 245). ....
....**Genus** *Apharyngostrigea* **Ciurea, 1927**

Key to species in Olsen (1940).

Life cycle: *A. pipientis—*

Strigea cercariae (Fig. 29) develop in daughter sporocysts in the freshwater planorbid snail, *Planorbula armigera.* The cercariae penetrate tadpoles of *Rana* and *Hyla* sp. and encyst in the coelom. The metacercaria is a tetracotyle (Fig. 49 c) (= *Tetracotyle pipientis*). The pharynx, present in the cercaria, is lost during development to the tetracotyle stage. The adult fluke was produced experimentally in pigeons. The natural definitive host is unknown (Olivier, 1940).

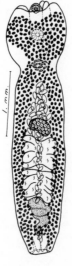

Fig. 245. *Apharyngostrigea bilobata.*

3b. Pharynx present. 4

4a. Forebody pyriform with lateral expansions, making it wider than hindbody. (Fig. 246). ....
.... **Genus** *Parastrigea*
Szidat, 1928

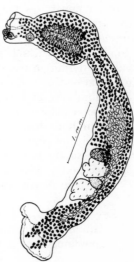

Fig. 246. *Parastrigea campanula.*

Key to species in Dubois (1955).
4b. Forebody cupshaped without lateral expansion (Fig. 247). ......
....Genus *Strigea* Abildgaard, 1790

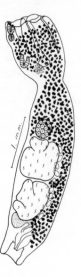

Fig. 247. *Strigea falconis.*

Key to species in Dubois (1968)
Life cycle: *S. elegans*—
Strigea cercariae (Fig. 29) develop in sporocysts in the fresh-water planorbid snail, *Gyraulus parvus*. After leaving the snail, the cercaria penetrates tadpoles of *Bufo* and *Rana* sp. and transforms to a mesocercaria (Fig. 47). The metacercaria, which is a tetra-cotyle (Fig. 49 c), is known to develop in the garter snake and domestic duck which probably devour the infected tadpoles. The natural definitive hosts are the snowy owl, *Nyctea nyctea* and the great-horned owl, *Bubo virginianus* (see Pearson, 1959).
5a. Hindbody at least four times longer than forebody which is spoon-shaped or heart-shaped. 6
5b. Hindbody less than four times longer than forebody which is ovoid or cupshaped. 7
6a. Hindbody four to eight times longer than the heart-shaped forebody; copulatory bursa and genital cone not unusually large in North American species (Fig. 248). ....
....Genus *Cardiocephalus* Szidat, 1928
Key to species in Dubois (1968).
6b. Hindbody filamentous, 8 to 20 times longer than forebody; copulatory bursa and genital cone large (Fig. 249). ....
....Genus *Nematostrigea* Sandground, 1934

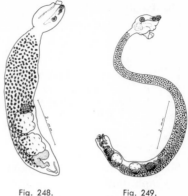

Fig. 248.   *Cardiocephalus brandesi.*
Fig. 249.   *Nematostrigea serpens annulata.*

Fig. 248.   Fig. 249.

7a. Genital bulb in copulatory bursa (Fig. 250). ....
....Genus *Cotylurus* Szidat, 1928

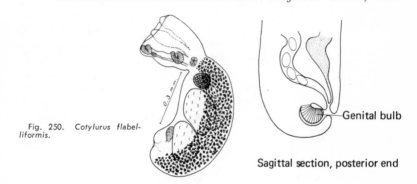

Fig. 250.   *Cotylurus flabelliformis.*

Genital bulb

Sagittal section, posterior end

Key to species in Dubois (1968).
Life cycle: *C. flabelliformis—*
Approximately three weeks are required for development and hatching of the miracidia after eggs are laid. The miracidia penetrate the freshwater snails, *Stagnicola emarginata angulata, Lymnaea stagnalis, Physa parkeri, P. sayii* and *Helisoma* spp. Longifurcate-pharyngeate cercariae (= *Cercaria flabelliformis*) develop in daughter sporocysts. The cercariae encyst in the same species of snail and develops into a tetracotyle (Fig. 49 c) (= *Tetracotyle flabelliformis*). Metacercariae of this species are very common in snails, sometimes encysting in the sporocysts or rediae of other species of trematodes. Snails that are infected with metacercariae of this species seem to develop an immunity to subsequent infections. Definitive hosts, such as birds of the genera *Nyroca, Marila, Anas, Querquedula* and *Spatula,* acquire the parasite by eating infected snails (Van Haitsma 1931; Cort *et al,* 1944).

7b. Genital bulb absent. 8

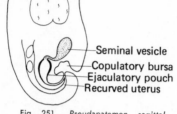

Fig. 251. *Pseudapatemon*, sagittal section, posterior end.

8a. Terminus of uterus curved forward, opening into posterior wall of copulatory bursa; genital pore directed toward dorsal body surface; ejaculatory pouch present (Fig. 251). ....
.... Genus *Pseudapatemon* **Dubois, 1936**

8b. Terminus of uterus united with ejaculatory duct to form hermaphroditic duct; genital pore terminal; ejaculatory pouch absent (Fig. 252). ....Genus *Apatemon* **Szidat, 1928**

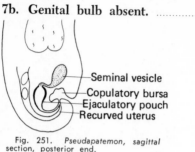

Fig. 252. *Apatemon gracilis*.

Key to species in Dubois (1968). Life cycle: *A. gracilis*—

Strigea cercariae (= *Cercaria burti*) develop in daughter sporocysts in the snails, *Helisoma trivolvis, H. antrosum* and *Bithynia tentaculata*. The metacercaria is a tetracotyle in leeches of the genera *Herpobdella* and *Haemopis*. The mature trematode inhabits the intestine of merganser and mallard ducks, becoming sexually mature within four days after metacercariae are ingested (Szidat, 1931; Stunkard *et al.*, 1941).

FAMILY DIPLOSTOMATIDAE Poirier, 1886

Body divided into a distinct fore- and hindbody, the forebody flat or spoon-shaped and containing the suckers and bulbous tribocytic organ; hindbody cylindrical, containing the reproductive organs; intestinal ceca long; testes tandem or opposite; cirrus sac absent; ovary pretesticular; copulatory bursa present, opening on dorsal surface near posterior end of body; vitelline follicles abundant, located in either fore- or hindbody or in both areas; uterus short; eggs few, large; intestinal parasites of birds and mammals.

KEY TO GENERA

1a. Vitelline follicles only in forebody; parasites of mammals. 2
1b. Vitelline follicles present in both fore- and hindbody or only in hindbody; parasites of birds and mammals. 6

2a. Pseudosuckers absent (Fig. 253). ....
....Genus *Fibricola* Dubois, 1932

Life cycle: *F. texensis—*

Miracidia develop and hatch within 12 days following oviposition. They penetrate the freshwater snail, *Physa anatina,* in which cercariae of the strigea type (Fig. 29) develop in daughter sporocysts. The metacercaria is a diplostomulum (Fig. 49 a.) in the coelom and muscles of tadpoles of the genus *Rana.* The diplostomula sometimes become enveloped by host connective tissue. The natural definitive host is the raccoon in which the parasite matures within 10 days. Experimental infections were established in chicks, mice, rats and hamsters (Chandler, 1942; Leigh, 1954).

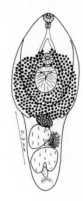

Fig. 253. *Fibricola cratera.*

2b. Pseudosuckers present. 3
3a. Testes tandem; parasites of mammals (Fig. 254). ....
....Genus *Alaria* Schrank, 1788

Life cycle: *A. canis—*

Adults are parasites of mammals of the family Canidae. Miracidia develop and hatch in two weeks. They penetrate snails of several species of *Helisoma* in which cercariae of the strigea type (Fig. 29) develop in daughter sporocysts. The cercariae penetrate the skin of tadpoles and metamorphose to the mesocercaria stage (Fig. 47). The cycle may now follow one of two courses:

1. The infected tadpole or frog is eaten by the definitive host such as a dog or fox in which the mesocercaria migrates through the diaphragm to the lung where it transforms to a metacercaria of the diplostomulum type (Fig. 49 a). After about five weeks these migrate up the trachea, are then swallowed and pass to the intestine where they mature, eggs appearing in the feces in about 35 days after the mesocercariae are eaten.

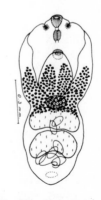

Fig. 254. *Alaria mustelae.*

2. A paratenic or "collector host," such as a snake, frog or mouse, eats the infected tadpole or frog. The mesocercariae then accumulate in the tissues of this host. Carnivorous mammals then devour the collector host (Pearson, 1956).

3b. Testes opposite. 4
4a. Ejaculatory pouch present; tribocytic organ ovoid (Fig. 255); parasites of raccoon. ....
..............................Genus *Pharyngostomoides* Harkema, 1942
4b. Ejaculatory pouch absent; tribocytic organ very elongate or bilobed; parasites of raccoon. 5
5a. Tribocytic organ elongate, contained in a pouch in the forebody; hindbody shorter than forebody; pseudosuckers on ventral body surface (Fig. 256). ....
..............................Genus *Procyotrema* Harkema and Miller, 1959

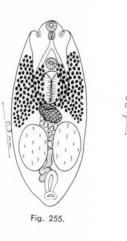

Fig. 255.

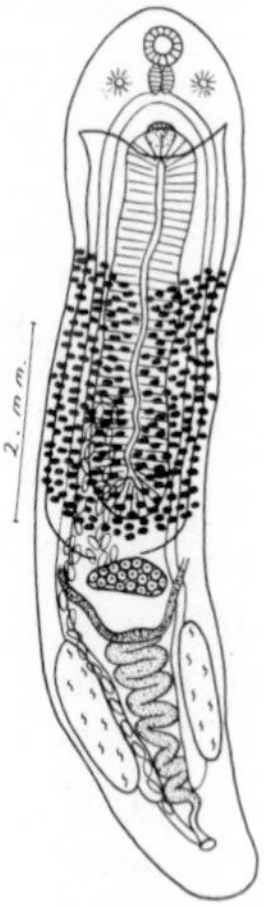

Fig. 256.

Fig. 255.   *Pharyngostomoides procyonis.*
Fig. 256.   *Procyotrema marsupiformis.*

5b. Tribocytic organ bilobed; hindbody longer than forebody; pseudosuckers at anterior edge of body; large copulatory bursa present, containing a ventral papilla (Fig. 257). ....
..........................Genus *Parallelorchis* Harkema and Miller, 1961
6a. Vitelline follicles only in hindbody. 7
6b. Vitelline follicles in fore- and hindbody. 8

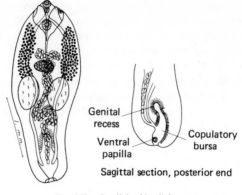

Genital recess

Ventral papilla

Copulatory bursa

Sagittal section, posterior end

Fig. 257. *Parallelorchis diglossus.*

7a. Genital bulb and ejaculatory pouch present; ventral sucker well developed but smaller than oral sucker; body elongate, not permanently arched dorsally; forebody much shorter than hindbody; parasites of birds (Fig. 258). ....
....Genus *Uvulifer* Yamaguti, 1934

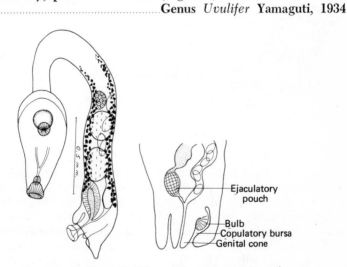

Ejaculatory pouch

Bulb
Copulatory bursa
Genital cone

Fig. 258. *Uvulifer ambloplitis,* sagittal section, posterior end.

Life cycle: *U. ambloplites*—
  Miracidia, which develop and hatch within three weeks follow-ing oviposition, penetrate the freshwater snails *Helisoma trivolvis* and *H. campanulatum* in which strigea cercariae (= *Cercaria bes-siae*) develop in daughter sporocysts. After leaving the snail, they

encyst in the muscles and skin of bass, perch, sunfish and pike, causing "black spot" disease, a condition arising from the deposition of black pigment in the cyst membrane. The metacercaria is a neascus (= *Neascus ambloplitis*). Kingfishers, *Ceryle alcyon*, become infected by eating the infected fish (many authors).

7b. **Genital bulb and ejaculatory pouch absent; ventral sucker vestigial or absent; body permanently arched dorsally (Fig. 259).**
....**Genus** *Crassiphiala* **Van Haitsma, 1925**

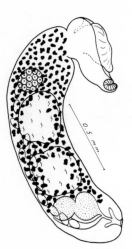

Fig. 259. *Crassiphiala bulboglossa*.

Life cycle: *C. bulboglossa*—
Miracidia develop and hatch within nine days after oviposition. After penetrating the planorbid snails, *Helisoma anceps* and *H. trivolvis,* longifurcate-pharyngeate cercariae of the strigea type develop in daughter sporocysts within 33 days. They encyst in the skin of freshwater fishes such as perch, pike, minnows and chub and cause "black spot" disease. The encysted metacercaria is a neascus (Fig. 49b). The Kingfisher, *Ceryle alcyon*, is definitive host (Hoffman, 1956).

8a. **Pseudosuckers present.** 9
8b. **Pseudosuckers absent.** 12
9a. **Boundary between fore- and hindbody distinct (Fig. 269).** 10
9b. **Boundary between fore- and hindbody indistinct (Fig. 271).**....11
10a. **Genital bulb present in copulatory bursa; testes H-shaped; parasites of birds (Fig. 260).** ....
.... **Genus** *Bolbophorus* **Dubois, 1935**

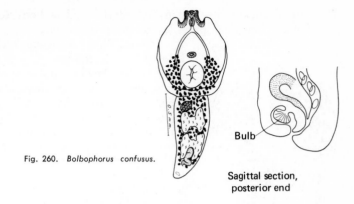

Fig. 260. *Bolbophorus confusus.*

Bulb

Sagittal section,
posterior end

10b. **Genital bulb absent; testes bilobed, concave ventrally; parasites of birds (Fig. 261).** ....
...................................**Genus** *Diplostomum* **von Nordmann, 1832**

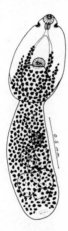

Fig. 261.   *Diplostomum huronense.*

Life cycle: *D. flexicaudum—*

The eggs are unembryonated when laid. Miracidia develop and hatch within three weeks and penetrate the freshwater snails *Stagnicola emarginata angulata* and *Lymnaea stagnalis* in which cercariae of the strigea type (Fig. 29) develop in daughter sporocysts. The cercaria (= *C. flexicauda*) penetrates the common sucker, *Catostomus commersoni* and develops into a diplostomulum type of metacercaria (= *Diplostomulum gigas*) in the lens of the eye. Natural definitive hosts are gulls and terns which feed upon the infected fish (Cort and Brooks, 1928; Hughes and Berkhout, 1929; Van Haitsma, 1931).

11a. Pseudosuckers deep, causing anterior end of body to be tri-lobed; intestinal parasites of birds (Fig. 262). ....
....Genus *Hysteromorpha* **Lutz, 1931**

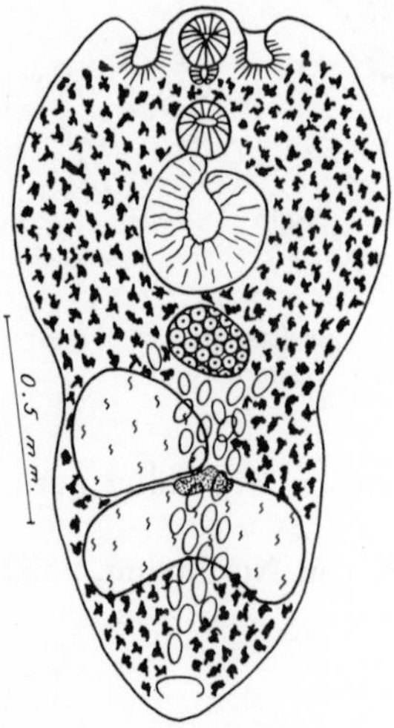

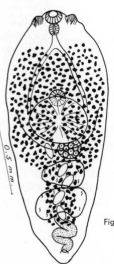

Life cycle: *H. triloba—*

Miracidia develop and hatch within seven days following oviposition and penetrate the freshwater snail *Gyraulus hirsutus* in which cercariae of the strigea type (Fig. 29) are produced in daughter sporocysts. The cercariae penetrate the bullheads, *Ameiurus melas* and *A. nebulosus*, in the muscles of which they transform into diplostomulum type of metacercaria (= *Diplostomulum corti*). Mature trematodes develop within 60 hours after metacercariae are eaten by piscivorous birds such as cormorants, herons, egrets or pelicans (Hugghins, 1954).

Fig. 262.   *Hysteromorpha triloba.*

11b. Pseudosuckers shallow; body not trilobed at anterior end; parasites of opossum (Fig. 263). ....
.... Genus *Didelphodiplostomum* **Dubois, 1944**

Fig. 263.   *Didelphodiplostomum variabile.*

12a. Ovary anterior to testes. 13
12b. Ovary between testes or opposite anterior testis. 14
13a. Genital cone surrounded by a prepuce; copulatory bursa
     evaginable; parasites of birds (Fig. 264). ....
     ....Genus *Posthodiplostomum* Dubois, 1936

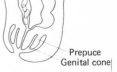

Prepuce
Genital cone

Sagittal section, posterior end

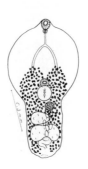

Fig. 264. *Posthodiplostomum
minimum.*

Prepuce

Dorsal view, posterior end

Life cycle: *P. minimum—*
Longifurcate-pharyngeate cercariae of the strigea type develop
in daughter sporocysts in *Physa gyrina* and *P. heterostropha.* The
metacercaria is a neascus (Fig. 49b) (= *Neascus vancleavei*) in
Lepomis gibbosus, L. megalotus and *Ambloplites rupestris.* The
mature flukes develop in the great blue heron, *Nycticorax nycticorax.* Experimental infections were established in chicks, the flukes
maturing within 32 hours after feeding metacercariae (Miller, 1954;
Hoffman, 1958a).
13b. **Prepuce absent; copulatory bursa not evaginable (Fig. 265).**
     ....**Genus *Neodiplostomum* Railliet, 1919**
     The genus contains many species and has been divided into two
subgenera:
     Subgenus *Neodiplostomum*: Genital cone absent; testes of un-
equal size.
     Subgenus *Conodiplostomum*: Genital cone present; testes of
equal size.
Life cycle: *N. intermedium—*
     Miracidia hatch in water and penetrate the freshwater limpet,
Pettancylus assimilis in which longifurcate pharyngeate cercariae
develop in daughter sporocysts. After emerging from the limpet,
the cercariae penetrate either tadpoles or adults of the tree frogs,

Hyla pearsoni or *H. caerula*. The natural definitive host is *Rattus assimilis*. The laboratory rat is a satisfactory experimental host. Eggs appear in the feces in seven to eight days (Pearson, 1961).

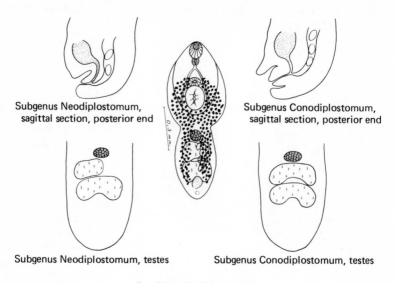

Subgenus Neodiplostomum, sagittal section, posterior end

Subgenus Conodiplostomum, sagittal section, posterior end

Subgenus Neodiplostomum, testes

Subgenus Conodiplostomum, testes

Fig. 265.   *Neodiplostomum* sp.

14a. **Ovary at one side of body, wedged between testes (Fig. 266).**
........................**Genus** *Mesophorodiplostomum* **Dubois, 1936**
14b. **Ovary opposite to anterior testis; hindbody progressively thicker toward posterior end (Fig. 267).** ....
.................................**Genus** *Ornithodiplostomum* **Dubois, 1936**
Life cycle: *O. ptychocheilus—*
Miracidia develop and hatch within ten days after eggs are laid. They penetrate the freshwater snail, *Physa anatina* in which strigea cercariae develop in daughter sporocysts. The cercariae penetrate chubs, shiners, squawfish, fatheads and Johnny darter. The metacercaria is a neascus. Natural definitive hosts are several species of ducks. Experimental infections were established in chicks (Hoffman, 1958b).

FAMILY PROTERODIPLOSTOMATIDAE Dubois, 1936

Body divided into a flat forebody, containing the suckers and a bulbous tribocytic organ, and a cylindrical hindbody which contains the reproductive organs; testes tandem or oblique, in middle third of hindbody; cirrus sac absent; seminal vesicles free in par-

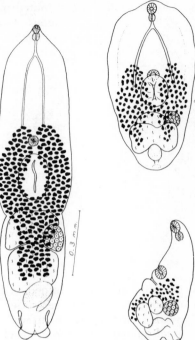

Fig. 266.   Mesoophorodiplostomum
pricei. Fig. 267.   Ornithodiplostomum
ptychocheilus.

Fig. 266.

O. ptychocheilus,
lateral view

Fig. 267.

enchyma; thick-walled paraprostate organ located posterior to
testes; genital atrium present, opening through a dorsal genital
pore near posterior end of body; hermaphroditic canal present;
vitelline follicles either confined to forebody or extending into
fore- and hindbody; intestinal parasites of reptiles, especially alligators. The species represented in North America are all parasites of the American alligator, *Alligator mississippiensis*.

KEY TO GENERA

1a. Body linguiform, division between fore- and hindbody indis-
     tinct; vitelline follicles confined to area between ventral sucker
     and ovary (Fig. 268). ....Genus *Crocodilicola* Poche, 1925
1b. Division between fore- and hindbody distinct. 2

2a. Vitelline follicles distributed in both fore- and hindbody (Fig. 269). ....Genus *Archaeodiplostomum* Dubois, 1944

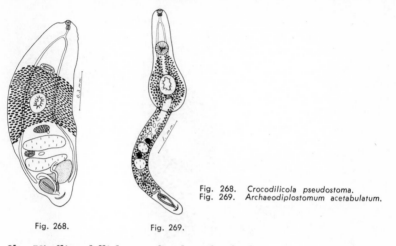

Fig. 268. *Crocodilicola pseudostoma.*
Fig. 269. *Archaeodiplostomum acetabulatum.*

Fig. 268.   Fig. 269.

2b. Vitelline follicles confined to forebody. 3
3a. Hindbody with a linear series of accessory suckers on dorsal surface; atrial sucker in wall of genital atrium; ejaculatory duct united with terminus of uterus; hermaphroditic canal thin-walled (Fig. 270). ....
..................................Genus *Polycotyle* Willemoes-Suhm, 1870
3b. Hindbody without accessory and atrial suckers; ejaculatory duct joined to side of paraprostate organ; hermaphroditic canal with thick, muscular wall (Fig. 271). ....
..................Genus *Pseudocrocodilicola* Byrd and Reiber, 1942

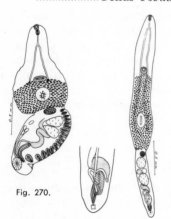

Fig. 270.

Fig. 271.

Fig. 270. *Polycotyle ornata.* Fig. 271. *Pseudo-crocodilicola americaniense.* (Redrawn from Byrd and Reiber, 1942.)

FAMILY CYATHOCOTYLIDAE Poche, 1926

Body round, pyriform, oval or elongate, usually not divided into distinct fore- and hindbody regions; bulbous tribocytic organ present in addition to oral and ventral suckers (ventral sucker absent in some genera); intestinal ceca extending to posterior end of body; testes usually tandem; cirrus sac present, near posterior end of body, base of sac usually directed toward anterior end of body; ovary between testes or opposite anterior testis; genital pore at posterior end of body; vitelline follicles variable in distribution; uterus short, eggs few and large; intestinal parasite of reptiles, birds and mammals, rarely in fishes.

KEY TO GENERA

1a. Body elongate, divided into a flat forebody and a conical hindbody (Figs. 272, 273). ....
.........................Genus *Neogogatea* Chandler and Rausch, 1947

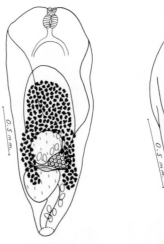

Fig. 272. *Neogogatea bubonis.* (Redrawn from Chandler and Rausch, 1947.) Fig. 273. *N. kentuckiensis.* (Redrawn from Myer, 1960.)

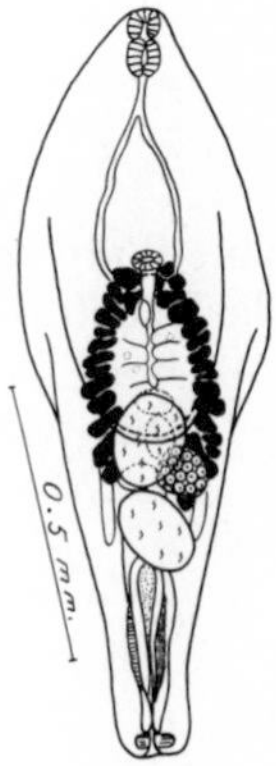

Fig. 273.

Fig. 272.

Life cycle: *N. kentuckiensis* (= *Mesostephanus kentuckiensis*)—
Longifurcate pharyngeate cercariae (= *C. kentuckiensis*) of the vivax group (Fig. 30) develop in daughter sporocysts in the operculate snails, *Anaplocamus dilatatus* and *Mudalia carinata*. They encyst in the muscles of at least 10 species of freshwater fishes. Infections with the adult fluke were established experimentally in young chicks, the parasite maturing in seven days after metacercariae were fed (Myer, 1960; Hoffman and Dunbar, 1963).

1b. Body oval or round in ventral view, not divided into distinct fore- and hindbody regions. **2**

2a. Body oval, concave ventrally; ventral sucker some distance posterior to oral sucker (Fig. 274). ....

....**Genus** *Prohemistomum* **Odhner, 1913**

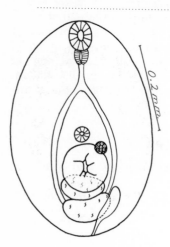

Life cycle: *P. chandleri*—

Longifurcate - pharyngeate cercariae of the vivax group (Fig. 30) develop in daughter sporocysts in the operculate snail, *Pleurocera acuta*. After leaving the snail, the cercariae encyst in the tissues of several species of bass. Immature adults were recoverd from the intestine of channel catfish, *Ictalurus punctata*, Northern sculpin, *Cottus bairdi*, and the water snake, *Natrix sipedon*, which had been fed metacercariae from bass (Vernberg, 1952).

The fishes and snakes are probably abnormal hosts for this parasite. The natural definitive hosts might be piscivorous birds.

Fig. 274. *Prohemistomum chandleri*. (Redrawn from Vernberg, 1952.)

2b. Body round; ventral sucker present or absent. **3**

3a. Ventral sucker absent; vitelline follicles fill lateral areas of body posterior to level of tribocytic organ; cirrus sac slender, thin-walled; eggs unusually large, few (Fig. 275). ....

....**Genus** *Linstowiella* **Szidat, 1933**

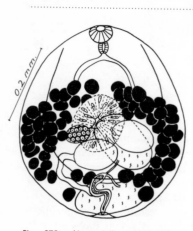

Life cycle: *L. szidati*—

Longifurcate-pharyngeate cercariae of the vivax group (= *Cercaria szidati*) develop in daughter sporocysts in the operculate snail, *Campeloma rufum*. The cercariae encyst in the muscles of common shiner, *Notropis cornutus*. The adult fluke was produced experimentally in young chicks in three days after feeding metacercariae (Anderson and Cable, 1950).

Fig. 275. *Linstowiella szidati*. (Redrawn from Anderson and Cable, 1950.)

3b. Ventral sucker present, immediately posterior to pharynx; body has well developed ventral pouch which contains tribocytic organ; cirrus sac large, thick-walled; eggs not unusually large; vitelline follicles in a wreath-like arrangement around body (Fig. 276). ....Genus *Holostephanus* Szidat, 1936

Life cycle: *H. ictaluri*—

Cercariae of the vivax group were obtained from the operculate snail, *Lioplax subcarinata*. They encysted in the tissues of shiner, *Notropis cornutus*. The adult fluke developed in the intestine of the catfish, *Ictalurus punctatus* (see Stang and Cable, 1966).

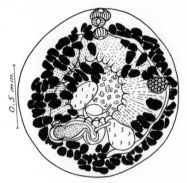

Fig. 276. *Holostephanus ictaluri*. (Redrawn from Vernberg, 1952.)

SUPERFAMILY SCHISTOSOMATOIDEA
Stiles and Hassall, 1926

Miracidia have two pairs of flame cells; cercariae of brevifurcate-apharyngeate or lophocercous-apharyngeate type, develop in sporocysts in aquatic snails; two hosts involved in life cycle; adults monoecious or dioecious; parasites in circulatory system of vertebrates.

FAMILY SCHISTOSOMATIDAE Poche, 1907
(Schistosomes)

Adult trematodes dioecious, exhibiting a distinct sexual dimorphism; suckers present or absent; pharynx absent; intestinal ceca fused in posterior part of body to form common cecum; body of male with edges curved ventrally to form gynaecophoric canal; testes four to many; body of female slender; ovary ovoid or spirally coiled; vitelline follicles abundant, distributed along common cecum; uterus usually short; eggs non-operculate, some have terminal spine, contain miracidium when laid; parasites in blood vessels of birds and mammals.

Several species of the genus *Schistosoma* are of considerable economic importance as parasites in the circulatory system of human beings and domestic animals, causing a disease known as schistosomiasis or bilharziasis. The adult parasites develop in the liver and in the veins associated with the digestive tract and urinary bladder of the host. Distressing pathological symptoms result from infection by these parasites.

In North America, a number of species of several other genera are the cause of schistosome dermatitis, the result of an allergic reaction to cercariae that penetrate the skin of human beings. Death of the cercariae in the skin provoke a skin reaction involving the formation of papules and severe itching, similar to the symptoms produced by poison ivy. The disease is more commonly known as "swimmers itch" due to its frequent occurrence around bathing beaches, especially in some of our north midwestern states. Species of the genera *Trichobilharzia*, *Schistosomatium* and *Gigantobilharzia* are most frequently involved in the epidemiology of the disease. Adults in these genera are normally parasites of wild birds and mammals. Effective control measures include destruction of the snails in which the sporocysts and cercariae of the schistosomes develop.

KEY TO GENERA

1a. Body of male with large gynaecophoric canal (Fig. 277), extending through at least half of length of body; testes anterior to common cecum; parasites of birds and mammals. 2

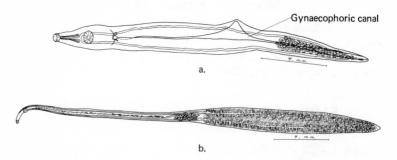

Fig. 277. *Heterobilharzia americanum* (a. male, b. female).

1b. Body of male with small gynaecophoric canal (Fig. 283), never extending through more than one-fifth of body length or gynaecophoric canal absent; testes located along common cecum; parasites of birds. 7

2a. Testes 28 or more (up to 250). 3

2b. Testes 20 or less. 4

3a. Parasites of mammals; uterus long; eggs abundant; ovary near middle of body; intestinal ceca of female with many lateral diverticula (Fig. 277); parasite of lynx and raccoon. ....**Genus** *Heterobilharzia* **Price, 1929**

Life cycle: *H. americana—*

Miracidia hatch in water and enter the freshwater snail, *Lymnaea cubensis* (natural host) and *Pseudosuccinea columella* (experimental host). Brevifurcate apharyngeate cercariae develop in daughter sporocysts. Following emergence the cercariae directly penetrate the skin of the definitive host which may be a raccoon, nutria, dog, rabbit or bobcat. Developmental stages migrate through the lungs. The mouse serves as a satisfactory experimental host (Lee, 1962).

3b. Parasites of birds; uterus short; one egg in uterus; ovary in anterior third of body; intestinal ceca of female without lateral diverticula (Fig. 278). ....Genus *Ornithobilharzia* **Odhner, 1912**

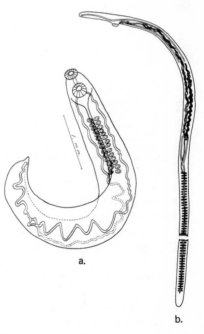

Fig. 278. *Ornithobilharzia pricei* (a. male, b. female). (Redrawn from Wetzel, 1930.)

a.

b.

Key to species in Price (1929) and Wetzel (1930).

4a. **Gynaecophoric canal extending from middle of body to posterior end; 14 to 18 testes; ceca with short diverticula; parasites of rodents (Fig. 279).** ....
....**Genus *Schistosomatium* Tanabe, 1923**

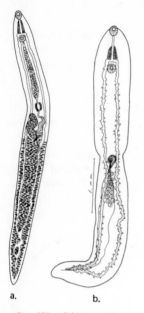

a.   b.

Fig. 279. *Schistosomatium douthitti* (a. female, b. male).

Life cycle: *S. douthitti*—

The mature male and female trematodes inhabit the mesenteric and hepatic portal veins of rodents. Embryonated eggs in the small veins in the wall of the intestine enter the lumen of this organ and pass in the feces. Miracidia hatch readily in water and penetrate the freshwater snails, *Lymnaea stagnalis, Stagnicola palustris; S. emarginata, Physa gyrina* and *P. parkeri.* Brevifurcate-apharyngeate cercariae (Fig. 26) develop in daughter sporocysts. After leaving the snail, the cercariae penetrate the skin of the definitive host, enter the circulating blood and grow to sexual maturity in the blood vessels of the liver and in the mesenteric veins. Natural definitive hosts are snowshoe rabbit, *Lepus americanus,* and Eastern meadow mouse, *Microtus pennsylvanicus.* Experimental infections have been established in rodents of the genera *Peromyscus, Mus, Rattus* and also in monkeys of the genus *Rhesus.* In the latter host, some sexually mature and some developing males and females were recovered from the mesenteric veins and the blood vessels of the liver. These observations are important because they tend to indicate some possibility of establishing infections with this species in human beings (Price, H. F., 1931; Kagan, 1953).

4b. **Gynaecophoric canal extending from ventral sucker to posterior end of body; intestinal ceca without lateral diverticula.**
....**5**

5a. **Testes 10 or less; ovary ovoid; parasites of mammals (Fig. 280).**
....**Genus *Schistosoma* Weinland, 1858**

Key to species in Price (1929).

Natural infections by species of this genus do not occur on the North American continent, however, endemic infections by S. *mansoni* occur in human beings in Puerto Rico and Jamaica as well as in some countries of South America. The sexually mature adults inhabit the mesenteric veins and lay eggs in the smaller branches in the wall of the intestine. Eggs are passed in the feces of the host and, when the fecal mass is diluted with water, the miracidia hatch and penetrate several different species of planorbid snails in which brevifurcate-apharyngeate cercariae (Fig. 26) develop in daughter sporocysts. The cercariae penetrate the skin of the de-

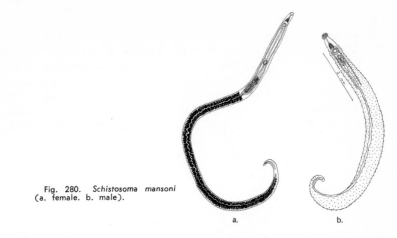

Fig. 280. *Schistosoma mansoni* (a. female. b. male).

a.   b.

finitive host, enter the blood vessels and migrate to the lungs, liver and heart. Those in the liver develop to sexual maturity and migrate to the mesenteric veins. Experimental infections have been established in rats, mice, hamsters, rabbits and monkeys.

5b. **Testes 18 to 20; ovary having an elongate spiral shape; parasites of birds.** 6

6a. **Ovary posterior to middle of body (Fig. 281).** ....
....**Genus** *Austrobilharzia* **Johnston, 1917**

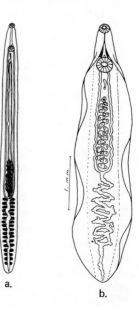

Fig. 281. *Austrobilharzia variglandis* (a. female, b. male). (Redrawn from Chu and Cutress, 1954.)

a.

b.

Life cycle: *A. variglandis*—

Brevifurcate-apharyngeate cercariae (Fig. 26) (= *Cercaria variglandis*) develop in daughter sporocysts in the marine snails, *Nassa obsoleta* and *Littorina pintado*. Cercariae penetrate the skin of the lesser scaup duck, *Marila affinis*, and the ruddy turnstone, *Arenaria interpres interpres*. The adult flukes inhabit the mesenteric veins. Experimental infections were established in canaries, pigeons, ducklings, chickens, gulls and terns (Stunkard and Hinchcliffe, 1951, 1952; Chu and Cutress, 1954).

6b. Ovary anterior to middle of body (Fig. 282). ....
.... **Genus** *Microbilharzia* **Price, 1929**

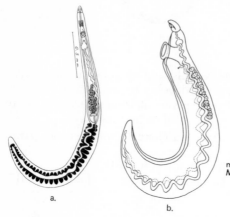

Fig. 282. *Microbilharzia lari* (a. female, b. male). (Redrawn from McLeod, 1937.)

Key to species in McLeod (1940).

7a. Body cylindrical, filamentous; gynaecophoric canal short, shallow (Fig. 293); posterior end of body with knob-like lateral projections. 8

7b. Body flat, large (up to 30 mm.) but not filamentous; gynaecophoric canal absent; posterior end of body tapered and rounded. 9

8a. Gynaecophoric canal narrow, slit-like, in anterior third of body; eggs ovoid; suckers absent (Fig. 283). ....
.... **Genus** *Gigantobilharzia* **Odhner, 1910**
Key to species in Brackett (1942).

Life cycle: *G. huronensis*—

Brevifurcate-apharyngeate cercariae are produced in daughter sporocysts in the freshwater snail, *Physa gyrina*. The cercariae have four pairs of flame cells in the body, cling to the surface film of water and penetrate the skin of the definitive host directly. Experimental infections were established in chickens and canaries. The natural hosts are cardinal and goldfinch (Najim, 1950).

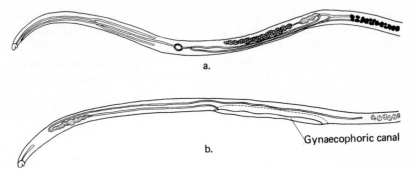

Fig. 283. *Gigantobilharzia gyrauli* (a. female, b. male). (Redrawn from Brackett, 1942.)

8b. **Gynaecophoric canal shallow, in the form of a widened area of the body (Fig. 284); eggs have a terminal spine; suckers present.** ....
................Genus *Trichobilharzia* Skrjabin and Zakharow, 1920

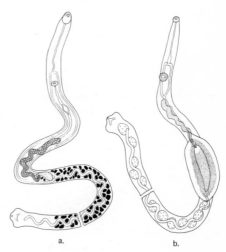

Fig. 284. *Trichobilharzia physellae* (a. female, b. male).

Life cycle: *T. physellae*—
Miracidia hatch in water and penetrate several species of physid snails. Brevifurcate-apharyngeate cercariae with six pairs of flame cells in the body develop in daughter sporocysts. The cercariae penetrate the skin of various species of ducks, in which they migrate by way of the circulatory system to the heart, lungs, liver and some other organs. Those that develop to mature adults in

the liver eventually migrate to the mesenteric veins. Natural definitive hosts are mallard, blue-winged teal, shoveller and pintail ducks (McLeod and Little, 1942; McMullen and Beaver, 1945).

9a. Intestinal ceca unite in anterior third of body, common cecum with many lateral diverticula; suckers absent; many eggs in uterus (Fig. 285). ....
..............Genus *Dendrobilharzia* (= *Dendritobilharzia*) **Skrjabin and Zakharow, 1920**

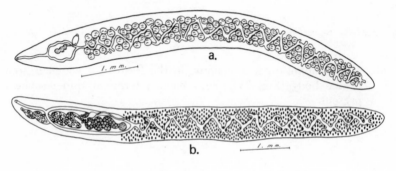

Fig. 285. *Dendrobilharzia anatinarum* (a. male, b. female).

Key to species in Skrjabin (1964).

9b. Intestinal ceca unite near middle of body, common cecum without diverticula; suckers present; one egg in uterus (Fig. 286). ....Genus *Bilharziella* **Looss, 1899**

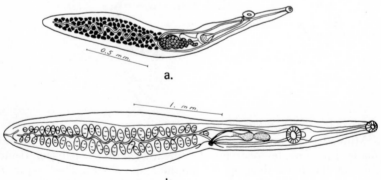

Fig. 286. *Bilharziella polonica* (a. female, b. male). (Redrawn from Price, 1929.)

FAMILY SPIRORCHIIDAE Stunkard, 1921

Body lanceolate, flat; oral sucker present; ventral sucker present or absent; pharynx absent; intestinal ceca long, sometimes fused part way to form a common cecum (one cecum in genus *Unicaecum*); testes one to many; genital pore in anterior or posterior third of body, ventral, lateral or dorsal; ovary between, anterior or posterior to testes; uterus short; eggs few, operculate; in blood vessels of turtles.

KEY TO GENERA

1a. Ventral sucker absent. 2
1b. Ventral sucker present. 5
2a. One intestinal cecum present; one testis; seminal vesicle and ovary elongate and spirally coiled; genital pore near posterior end of testis; parasites of freshwater turtles (Fig. 287). ....
....Genus *Unicaecum* Stunkard, 1925

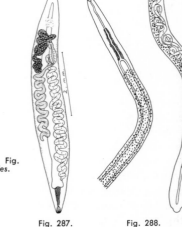

Fig. 287. *Unicaecum ruszkowskii.* Fig. 288. *Neospirorchis schistosomatoides.*

Fig. 287.   Fig. 288.

2b. Two intestinal ceca present, sometimes fused to form common cecum in posterior part of body; testes numerous or a single spirally-coiled testis. 3
3a. Intestinal ceca united in midbody region to form a common cecum which extends to posterior end of body; testis and ovary elongate, spirally coiled; ovary posterior to testis; parasites of marine turtles (Fig. 288). ....
....Genus *Neospirorchis* Price, 1934

3b. Intestinal ceca separate throughout their length; testes numerous; ovary not elongate; parasites of freshwater turtles. 4
4a. Testes anterior to ovary (Fig. 289, 290). ....
....Genus *Spirorchis* MacCallum, 1919

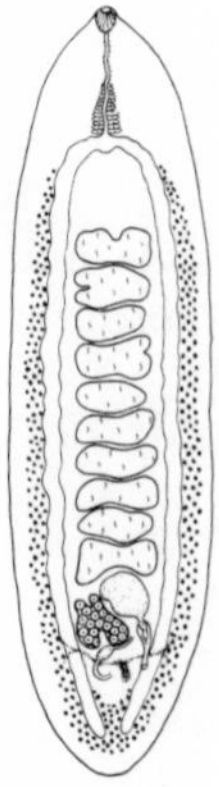

Fig. 289.   *Spirorchis* (*Spirorchis*) *artericola.*
Fig. 290.   *Spirorchis* (*Henotosoma*) *haematobium.*

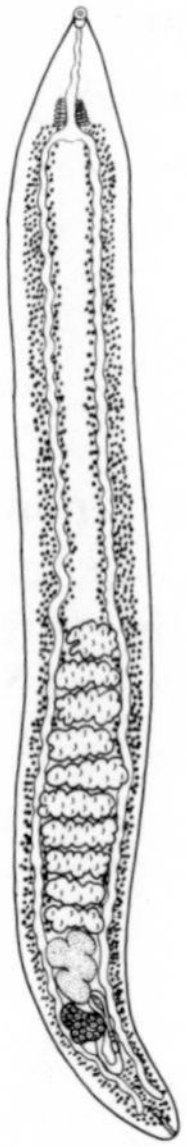

Fig. 289.

Fig. 290.

Key to species in Byrd (1939).
Life cycle: *S. elegans*—
Embryonated eggs in the feces of turtles were incubated several
days before miracidia hatched. The miracidia penetrate the freshwater snails, *Menetus dilatatus buchanensis* and *Helisoma anceps.*
Brevifurcate-apharyngeate cercariae (Fig. 26) develop in daughter
sporocysts. After leaving the snail, the cercariae penetrate the
mucous membranes of the eye, nose, mouth and cloaca of turtles
of the genera *Chrysemys* and *Pseudemys.* Development to sexual
maturity requires six to ten weeks. Most of the parasites occur
in the heart and large arteries (Goodchild and Kirk, 1960).
    The life cycles of *S. artericola* and *S. parvus* are similar to that
of *S. elegans.*

4b. One testis posterior to ovary, the others anterior to ovary
(Fig. 291). ....Genus *Diarmostorchis* Ejsmont, 1927
5a. Testes numerous, filling intercecal area; parasites of marine
turtles. 6
5b. One elongate spirally-coiled testis or two testes. 10

6a. Testes separated into two groups by ovary; genital pore lateral
     to ovary and enclosed in a muscular genital sucker (Fig. 292).
     ....Genus *Hapalotrema* Looss, 1899

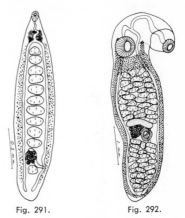

Fig. 291. *Diarmostorchis blandingi.* Fig. 292.
Hapalotrema synorchis. (Redrawn from Luhman,
1935.)

Fig. 291.   Fig. 292.

Key to species in Byrd (1939) and Skrjabin (1964).
6b. Testes not separated by ovary; genital sucker absent. 7
7a. Ovary posterior to testes. 8
7b. Ovary anterior to testes. 9
8a. Testes numerous (20 or more); esophagus at least one-third
     as long as body (Fig. 293). ....Genus *Learedius* Price, 1934
     Key to species in Byrd (1939).
8b. Testes 5 to 12; esophagus about one-fifth as long as body
     (Fig. 294). ....Genus *Monticellius* Mehra, 1939

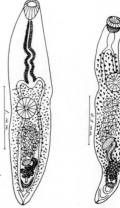

Fig. 293. *Learedius learedi.* Fig. 294. Monticellius *similis.*

Fig. 293.   Fig. 294.

9a. Muscular vagina present, posterior to ovary; testes in a single linear series between ceca (Fig. 295). ....
....Genus *Carettacola* Manter and Larson, 1950

9b. Muscular vagina absent; testes in a zigzag linear series (Fig. 296). ....Genus *Haemoxenicon* Martin and Bamberger, 1952

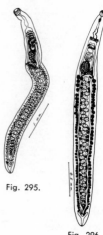

Fig. 295.

Fig. 296.

Fig. 295. *Carettacola bipora.* Fig. 296. Haemoxenicon *stunkardi.* (Redrawn from Martin and Bamberger, 1952.)

10a. One elongate, spirally-coiled testis filling intercecal area; ovary pretesticular; parasites of freshwater turtles (Figs. 297, 298). ....Genus *Vasotrema* Stunkard, 1928

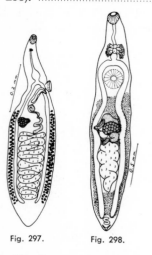

Fig. 297.   Fig. 298.

Fig. 297. *Vasotrema longitestis.* Fig. 298. *Vasotrema robustum.* (Redrawn from Stunkard, 1928.)

Key to species in Skrjabin (1964).

Life cycle: *V. robustum*—

Embryonated eggs are passed in the feces of the host. Miracidia hatch and penetrate the aquatic snails, *Physa gyrina* and *P. integra,* in which brevi-furcate-apharyngeate cercariae (Fig. 26) develop in daughter sporocysts. After leaving the snail, the cercariae penetrate the mucous membranes of the mouth, nose and cloaca of turtles. Development to sexual maturity occurs in the heart and large arteries within 10 to 12 months. Turtles in the Genus *Amyda* serve as definitive host (Wall, 1951).

10b. Two testes present; ovary between testes. 11
11a. Ovary, seminal vesicle and cirrus sac between testes; parasites of marine turtles (Fig. 299). ....
....**Genus** *Amphiorchis* **Price, 1934**
11b. Testes separated only by ovary; cirrus sac and seminal vesicle anterior to testes; parasites of freshwater turtles (Fig. 300).
....**Genus** *Hapalorhynchus* **Stunkard, 1922**
Key to species in Byrd (1939).

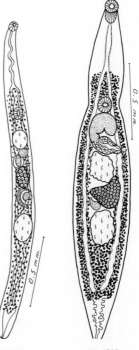

Fig. 299. *Amphiorchis amphiorchis.* Fig. 300. *Hapalorhynchus gracilis.*

Fig. 299.   Fig. 300.

FAMILY SANGUINICOLIDAE Graff, 1907

Body small, flat, delicate; a posterior lobe sometimes present; suckers and pharynx absent; intestinal ceca X- or H-shaped; one or many testes present, sometimes indistinct (diffuse); cirrus sac usually absent; ovary posttesticular, in posterior third of body; male and female genital pores separate, opening on dorsal surface of posterior third of body; vitelline follicles small and variable in extent; uterus usually short; eggs non-operculate, shells thin; parasites in blood vessels and heart of freshwater and marine fishes.

KEY TO GENERA

1a. Many small testes present. 2
1b. One large testis present or testes diffuse (indistinct). 3
2a. Intestinal ceca long, H-shaped; ovary lobed; patch of spines at posterior end of body; exclusively parasites of marine fishes (Fig. 301). ....Genus *Paradeontacylix* McIntosh, 1934

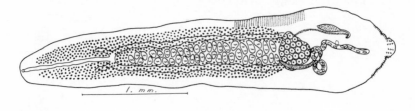

Fig. 301.   *Paradeontacylix sanguinicoloides.*

Key to species in McIntosh (1934a).

2b. Intestinal ceca short, X-shaped; ovary H-shaped or rectangular; no spines at posterior end of body (Fig. 302). ....
....Genus *Sanguinicola* Plehn, 1905

Key to species in Erickson and Wallace (1959).
Life cycle: *S. inermis*—

The adult is a parasite in the blood vessels of carp, *Cyprinus carpio*, in Europe. Miracidia hatch from eggs that are in the blood vessels of the gills. They apparently penetrate aquatic snails of the Genus *Lymnaea* in which lophocercous-apharyngeate cercariae (Fig. 25). (= *C. sanguinicolae inermis*) develop in sporocysts (Scheuring, 1922).

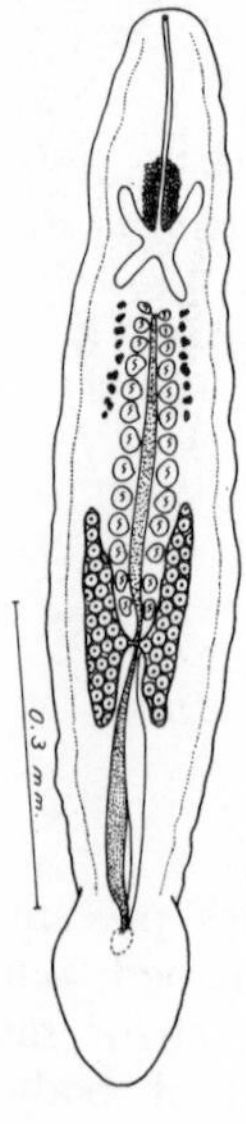

Fig. 302.   *Sanguinicola occidentalis.*

3a. Testes diffuse (indistinct) around ceca; ovary near right margin of body; uterus extending anterior to ovary (Fig. 303). ....
....Genus *Deontacylix* Linton, 1910

3b. One large testis present; ovary near median line; uterus entirely posterior to ovary. 4

4a. Intestinal ceca short, X-shaped; parasites in blood vessels of sharks (Fig. 304). ....Genus *Selachohemecus* Short, 1954

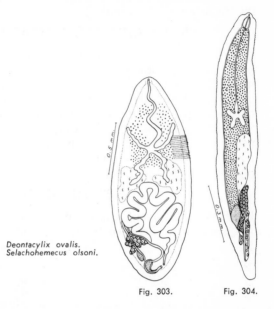

Fig. 303. *Deontacylix ovalis.*
Fig. 304. *Selachohemecus olsoni.*

Fig. 303.   Fig. 304.

4b. Intestinal ceca long, H-shaped; parasites of teleost fishes (Fig. 305). ....Genus *Cardicola* Short, 1953

Life cycle: *C. alseae—*

The adults are parasites in the blood vessels of cutthroat trout, *Salmo clarkii* and rainbow trout, *S. gairdnerii.* The eggs are non-operculate with thin shell. Miracidia hatch in the blood vessels of the gills. After leaving the gills they are probably eaten by the operculate snail *Oxytrema silicula* in which lophocercous-apharyngeate cercariae (Fig. 25) develop in sporocysts. After leaving the snail, the cercariae penetrate the tissues of the definitive host and develop to sexual maturity in the blood vessels of the gills, liver, mesenteries and kidneys (Meade and Pratt, 1965).

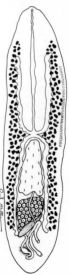

Fig. 305. *Cardicola laruei.*

SUPERFAMILY CLINOSTOMATOIDEA Dollfus, 1931

Miracidia have two pairs of flame cells; cercariae of brevifurcate-pharyngeate (clinostomoid) type, develop in rediae in aquatic snails; three hosts involved in life cycle; adults in mouth and esophagus of reptiles and birds.

FAMILY CLINOSTOMATIDAE Lühe, 1901

Body large, flat; oral sucker small or vestigial; anterior end of body retractile, forming a collar-like fold at anterior end of body; intestinal ceca long, sometimes sinuous; ventral sucker very large, in anterior third of body; testes tandem, in posterior third of body; cirrus sac and genital pore in posterior third of body; ovary between testes; uterus with ascending and descending limbs, entirely posterior to ventral sucker; vitelline follicles in lateral area of body, posterior to level of ventral sucker; parasites in mouth and esophagus of reptiles and birds.

KEY TO GENERA

1a. Parasites in mouth and esophagus of alligators; cirrus sac and genital pore between testes (Fig. 306). ....
....Genus *Odhneriotrema* Travassos, 1928

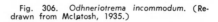

Fig. 306. *Odhneriotrema incommodum.* (Redrawn from McIntosh, 1935.)

1b. **Parasites in mouth and esophagus of birds; cirrus sac and genital pore anterior to testes or opposite anterior testis (Fig. 307).** ....Genus *Clinostomum* Leidy, 1856

Key to species in Skrjabin (1964).
Life cycle: *C. marginatum*—
Embryonated eggs pass in the feces or are washed into the water when the bird drinks or eats. The miracidia hatch in the water and penetrate the freshwater snails, *Helisoma antrosum* and *H. campanulatum* in which a sporocyst and two redial generations develop, the daughter rediae producing brevifurcate-clinostomatoid cercariae (Fig. 27) which have a dorsal finfold on the body. The cercariae encyst in the muscles and connective tissue of freshwater fishes. The metacercariae are large, yellow or cream colored. Their presence results in "yellow grub" disease of fishes. The mature trematode develops in the mouth and esophagus of herons, gulls and bitterns which eat infected fish. The metacercaria is thought to be precocial as only a few days are required for development to sexual maturity in the birds (Hopkins, 1933; Hunter and Hunter, 1934; Cameron, 1945).

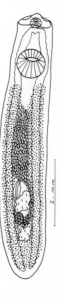

Fig. 307. *Clinostomum marginatum.*

The cercaria of *C. attenuatum* tends to encyst in the tissues of frogs instead of fish. The adult fluke develops in the mouth of bitterns.

SUPERFAMILY AZYGIOIDEA Skrjabin and Guschanskaja, 1956

Miracidia have one pair of flame cells; cercariae of furcocystocercous type, develop in rediae in aquatic snails; two hosts involved in life cycle or progenetic and involving only one host; parasites in the digestive tract of fishes.

FAMILY AZYGIIDAE Odhner, 1911

Body muscular, nonspinous, elongate or oval; suckers large; intestinal ceca long; testes tandem, oblique or opposite; ovary pre- or posttesticular; seminal receptacle absent; vitelline follicles in narrow bands lateral to ceca and usually restricted to area posterior to ventral sucker; excretory vesicle Y-shaped; parasites in stomach and intestine of fishes.

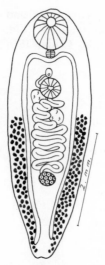

KEY TO GENERA

1a. Ovary posterior to testes (Fig. 308). ....
   ....Genus *Leuceruthrus* Marshall and
   Gilbert, 1905
1b. Ovary anterior to testes. 2

Fig. 308. *Leuceruthrus micropteri.*

2a. Vitelline follicles and uterus extend anterior to ventral sucker;
   body oval (Fig. 309). ....Genus *Proterometra* Horsfall, 1933

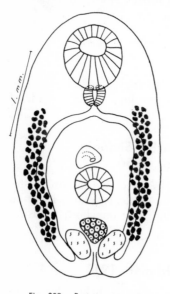

Life cycle: *P. macrostoma*—

Embryonated eggs are eaten by the operculate snails *Goniobasis livescens* and *Pleurocera acuta*. Miracidia hatch in the snail and metamorphose to a sporocyst which produces a generation of rediae in which furcocystocercous cercariae (Fig. 23) develop. The cercariae leave the snail and are eaten directly by the definitive host which can be one of several species of freshwater fishes (Horsfall, 1933, 1934; Dickerman, 1934, 1945).

The life cycle of *P. dickermani* is similar except that the cercariae are known to develop to sexually mature adults in the host snail. Embryonated eggs are produced and miracidia hatch here. The cycle can not only be completed in a single host but can be repeated in the

Fig. 309. *Proterometra macrostoma.*

same individual host. The cycle can pursue an alternate course by having the cercariae leave the snail and enter another snail (Anderson and Anderson, 1963).

For life cycles of other species of *Proterometra* see Anderson and Anderson (1967).

2b. Vitelline follicles and uterus entirely posterior to ventral sucker. 3

3a. Vitelline follicles invade median area of body posterior to testes; arms of excretory vesicle pass anterior and unite dorsal to oral sucker; parasites in stomach of elasmobranchs (Fig. 310). ....Genus *Otodistomum* **Stafford, 1904**

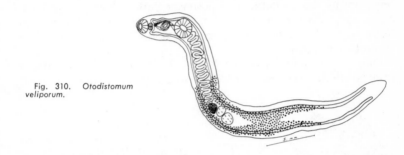

Fig. 310.   *Otodistomum veliporum.*

Key to species in Dollfus (1937).

3b. Vitelline follicles restricted to lateral areas of body posterior to testes; arms of excretory vesicle long but not united dorsal to oral sucker; parasites in stomach of teleost fishes (Figs. 311, 312). ....Genus *Azygia* **Looss, 1899**

Life cycle: A. *longa*—

Embryonated eggs, passed in the feces of the host, are eaten by the operculate snail, *Amnicola limosa*, in which furco-cystocercous cercariae (Fig. 23) develop in rediae. The cercariae are ingested directly by the definitive host in which the mature trematode develops. This parasite has been reported from many species of fish (Sillman, 1962).

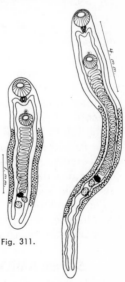

Fig. 311.

Fig. 311.   *Azygia angusticauda.* Fig. 312.
Azygia longa.

Fig. 312.

FAMILY BIVESICULIDAE Yamaguti, 1939

Body small (1 mm. or less) fusiform, partly spinous; pigmented eyespots present; oral and ventral suckers absent; pharynx present; intestinal ceca half body length; one testis; cirrus sac large, ovoid in midbody region, the base directed toward anterior end of body; internal and external seminal vesicles present; ovary anterior to testis and lateral to cirrus sac; genital pore median, near midbody region; seminal receptacle present; vitelline follicles surrounding ceca; uterus short, confined to posterior part of body, posterior to cirrus sac; two excretory vesicles, the arm of each extending anterior to level of esophagus; parasites in the intestine and pyloric ceca of marine fishes.

Only the Genus *Bivesicula* Yamaguti, 1934 has been reported from North America. Key to species in Cable and Nahhas, (1962b).

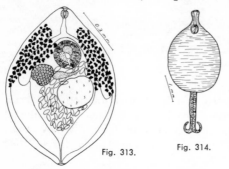

Fig. 313.

Fig. 314.

Fig. 313. *Bivesicula caribbensis.* Fig. 314. B. *caribbensis, cercaria.* (Redrawn from Cable and Nahhas, 1962b.)

Life cycle: *B. hepsetiae—*

Following oviposition, two weeks are required for development of the miracidia. It is not known whether the miracidia hatch and penetrate the host snail or whether the embryonated eggs are eaten. Furcocystocercous cercariae develop in forktailed rediae in several species of marine snails of the Genus *Cerithium.* The cercariae are eaten by the host fish which is the hardhead silverside, *Atherinomorus stipes.* During the development of the cercarial excretory system, the two tubule primordia fail to fuse, resulting in two excretory vesicles in the posterior part of the body (LeZotte, 1954).

The life cycle of *B. caribbensis* (Fig. 313) is similar to the above with furcocystocercous cercariae (Fig. 314) developing in forktailed rediae in the snail, *Cerithium literatum.* The large cercariae are eaten by the big-eyed squirrel fish, *Myripristis jacobus* (see Cable and Nahhas, 1962b).

The development of furcocystocercous cercariae in a redia and the absence of a second intermediate host in the life cycle indicates relationship to the Family Azygiidae.

SUPERFAMILY CYCLOCOELOIDEA Nicoll, 1934

Miracidia have one pair of flame cells and contain a redia; cercariae tailless, develop in rediae in aquatic snails; three hosts involved in life cycle; intestinal ceca of cercaria, metacercaria and adult fused posteriorly to form a cyclocoel; parasites in respiratory tract of birds.

FAMILY CYCLOCOELIDAE Kossack, 1911

Body large and flat, oval or fusiform; suckers vestigial or absent; intestinal ceca fused posteriorly to form cyclocoel and somtimes having lateral diverticula; testes near posterior end of body, oblique or opposite; genital pore median, near anterior end of body; ovary between testes or opposite anterior testis; uterus composed of many transverse folds, at least filling intercecal area; vitelline follicles distributed along ceca; parasites in respiratory system and air sacs of birds.

KEY TO GENERA

1a. Intestinal ceca have lateral diverticula. 2
1b. Intestinal ceca without lateral diverticula. 3
2a. Some folds of uterus between testes (Fig. 315). ....
......................................Genus *Tracheophilus* Skrjabin, 1913

Life cycle: *T. cymbius—*
Eggs are embryonated at time of oviposition. Miracidia, which already contain a redia, hatch as soon as eggs enter water. The miracidia penetrate the aquatic snail *Helisoma trivolvis* in which tailless cercariae develop in rediae. The cercariae leave the redia and encyst in the tissues of the same species of snail. The intestinal ceca of the cercaria and metacercaria are fused caudally like that of the adult fluke. The ventral sucker is lost in the metacercarial stage. The definitive host acquires the infection by eating infected snails. The adult parasite inhabits the mouth, nose, trachea and bronchi of ducks, geese and grebes (Stunkard, 1934).

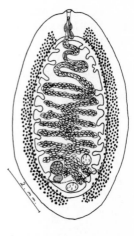

Fig. 315. *Tracheophilus cymbius.*

2b. No uterine folds between testes (Fig. 316). ....
...............................Genus *Typhlocoelum* Stossich, 1902

Key to species in Skrjabin (1964).

3a. Vitelline follicles confluent across posterior end of body; testes and ovary form a triangle; uterine folds extend laterally beyond ceca (Fig. 317). ....Genus *Uvitellina* Witenberg, 1926

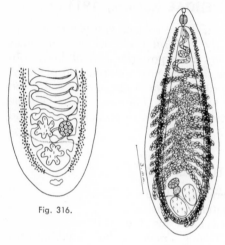

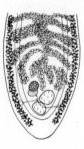

Fig. 316.

Fig. 316. *Typhlocoelum cucumerinum*. Fig. 317. *Uvitellina macroisophaga*.

Fig. 317.

3b. Vitelline follicles not confluent across posterior end of body....4
4a. Uterine folds extend laterally beyond ceca. 5
4b. Uterine folds do not extend laterally beyond ceca. 6
5a. Uterine folds extend laterally beyond ceca and vitelline follicles, nearly to lateral margins of body; no uterine folds between testes (Fig. 318). ....
....Genus *Haematotrephus* Stossich, 1902
5b. Uterine folds extend laterally only beyond ceca; some uterine folds between testes (Fig. 319). ....
....Genus *Harrahium* Witenberg, 1926

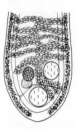

Fig. 318. *Haematotrephus nittanyense*. Fig. 319. *Harrahium halli*.

Fig. 318.   Fig. 319.

6a. Testes tandem; ovary between testes (Fig. 320). ....
....Genus *Morishitium* Witenberg, 1928

6b. Testes opposite or oblique; ovary pretesticular or opposite an-
terior testis. 7

7a. Testes opposite; ovary pretesticular; no uterine folds between
testes (Fig. 321). ....Genus *Wardianum* Witenberg, 1923

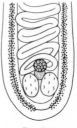

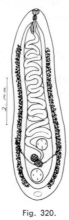

Fig. 320.   *Morishitium dumetellae.*
Fig. 321.   *Wardianum triangulare.*

Fig. 321.

Fig. 320.

7b. Testes oblique; ovary opposite anterior
testis; some uterine folds between testes
(Fig. 322). ....
.......Genus *Cyclocoelum* Brandes, 1892
Key to species in Skrjabin (1964).

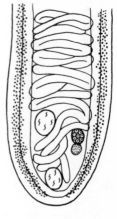

Fig. 322.   *Cyclocoelum mutabile.*

SUPERFAMILY BRACHYLAIMOIDEA Allison, 1943

Cercariae microcercous, furcocercous or tailless, develop in
branched sporocysts in terrestrial or aquatic snails; two or three
hosts involved in life cycle; adults in intestine of birds and mammals.

FAMILY BRACHYLAIMIDAE Joyeux and Foley, 1930

Body usually elongate, rarely oval, spinous or nonspinous; intestinal ceca long, sometimes sinuous; testes tandem or oblique, usually near posterior end of body; genital pore and cirrus sac in posterior third of body; ovary anterior to testes, between testes or opposite anterior testis; vitelline follicles in narrow lateral rows; uterus long, with ascending and descending limbs; intestinal parasites of birds and mammals.

KEY TO GENERA

1a. Cirrus sac and genital pore at posterior end of body; parasites in cloaca and bursa Fabricii of birds. 2
1b. Cirrus sac and genital pore some distance from posterior end of body; intestinal parasites of birds and mammals. 3

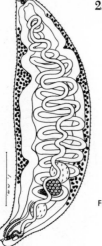

2a. Body linguiform; suckers vestigial or absent (Fig. 323). ....Genus *Urotocus* Looss, 1899

Fig. 323.   *Urotocus fusiformis.*

2b. Body short, oval; suckers large (Fig. 324). ....
....Genus *Leucochloridium* Carus, 1835
Keys to species in McIntosh (1932) and Kagan (1951, 1952b).
Life cycle: *L. problematicum*—
Embryonated eggs, passed in the feces of the host, are ingested by the amphibious snail, *Oxyloma retusa*. Tailless cercariae develop in branched sporocysts. One or more branches of the sporocyst become pigmented brood sacs (Fig. 9b) which are located in the tentacles of the snail. Cercariae migrate into the brood sacs. The brood sacs pulsate when light intensity or temperature in-

crease. Tentacles, containing brood sacs, become greatly distended and sometimes rupture, exposing the brightly-colored sacs which are thought to attract birds that eat the infected snails. Definitive hosts are bords of the family Rallidae. Trematodes become sexually mature within five to eight days in the cloaca of the birds (Kagan 1951, 1952a).

3a. **Body linguiform or oval; testes opposite or oblique; ovary opposite anterior testis or anterior to both testes.** **4**

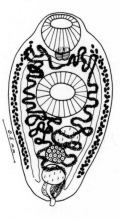

Fig. 324.   *Leucochloridium certhiae.*

3b. **Body elongate or oval; testes tandem; ovary between testes.**....**7**

4a. **Intestinal ceca sinuous; body linguiform; parasites in cecum and large intestine of birds and mammals (Fig. 325).** ....
...................................**Genus** *Postharmostomum* **Witenberg, 1923**

Key to species in McIntosh (1934b).

Life cycle: *P. helicis—*

Embryonated eggs, passed in the feces of the host, are ingested by the terrestrial snails, *Anguispira alternata, Deroceras laeve* and *Polygyra* spp. Obscuromicrocercous cercariae (Fig. 17) develop in branched daughter sporocysts. The cercariae enter the pericardial cavity of another snail of the same species or a different species and develop into metacercariae without encysting. The latter apparently cannot develop in the snail that produced the sporocysts. Mature trematodes develop in about eight days in the cecum of Eastern chipmunk, *Tamias striatus,* and deer mouse, *Peromyscus maniculatus* (see Ulmer, 1951).

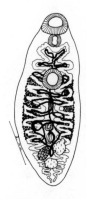

Fig. 325.   *Postharmostomum gallinum.*

4b. Intestinal ceca straight; body oval. **5**

5a. Vitelline follciles in lateral clusters, anterior to level of ventral sucker; parasites in bursa Fabricii of birds (Fig. 326). ....
....Genus *Leucochloridiomorpha* Gower, 1938

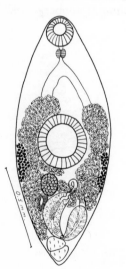

Life cycle: *L. constantiae*—

Embryonated eggs are ingested by the operculate snail, *Campeloma decisum.* Furcocercous cercariae resembling the dichotoma type (Fig. 28), develop in branched sporocysts. The cercariae, upon leaving one snail, may be swept into the respiratory chamber of another snail of the same species. Metacercariae accumulate in the uterus of the snail. The mature trematode has been produced experimentally in chickens, ducks and raccoon. Natural infections occur in the bursa Fabricii of the black duck, *Anas rubripes* (see Allison, 1943).

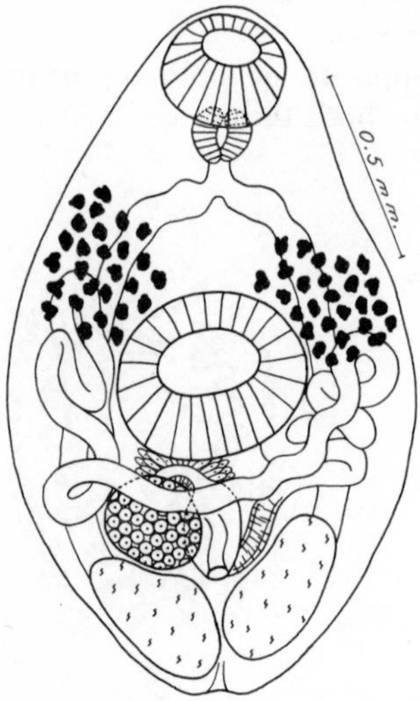

Fig. 326.   *Leucochloridiomorpha constantiae.*

5b. Vitelline follicles in narrow lateral rows, largely lateral to intestinal ceca; parasites of rodents. **6**

6a. Vitelline follicles entirely posterior to level of ventral sucker; ovary anterior to both testes; parasites in salivary glands of muskrat (Fig. 327). ....
...........Genus *Ptyalincola* Wootton and Murrell, 1967

Fig. 327.   *Ptyalincola ondatrae.*

6b. Vitelline follicles anterior and posterior to ventral sucker; ovary opposite anterior testis; intestinal parasites of rabbits (Fig. 328). ....Genus *Hasstilesia* Hall, 1916

Key to species in Rowan (1955).

Life cycle: *H. tricolor—*
Embryonated eggs are eaten by the pupillid terrestrial snails, *Vertigo ventricosa* and *V. ovata*. The miracidia hatch in the snail intestine. Microcercous cercariae develop in branched sporocysts. The cercariae lose their tail and develop into metacercariae in the sporocyst without encysting. Rabbits probably ingest infected snails with their forage. Natural definitive hosts are the cottontail, *Sylvilagus floridanus* and the black-tailed jackrabbit, *Lepus californicus* (see Rowan 1955).

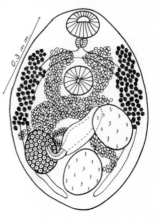

Fig. 328. *Hasstilesia tricolor.*

7a. Genital pore and cirrus sac anterior to both testes. 8
7b. Genital pore and cirrus sac between testes or posterior to testes. 11
8a. Body oval; vitelline follicles confined to lateral regions in posterior half of body; intestinal ceca slightly sinuous; intestinal parasites of mammals (Fig. 329). ....
....Genus *Ectosiphonus* Sinitzin, 1931

Life cycle: *E. rhomboideus—*
Embryonated eggs were fed to the land snail, *Ventridens ligera*. Microcercous cercariae developed in branched daughter sporocysts in 52 to 60 days. Cercariae transform to metacercariae in the same snail or in a different one. Transfer of cercariae occurs in abundant mucous secretions. About three months are required for metacercariae to become infective for the definitive host. Sexually mature trematodes develop experimentally in hamsters in 21 days. The short-tailed shrew, *Blarina brevicauda*, is the natural definitive host (Villella, 1953b, 1954).

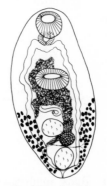

Fig. 329. *Ectosiphonus ovatus.* (Redrawn from Sinitsin, 1931.)

8b. Body elongate; vitelline follicles in lateral rows along most of length of body or restricted to midbody region. 9
9a. Muscular prepharynx present; vitelline follicles restricted to midbody region (Fig. 330). ....

....Genus *Entosiphonus* Sinitzin, 1931

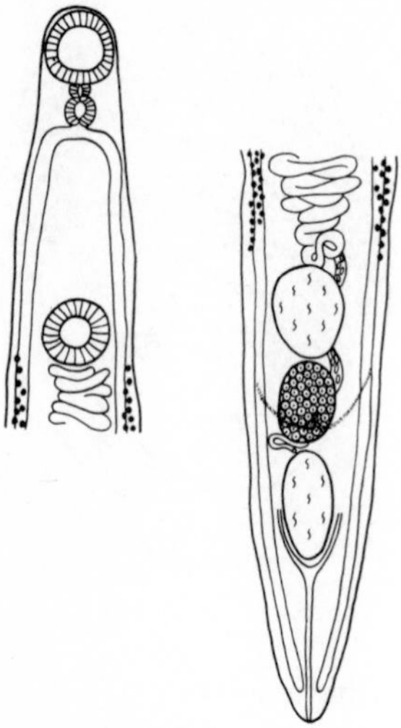

Life cycle: *E. thompsoni*—

Embryonated eggs are ingested by the terrestrial snails, *Retinella indentata, Succinea ovalis, Ventridens ligera* and *Zonitoides nitidus.* Mother and daughter branched sporocysts develop, the latter producing microcercous cercariae in about 70 days. Infective metacercariae are known to develop in *R. indentata, V. ligera, S. ovalis* and also in the slug, *Deroceras laeve.* The adult trematode develops in the short-tailed shrew, *Blarina brevicauda,* and in the white-footed mouse, *Peromyscus leucopus noveboracensis.* Eggs were found in the feces of the latter within 15 days (Villella, 1953a).

Fig. 330. *Entosiphonus thompsoni.* (Redrawn from Sinitsin, 1931.)

9b. Muscular prepharynx absent; vitelline follicles more extensive than described above. **10**
10a. Body very elongate, filiform; uterus not extending anterior to ventral sucker (Fig. 331). ....

....Genus *Scaphiostomum* Braun, 1901

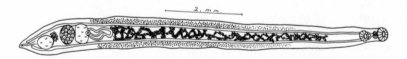

Fig. 331. *Scaphiostomum pancreaticum.*

10b. Body moderately elongate; part of uterus extends anterior to ventral sucker (Fig. 332). ....

....Genus *Brachylaima* Dujardin, 1843

Life cycle: *B. virginiana*—

Embryonated eggs are eaten by the land snail *Polygyra thyroides* which can serve as both first and second intermediate host. Obscuromicrocerous cercariae (Fig. 17) develop in branched sporocysts, leave the sporocyst, creep over the surface of the snail and are transferred when snails contact each other. Encystment and development to the metacercarial stage occurs in the kidney of the snail. Other suitable second intermediate hosts besides *P. thyroides* are the slugs, *Deroceras laeve* and *Agriolimax columbianus;* the aquatic snails *Helisoma trivolvis* and *Pseudosuccinea columella* and the land snails *Helix pomatia, Mesomphix cupreus* and *Succinea* spp. The adult fluke develops in the large intestine of the opossum (Krull, 1934a, 1935a, 1936; Hand and Voge, 1952; Ulmer, 1952).

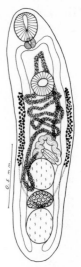

Fig. 332. *Brachylaima virginiana.*

11a. **Genital pore posterior to testes; uterus not extending anterior to ventral sucker; intestinal parasites of mammals (Fig. 333).**
....Genus *Panopistus* Sinitzin, 1931

Life cycle: *P. pricei*—

Embryonated eggs, passed in the feces of the host, are ingested by the terrestrial snails *Ventridens ligera, Zonitoides arboreus* and the slug *Agriolimax agrestis.* Obscuromicrocercous cercariae (Fig. 17) are produced in branched sporocysts. Snails shed cercariae which creep over the surface of the snail and are transferred to another snail upon contact. Metacercariae develop in the pericardial cavity of the land snails *Stenotrema monodon, Deroceras laeve, Zonitoides* spp. and *Ventridens* spp. The short-tailed shrew, *Blarina brevicauda* is the definitive host (Krull, 1934b, 1935b; Reynolds, 1938; Villella, 1954).

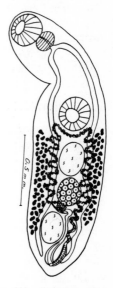

Fig. 333. *Panopistus pricei.*

11b. Genital pore between testes; uterus extends anterior to ventral sucker; intestinal parasites of birds (Fig. 334). ....

....**Genus** *Glaphyrostomum* **Braun, 1901**

Life cycle: *G. mcintoshi*—

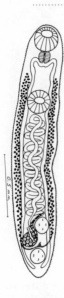

Embryonated eggs are eaten by the land snail *Zonitoides arboreus*. Tailless cercariae develop in branched sporocysts. The cercariae do not encyst and do not leave the sporocyst. Experimental infections were established in chicks. The adult fluke normally develops in the digestive tract of the ovenbird (Krull, 1935c).

Fig. 334.   *Glaphyrostomum mcintoshi.*

SUPERFAMILY FELLODISTOMATOIDEA Larue, 1957

Cercariae of the furocercous dichotoma type and possibly of the non-oculate trichocercous type; excretory vesicle of cercaria large and U-shaped; larval stages develop in marine lamellibranch or gastropod molluscs; cercariae encyst in the same or a different mollusc; two or three hosts involved in the life cycle; parasites of marine fishes or shore birds.

FAMILY FELLODISTOMATIDAE Nicoll, 1913

Body muscular, thick, usually nonspinous, either oval, fusiform or elongate; oral and ventral suckers of about equal size or the ventral larger than the oral; intestinal ceca short or extending to posterior end of body; testes oblique, opposite or tandem; cirrus sac anterior or dorsal to ventral sucker; seminal vesicle usually bipartite; ovary between, anterior or posterior to testes; genital pore median or sublateral; vitelline follicles usually restricted to small lateral clusters in middle third of body but more extensive in a few genera; uterus has descending and ascending limbs; excretory vesicle Y- or V-shaped with arms long, extending forward as far as pharynx in some genera; intestinal parasites of marine fishes.

Cable (1954a) discussed the possibility of non-oculate trichocerous cercariae (Fig. 40) being the cercarial type for trematodes in this family. He described *Cercaria laevicardii* which develops in simple sporocysts in the marine lamellibranch, *Laevicardium mortoni* and resembles the cercaria of *Bacciger bacciger* as described by Palombi (1934a). The excretory vesicle is large and U-shaped, like that of the furcocercous dichotoma type of cercaria of the trematodes of the Family Gymnophallidae.

KEY TO GENERA

1a. Conical muscular papillae around oral sucker; neck region of body with lateral muscular papillae; body elongate; testes tandem or oblique (Fig. 335). ....
....Genus *Tergestia* Stossich, 1899
Key to species in Manter (1954) and in Skrjabin (1964).
1b. Body without muscular papillae. 2
2a. Testes tandem; body elongate; vitelline follicles lateral to intestinal ceca between level of ventral sucker and anterior testis; intestinal ceca long; parasites of parrotfishes (Fig. 336).
....Genus *Mesolecitha* Linton, 1910

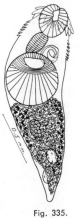
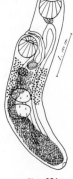

Fig. 335.   *Tergestia acuta.*
Fig. 336.   *Mesolecitha linearis.*

Fig. 335.   Fig. 336.

2b. Testes opposite to slightly oblique; body oval or fusiform..... 3
3a. Body fusiform; oral sucker cup-shaped, directed anteriad; testes opposite; ceca short, extending only to testes; vitelline follicles restricted to forebody, lateral to ceca (Fig. 337). ....
....Genus *Antorchis* Linton, 1911
3b. Body broadly oval; other features not as descirbed above. 4

4a. Body thick, muscular; oral sucker with zone of circular muscular fibers close to mouth; ventral muscle fibers extending
from sides of oral sucker to posterior margin of ventral sucker;
genital atrium tubular with a spinous diverticulum; cirrus
spiny; parasites of hogfishes (Fig. 338). ....
....Genus *Megalomyzon* Manter, 1947

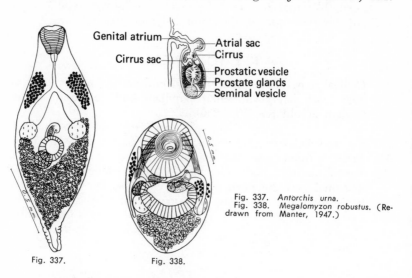

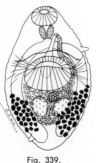

Fig. 337. *Antorchis urna.*
Fig. 338. *Megalomyzon robustus.* (Redrawn from Manter, 1947.)

Fig. 337.   Fig. 338.

4b. Oral sucker, cirrus and genital atrium not as described above;
ventral muscle fibers absent. 5
5a. Vitelline follicles extend posterior to testes; parasites of
porgies. 6
5b. Vitelline follicles not extending posterior to testes. 7
6a. Vitelline follicles confined to hindbody; genital pore to left
of pharynx (Fig. 339). ....
....Genus *Pycnadenoides* Yamaguti, 1938

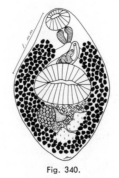

Fig. 339. *Pycnadenoides calami.*
Fig. 340. *Pycnadena lata.*

Fig. 339.   Fig. 340.

6b. Vitelline follicles in fore- and hindbody; genital pore median or slightly sinistral, at level of cecal bifurcation (Fig. 340).
....Genus *Pycnadena* Linton, 1910

7a. Vitelline follicles in compact clusters in forebody, lateral to ceca; ceca short (Fig. 341). ....
....Genus *Bacciger* Nicoll, 1914

Key to species in Skrjabin (1964).
Life cycle: *B. bacciger—*
The cercaria is of the nonoculate trichocercous type (Fig. 40) which develops in daughter sporocysts in the marine lamellibranchs, *Donax vittatus, Pholas candida* and several species of the genus *Tapes* and encyst in the marine amphipod, *Erichthonius difformis.* The adult fluke develops in the intestine of the silverside, *Atherina hepsetus* (see Palombi, 1934a).

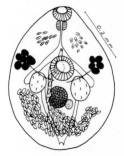

Fig. 341.   *Bacciger   harengulae.*

7b. Vitelline follicles in region of ventral sucker and testes. 8

8a. Excretory vesicle Y-shaped (Fig. 342). ....
...........Genus *Fellodistomum* Stafford, 1904 (= *Steringophorus* Odhner, 1905)

Life cycle: *F. fellis—*
Furcocercous cercariae, having a large V-shaped excretory vesicle, develop in sporocysts in the nut clam, *Nucula tenuis.* After leaving the clam, the cercariae enter the brittle star, *Ophiura sarci*, in which they metamorphose to the metacercarial stage. Infected brittle stars are eaten by wolffishes in which the adult trematode develops (Chubrik, G. K., 1952. Zoologicheski Zhurnal 31:653-658).

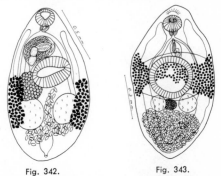

Fig. 342.   *Fellodistomum   brevum.*
Fig. 343. *Steringotrema corpulentum.*
(Redrawn   from   Manter,   1931.)

Fig. 342.   Fig. 343.

8b. Excretory vesicle V-shaped (Fig. 343). ....
....Genus *Steringotrema* Odhner, 1911
Key to species in Skrjabin (1964).

FAMILY GYMNOPHALLIDAE Morozov, 1955 EMEND.

Body small, oval, spinous; oral sucker larger than ventral sucker; intestinal ceca short, divergent; testes opposite, near lateral margins of body at about level of ventral sucker; cirrus and cirrus sac absent; genital atrium present, anterior to ventral sucker; ovary lateral, anterior to either right or left testis; vitelline glands in the form of one or two compact clusters of follicles; uterus has descending and ascending limbs; eggs large, not very abundant; excretory vesicle V- or Y-shaped, arms long, extending forward to pharynx; parasites in intestine, bursa Fabricii or gall bladder of shore birds.

KEY TO GENERA

1a. Body usually larger than 1 mm.; oral sucker moderately large; genital pore small, located at anterior edge of ventral sucker or within it; genital atrium tubular; prostate glands open into pars prostatica, not directly into genital atrium; pharynx small; excretory vesicle Y-shaped; parasites in intestine, gall bladder or bursa Fabricii of birds (Fig. 344). ....
....Genus *Gymnophallus* **Odhner, 1900**

Key to species in James (1964).
Life cycle: *G. australis*—
Szidat (1962) discovered that the metacercaria of this species from the mussel, *Mytilus platensis,* in the South Atlantic developed testes and ovary. After the testes atrophied, the ovary persisted as

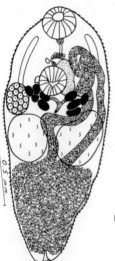

Fig. 344. *Gymnophallus deliciosus.*

a source of germinal cells that eventually developed to cercariae. He regarded this as parthenogenetic reproduction and attributed this type of regression to the low temperature of water in which the mussels occur.

1b. **Body very small (less than 1 mm.); oral sucker very large; genital pore large, located distinctly anterior to very small ventral sucker; prostate glands open into shallow genital atrium; pharynx well developed; excretory vesicle V-shaped; intestinal parasites of birds (Figs. 345, 346).** ....
....**Genus** *Parvatrema* **Cable, 1953**

Fig. 345. *Parvatrema borinquenae.*
Fig. 346. *P. obscurum.*

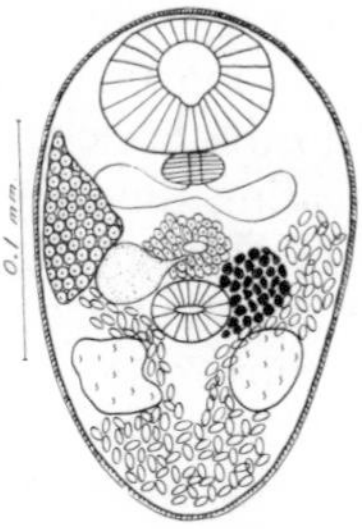

Fig. 345. 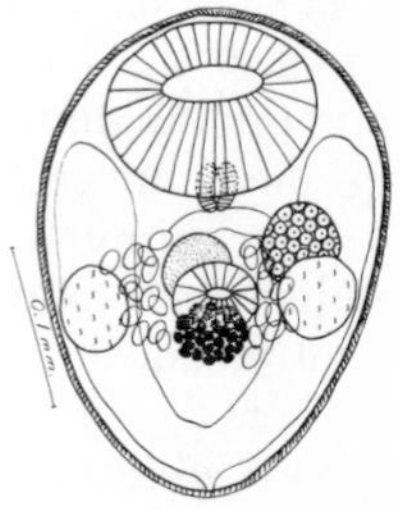   Fig. 346.

Key to species in James (1964).
Life cycle: *P. borinquenae*—

Furcocercous cercariae of the dichotoma type (Fig. 28) develop in sporocysts in the marine lamellibranch, *Gemma purpurea*. The cercariae penetrate the marine snail, *Cerithidea costata* and develop to infective metacercariae without encysting. The adult trematode develops in chicks of *Gallus domesticus* that are fed metacercariae. The natural definitive host is unknown (Cable, 1953).

James (1964) described the life cycle of *P. homoeotecnum*, a parasite of the oystercatcher, *Haematopus ostralegus occidentalis.* Embryonated eggs are ingested by the marine snail, *Littorina saxatilis tenebrosa*, in which primary germinal sacs (Fig. 347) develop

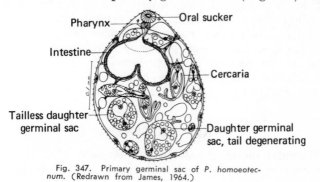

Pharynx
Oral sucker
Intestine
Cercaria
Tailless daughter germinal sac
Daughter germinal sac, tail degenerating

Fig. 347. Primary germinal sac of *P. homoeotecnum.* (Redrawn from James, 1964.)

and produce a generation of similar daughter germinal sacs. The young daughter germinal sacs are at first furcocercous, resembling dichotoma cercariae, but the tail gradually degenerates. When the primary germinal sacs rupture, the daughter germinal sacs are released. From here the cycle can follow one of three courses:

1. Daughter germinal sacs produce furcocercous cercariae and subsequently metacercariae after degeneration of the forked tail.

2. Daughter germinal sacs produce a second generation of daughter germinal sacs which can in turn produce either cercariae or a third generation of daughter germinal sacs.

3. Daughter germinal sacs produce cercariae, metacercariae and a generation of daughter germinal sacs simultaneously.

All of the larval stages remain in the host snail, there being but one intermediate host in the life cycle. The definitive host probably becomes infected by eating the metacercariae in infected snails.

The germinal sacs of this species differ from the conventional rediae and sporocysts of other trematodes in having an oral and ventral sucker, a pharynx and a bilobed intestine. The ventral sucker degenerates in the older germinal sacs. This is the first record of a gymnophallid trematode developing in a gastropod mollusc. The larvae of all other species in which the life cycle is known, develop in sporocysts in lamellibranch molluscs.

SUPERFAMILY BUCEPHALOIDEA Larue, 1926

Cercariae of the gasterostome (bucephaloid) type, develop in branched sporocysts in lamellibranch molluscs; three hosts involved in the life cycle; aduts have oral opening on midventral body surface; parasites of fishes.

FAMILY BUCEPHALIDAE Poche, 1907

Mouth on midventral body surface, leading to pharynx and sac-shaped intestine; muscular sucker or a conical rhynchus at anterior end of body; two testes, tandem or oblique, in posterior half of body; cirrus sac and genital pore near posterior end of body; genital atrium present; ovary pretesticular or opposite anterior testis; vitelline follicles in small clusters in anterior half of body; parasites in digestive tract or coelom of fishes.

KEY TO GENERA

1a. Muscular sucker at anterior end of body. 2
1b. Muscular conical rhynchus at anterior end of body. 4

2a. Sucker surmounted by a flat hood; in marine and freshwater fishes (Fig. 348). ....Genus *Rhipidocotyle*

Life cycle: *R. septpapillata*—
The adult fluke is a parasite of pumpkinseed and small mouth bass. Freshly-laid eggs contain miracidia which hatch in water and are then probably swept into the incurrent siphon of the freshwater mussel, *Lampsilis siliquoidea,* in the gonads of which bucephaloid cercariae develop in branched sporocysts. The cercariae are known to encyst in tissues of pumpkinseed, creek chub and large mouth bass (Krull 1934c; Kniskern, 1952).

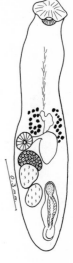

Fig. 348. *Rhipidocotyle barracudae.* (Redrawn from Manter, 1940b.)

2b. Sucker not surmounted by hood. 3
3a. Sucker provided with tentacles (fimbriae); in marine and freshwater fishes (Fig. 349). ....Genus *Bucephalus* Baer, 1826

Life cycle: *B. polymorphus*—
Eggs in the feces of the host contain miracidia which hatch in water. Bucephaloid cercariae develop in branched sporocysts in the gonads of the freshwater clams, *Lampsilis iris* and *Anodonta* spp. After losing the tail, the cercariae penetrate the fins of freshwater fishes and encyst in the subcutaneous connective tissue and muscles. The adult trematode develops in bluegill, bass, perch, pike, burbot and gudgeon (Woodhead, 1929, 1930).

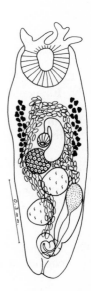

Fig. 349. *Bucephalus elegans.*

3b. Sucker without tentacles (Figs. 350, 351). ....
....Genus *Bucephaloides* Hopkins, 1954

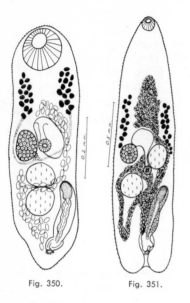

Life cycle: *B. haemeanus—*
Bucephaloid cercariae develop in branched sporocysts in the liver, gonads, gills and pericardium of the oyster, *Ostrea edulis,* and the cockle, *Cardium rusticum.* The developing sporocysts interfere with the sexual reproduction of the molluscs. Cercariae encyst in the Atlantic silverside, *Menidia menidia.* The garfish, *Tylosurus marinus,* is the natural definitive host (Tennent, 1906; Palombi, 1934b).

Fig. 350.   Fig. 351.

Fig. 350. *Bucephaloides pusilla.*
Fig. 351. *B. longovifera.*

4a. Rhynchus provided with several transverse rows of spines; parasites of marine fishes (Fig. 352). ....
....Genus *Dollfustrema* Eckmann, 1934

4b. Rhynchus without spines. 5

5a. Rhynchus elongate and provided with tentacles; in marine fishes (Fig. 353). .... Genus *Alcicornis* MacCallum, 1917

5b. Rhynchus not elongate, without tentacles. 6

6a. Rhynchus well developed; testes round or oval; in digestive tract of fishes (Fig. 354). ....
....Genus *Prosorhynchus* Odhner, 1905

6b. Rhynchus small, weakly developed; testes deeply lobed; in coelom of freshwater fishes (Fig. 355). ....
....Genus *Paurorhynchus* Dickerman, 1954

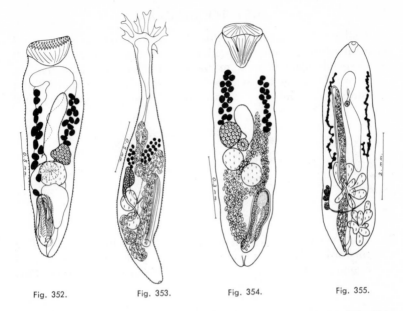

Fig. 352.   Fig. 353.   Fig. 354.   Fig. 355.

Fig. 352. *Dollfustrema macracanthum.* (Redrawn from Hanson, 1950.) Fig. 353. *Alcicornis carangis.* (Redrawn from MacCallum, 1917.) Fig. 354. *Prosorhynchus pacificus.* Fig. 355. *Paurorhynchus hiodontis.* (Redrawn from Dickerman, 1954.)

ORDER ECHINOSTOMIDA Larue, 1957
SUPERFAMILY ECHINOSTOMATOIDEA Faust, 1929

Cercariae of echinostome, echinostome-like, gymnocephalous or megalurous type, having stenostomate excretory system and develop in rediae having a collar and procrusculi; two or three hosts involved in the life cycle; parasites in the intestine, bile ducts, cloaca, bursa Fabricii or eyes of reptiles, birds and mammals.

FAMILY ECHINOSTOMATIDAE Looss, 1902

Body spinous, provided with a head collar which surrounds oral sucker and contains a single or double row of large spines; ventral sucker usually much larger than oral sucker; intestinal ceca extending to posterior end of body; testes tandem, variable in shape; cirrus sac present; genital pore median, anterior to ventral sucker; ovary pretesticular; seminal receptacle absent; vitelline follicles abundant, distributed along ceca, confined to region posterior to ventral sucker; uterus entirely anterior to ovary; eggs large; intestinal parasites of reptiles, birds and mammals.

KEY TO GENERA

1a. Collar spines interrupted dorsal to oral sucker. 2
1b. Collar spines uninterrupted dorsal to oral sucker. 3
2a. Body elongate (3 mm. or more); vitelline follicles extending forward only as far as anterior testis; parasites of reptiles and birds (Fig. 356). ....Genus *Stephanoprora* Odhner, 1902

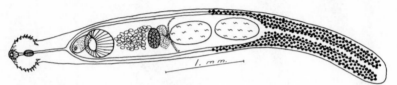

Fig. 356. *Stephanoprora pseudoechinata.*

2b. Body small, oval (less than 3 mm.); vitelline follicles extending forward to level of ventral sucker; parasites of birds and mammals (Fig. 357). ....Genus *Echinochasmus* Dietz, 1909

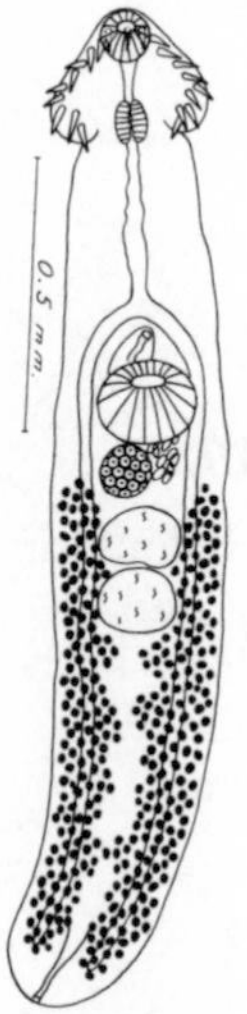

Life cycle: *E. donaldsoni—*

Echinostome cercariae develop in rediae in the operculate snails, *Amnicola limosa* and *A. lustrica*. The cercariae encyst on the gills of several species of freshwater fishes. Metacercariae are infective after the third week of encystment. Experimental infections were established by feeding metacercariae to pigeons but the natural definitive host is the pied-billed grebe (Beaver 1941b).

Fig. 357. *Echinochasmus donaldsoni.*

3a. Body very elongate; testes close to posterior end of body; uterus very long, extending through at least two-thirds of body length; parasites of birds. 4
3b. Body moderately elongate; testes some distance from posterior end of body; uterus short, occupying one-third or less of body length. 5
4a. No vitelline follicles posterior to testes; eggs have unipolar filament (Fig. 358). ....Genus *Aporchis* Stossich, 1905

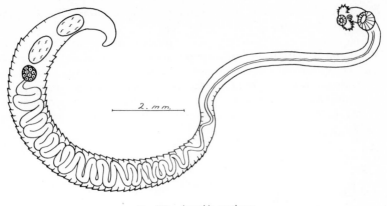

Fig. 358. *Aporchis continuus.*

4b. Some vitelline follicles posterior to testes; eggs without polar filament (Fig. 359). ....Genus *Himasthla* **Dietz, 1909**

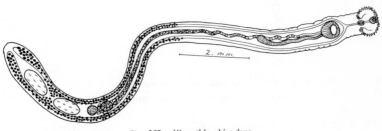

Fig. 359. *Himasthla rhigedana.*

Key to species in Skrjabin (1964).

Life cycle: *H. rhigedana*—

Eggs are unembryonated when laid. Miracidia developed within 18 days in eggs kept in seawater at room temperature. After hatching, they penetrate the brackish water snail, *Cerithidia californica* in which echinostome cercariae are produced in rediae. After leaving the snail, the cercariae encyst on vegetation or any solid objects. Metacercariae are infective immediately for chicks. The natural definitive host is the curlew (Adams and Martin, 1963).

The life cycle of *H. quissetensis* was described by Stunkard (1938a). The cercariae are produced in daughter rediae in the snail, *Nassa obsoleta* and encyst in the gills, mantle and foot of marine molluscs of the genera *Mya, Modiolus, Mytilus, Cumingia, Pecten, Ensis* and *Crepidula*. The definitive host is the herring gull.

5a. Lateral margins of body serrated; collar reniform; testes elongate; parasites of birds (Fig. 360). ....
....Genus *Prionosoma* **Dietz**, 1909
5b. Lateral margins of body nonserrated; testes oval or lobed. 6
6a. Testes lobed; corner spines of collar much larger than the others; body tapered gradually toward posterior end; some vitelline follicles anterior to testes; parasites of cormorants (Fig. 361). ....Genus *Drepanocephalus* **Dietz**, 1909

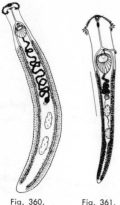

Fig. 360. *Prionosoma serratum.* Fig. 361. *Drepanocephalus spathans.*

Fig. 360.   Fig. 361.

6b. Testes oval; collar spines all of same size. 7
7a. Collar weakly developed; collar spines very small, deciduous. 8
7b. Collar well developed; collar spines large, usually present. 9
8a. Suckers of about equal size; ventral sucker near midbody region; uterus short; eggs few (Fig. 362). ....
....Genus *Protechinostoma* **Beaver**, 1943
Life cycle: *P. mucronisertulatum*—
Echinostome-like cercariae develop in rediae in the freshwater snail, *Stagnicola reflexae*. These cercariae have a dorso-ventral finfold on the tail, are without a collar but have an excretory system like that of the echinostomes. They encyst in the mantle cavity of *Physa gyrina* and *Stagnicola reflexae*. Experimental infections were established in chicks, the flukes attaining sexual maturity within five days (Feldman, 1941).

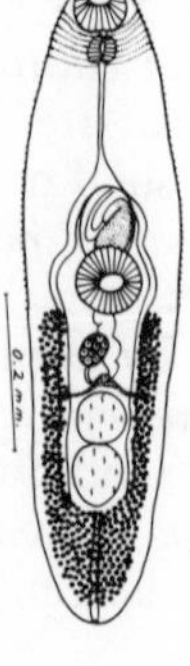

Fig. 362. *Protechinostoma mucronisertulatum.* (Redrawn from Beaver, 1943.)

8b. **Ventral sucker much larger than oral sucker and located close to oral sucker; uterus long; eggs abundant (Fig. 363).** ....
....**Genus** *Hypoderaeum* **Dietz, 1909**

Key to species in Skrjabin (1964).
Life cycle: *H. conoideum*—
Eggs are unembryonated when laid. About three weeks are required for development and hatching of the miracidia which penetrate the freshwater snail, *Lymnaea stagnalis* and *L. limosa* in which a generation of sporocysts and mother and daughter rediae develop. Echinostome cercariae develop in the latter. After leaving the snail, the cercariae again enter a snail to encyst. The mature flukes develop in the intestine of ducks, geese and swans. Completion of the life cycle requires about four months at 20° C (Mathias, 1925).

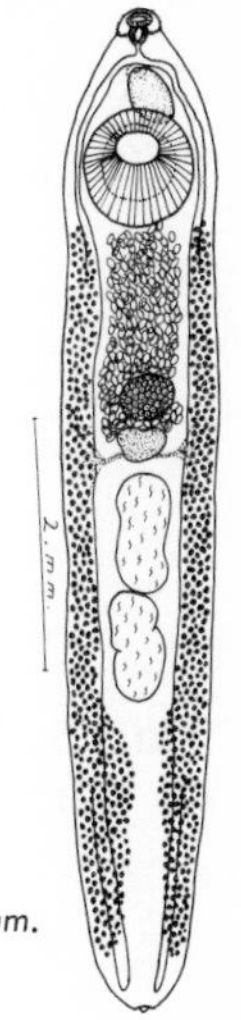

Fig. 363. *Hypoderaeum conoideum.*

9a. **Body elongate (8 to 20 mm.); eggs abundant.** **10**
9b. **Body short (4 mm. or less); eggs few.** **11**
10a. **Some vitelline follicles extend anterior to level of testes; intestinal parasites of birds and mammals (Fig. 364).** ....
....**Genus** *Echinostoma* **Rudolphi, 1809**

Key to species in Skrjabin (1964).
Life cycle: *E. revolutum*—
Three to four weeks are required for development of the miracidium after the eggs are laid. They hatch and penetrate snails of the genera *Physa, Lymnaea, Stagnicola, Helisoma* and *Pseudosuccinea*, in which a generation of sporocysts and mother and daughter rediae develop. The latter produce echinostome cercariae (Fig. 39) which, after emerging from the snail, encyst in the same or a different species of snail, in clams or in larval amphibians. The adult fluke is a parasite of ducks. It has been reported rarely as a parasite of human beings (Beaver, 1937).

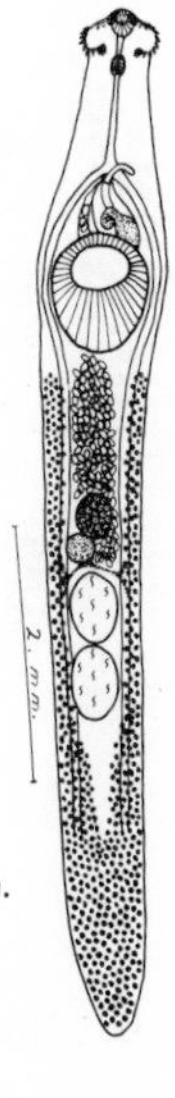

Fig. 364. *Echinostoma revolutum.*

10b. Vitelline follicles confined to testicular and posttesticular region; intestinal parasites of otter (Fig. 365). ....
....Genus *Baschkirovitrema* Skrjabin, 1944

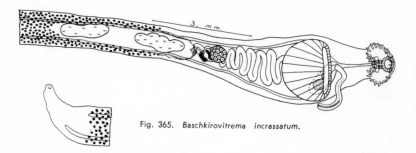

Fig. 365. *Baschkirovitrema incrassatum.*

11a. Body short, plump; ventral sucker near middle of body or posterior to middle; parasites of birds (Fig. 366). ....
....Genus *Petasiger* Dietz, 1909

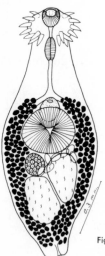

Fig. 366. *Petasiger nitidus.*

Key to species in Skrjabin (1964).
Life cycle: *P. nitidus—*
Echinostome cercariae, having an enormous tail, are produced in rediae in the planorbid snail, *Helisoma antrosum percarinatum.* After the cercariae leave the snail, they are eaten by several different species of freshwater fishes in which they encyst. Experimental infections were established in canaries. The horned grebe, *Colymbus auritus,* is the natural definitive host (Beaver, 1939a).

11b. Body slender; ventral sucker anterior to middle of body. 12

12a. Cirrus sac long, extending far posterior to ventral sucker; testes spherical or lobed; collar spines 24 or less (Fig. 367).
...................................Genus *Acanthoparyphium* Dietz, 1909

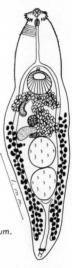

Key to species in Skrjabin (1964).
Life cycle: *A. spinulosum*—
Eggs are unembryonated at time of oviposition. Miracidia develop and hatch within 16 to 27 days and penetrate the brackish water snail, *Cerithidea hegewishi californica* in which echinostome cercariae (Fig. 39) develop in daughter rediae. The cercariae encyst in the tissues of the same species of snail. The natural definitive hosts are plover and avocet which acquire the parasite by eating the infected snails (Martin and Adams, 1961).

Fig. 367. *Acanthoparyphium spinulosum.*

12b. Cirrus sac short, not extending posterior to ventral sucker; testes elongate or oval; collar spines 25 or more. 13
13a. Testes elongate with wavy margins; collar spines 25 to 30 (Fig. 368). ....Genus *Euparyphium* Dietz, 1909

Key to species in Skrjabin (1964).
Life cycle: *E. beaveri*—
Echinostome cercariae develop in rediae in the freshwater snail, *Stagnicola emarginata angulata*. The cercariae enter the cloaca of tadpoles and encyst in the cloacal wall. The definitive hosts, such as mink, American otter, and snowshoe hare eat infected tadpoles or newly metamorphosed frogs (Beaver, 1941a).

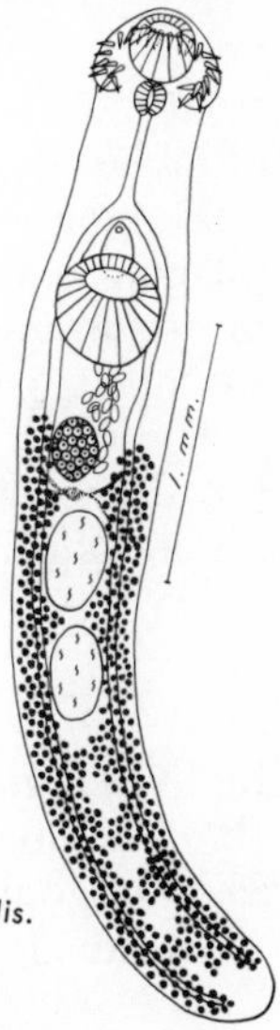

Fig. 368. *Euparyphium melis.*

13b. Testes oval margins smooth; collar spines 40 to 45 (Fig. 369).
....Genus *Echinoparyphium* Dietz, 1909

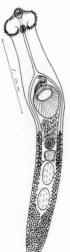

Key to species in Skrjabin (1964).
Life cycle: *E. flexum—*
Miracidia develop and hatch within 14 days and penetrate the freshwater snail, *Stagnicola palustris,* in which a generation of sporocysts and two of rediae develop. Echinostome cercariae develop in the daughter rediae and after leaving the snail in which they were produced, encyst in the heart and kidneys of the aquatic snails, *Helisoma trivolvis, Physa integra* and *Stagnicola palustris* and the kidneys of tadpoles of *Rana, Hyla* and *Pseudacris* spp. The metacercariae survive in the newly metamorphosed frogs. Natural definitive hosts are blue-winged teal and American scoter ducks which probably acquire the parasite by eating infected snails and tadpoles (McCoy 1927; Najarian 1953, 1954).

Fig. 369. *Echinoparyphium recurvatum.*

FAMILY PSILOSTOMATIDAE Odhner, 1913

Body oval or elongate, spinous or nonspinous; suckers well developed, ventral sucker larger than oral (ventral sucker pedunculate in *Stephanoproraoides*); intestinal ceca long; testes tandem or oblique, in posterior half of body; cirrus sac present; genital pore either anterior to ventral sucker or lateral to pharynx or esophagus; ovary pretesticular; vitelline follicles abundant, variable in extent; uterus entirely anterior to ovary; excretory vesicle usually Y-shaped; parasites of birds and mammals.

The adult psilostomes bear some resemblance to echinostomes but do not have a spiny collar. The cercariae of both groups have a stenostomate type of excretory system.

KEY TO GENERA

1a. Vitelline follicles only in hindbody. 2
1b. Vitelline follicles in fore- and hindbody. 3
2a. Body elongate, cylindrical; ventral sucker pedunculate; intestinal parasites of beaver (Fig. 370). ....
....................................Genus *Stephanoproraoides* Price, 1934

2b. Body oval to elongate, flat; ventral sucker sessile; intestinal parasites of birds (Fig. 371). ....
....Genus *Psilostomum* Looss, 1899

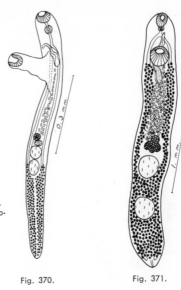

Fig. 370. *Stephanoproraoides lawi*. (Redrawn from Price, 1934.) Fig. 371. *Psilostomum lineatum*.

Fig. 370.   Fig. 371.

3a. Esophagus with a pair of lateral diverticula; parasites of birds (Fig. 372). ....Genus *Ribeiroia* Travassos, 1939

Life cycle: *R. thomasi*.

Eggs are unembryonated when laid. Miracidia develop and hatch in two to three weeks and penetrate the planorbid snail, *Helisoma antrosum percarinatum* in which echinostome-like cercariae (= *Cercaria thomasi*) are produced in daughter rediae. The cercariae encyst in the lateral line canal, nasal cavities and beneath scales of perch, bluegill, pumpkinseed and bass. The cercariae and metacercariae have esophageal diverticula like those of the adult fluke which develops in the intestine of ducks, gulls, osprey and hawk. Experimental infections were established in ducks, chicks, pigeons and canaries (Beaver, 1939b).

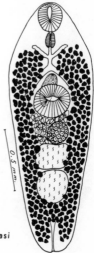

Fig. 372. *Ribeiroia thomasi*

3b. Esophagus without lateral diverticula. 4
4a. Body broadly oval; ventral sucker about three times as large
     as oral sucker; genital pore sinistral; testes and ovary close
     to posterior end of body. 5
4b. Body narrowly oval; ventral sucker only slightly larger than
     oral sucker; genital pore median; testes and ovary usually
     some distance from posterior end of body. 6
5a. Genital pore posterior to intestinal bifurcation; cirrus sac long,
     bipartite; testes oblique or nearly opposite (Fig. 373). ....

............................Genus *Astacatrematula* Macy and Bell, 1968

Life cycle: *A. macrocotyla*—

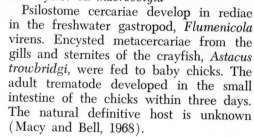

Psilostome cercariae develop in rediae
in the freshwater gastropod, *Flumenicola
virens*. Encysted metacercariae from the
gills and sternites of the crayfish, *Astacus
trowbridgi,* were fed to baby chicks. The
adult trematode developed in the small
intestine of the chicks within three days.
The natural definitive host is unknown
(Macy and Bell, 1968).

Fig. 373. *Astacatrematula macrocotyla*. (Redrawn
from Macy and Bell, 1968.)

5b. Genital pore anterior to intestinal bifurcation; cirrus sac short,
     oval; testes tandem (Fig. 374). ....

............................Genus *Sphaeridiotrema* Odhner, 1913

Life cycle: *S. globulus*—

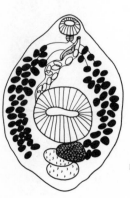

Echinostome-like cercariae (= *Cercaria
helvetica* XVII) develop in rediae in the
snail, *Bithynia tentaculata*. They escape
from the snail, swim for a brief period,
then return to a snail of the same species
and encyst between the mantle and the
shell. The adult trematode develops in the
intestine of merganser, scaup, old squaw
and domestic ducks which eat the infected
snails (Szidat, 1937).

Fig. 374. *Sphaeridiotrema globulus.*

Macy and Ford (1964) obtained encysted metacercariae from the snail, *Fluminicola virens*, fed them to ducks and recovered the adults of *S. globulus*.

Burns (1961a) investigated the life cycle of *S. spinoacetabulum* which is also a parasite of ducks. The cycle is similar to that of *S. globulus* except that the host snail is *Fluminicola virens* and the adult inhabits the ceca of the duck.

6a. Vitelline follicles confluent posterior to testes; testes near posterior end of body; eggs abundant, small (Fig. 375). ....
.................................Genus *Pseudopsilostoma* Yamaguti, 1958

6b. Vitelline follicles not confluent posterior to testes; testes some distance from posterior end of body; usually one large egg in uterus (Fig. 376). ....
.....................Genus *Grysoma* Byrd, Bogitsh and Maples, 1961

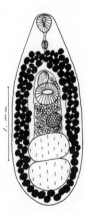 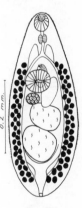

Fig. 375. *Pseudopsilostoma ondatrae.*
Fig. 376. *Grysoma singularis.*

Fig. 375.   Fig. 376.

FAMILY RHYTIDODIDAE Odhner, 1926

Body elongate, nonspinous; oral sucker has one dorsal and two subventral muscular papillae; ventral sucker in anterior third of body; pharynx present; intestinal ceca long; two tandem testes, in middle third of body; cirrus sac present; genital pore anterior to ventral sucker; ovary pretesticular; seminal receptacle absent; vitelline follicles restricted to hindbody; uterus entirely anterior to ovary; excretory vesicle Y-shaped; the arms having numerous lateral diverticula; intestinal parasites of turtles.

The Genus *Rhytidodes* Looss, 1901 is represented in North America by the species *R. secunda* Pratt, 1914 from the intestine of *Caretta caretta* from the Gulf of Mexico (Fig. 377).

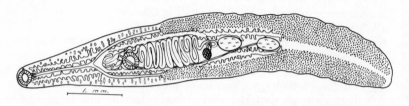

Fig. 377. *Rhytidodes secundus.* (Redrawn from Pratt, 1914.)

FAMILY CATHAEMASIIDAE Fuhrmann, 1928

Body elongate, usually spinous; suckers well developed, the ventral sucker larger than the oral; intestinal ceca long, end blindly; testes tandem, lobed or ovoid; cirrus sac present; ovary anterior to testes; genital pore median, anterior to ventral sucker; vitelline follicles in lateral areas of hind body; uterus entirely anterior to ovary; intestinal parasites of birds.

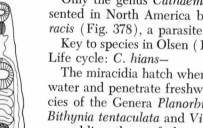

Only the genus *Cathaemasia* Looss, 1899 is represented in North America by the species *C. nycticoracis* (Fig. 378), a parasite of herons.

Key to species in Olsen (1940) and Skrjabin (1964). Life cycle: *C. hians*—

The miracidia hatch when embryonated eggs enter water and penetrate freshwater snails of several species of the Genera *Planorbis* and *Lymnaea* and also *Bithynia tentaculata* and *Vivipara fasciata*. Cercariae resembling those of the echinostome type develop in daughter rediae and encyst in tadpoles of *Rana esculenta*. The adult trematode develops in storks and herons (Szidat, 1939).

Fig. 378. *Cathaemasia nycticoracis.*

FAMILY CAMPULIDAE Odhner, 1926

Body elongate, fusiform or linguiform; intestinal ceca with a pair of anterior diverticula and in some genera lateral diverticula; testes tandem, usually lobed or dendritic; cirrus sac present; genital pore anterior to ventral sucker; ovary pretesticular; vitelline follicles variable in extent and shape, sometimes in form of rosettes; uterus entirely anterior to ovary; eggs triangular in cross section; parasites in bile duct or small intestine of marine mammals.

KEY TO GENERA

1a. Intestinal ceca with only anterior diverticula; vitelline glands in the form of rosettes and restricted to posttesticular region; body large (27 to 60 mm.); parasites of Cetacea (Fig. 379). ....Genus *Hadwenius* Price, 1932

1b. Intestinal ceca with anterior and lateral diverticula; vitelline follicles distributed all along ceca; parasites in bile duct of Cetacea and Pinnipedia. 2

2a. Body 25 to 45 mm. long; ventral sucker located in midbody region; vitelline follicles in quadrangular masses, all along ceca (Fig. 380). ....Genus *Lecithodesmus* Braun, 1902

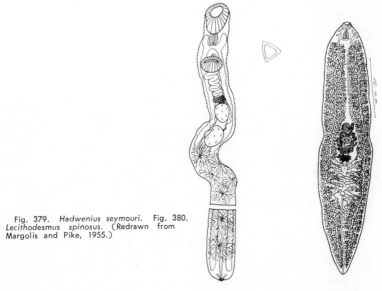

Fig. 379. *Hadwenius seymouri.* Fig. 380. *Lecithodesmus spinosus.* (Redrawn from Margolis and Pike, 1955.)

Fig. 379.   Fig. 380.

2b. Body 10 to 15 mm. long; ventral sucker close to oral sucker; vitelline follicles small, evenly distributed along ceca. 3

3a. Cloaca present; eggs triangular in cross section; parasite of porpoise (Fig. 381). ....Genus *Campula* Cobbold, 1858
Key to species in Price (1932) and Skrjabin (1964).

3b. Cloaca absent; eggs round in cross section; parasite of seals (Fig. 382). ......Genus *Zalophotrema* Stunkard and Alvey, 1929

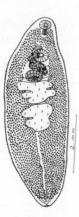
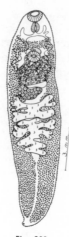

Fig. 381. *Campula oblonga*. Fig. 382.
Zalophotrema hepaticum.

Fig. 381.　　　Fig. 382.

FAMILY FASCIOLIDAE Railliet, 1895

Body very large, leaflike; suckers close together at anterior end of body; intestinal ceca usually with numerous diverticula (no diverticula in *Fasciolopsis*); testes tandem, dendritic; ovary dendritic, pretesticular; genital pore median, anterior to ventral sucker; cirrus sac present; vitelline follicles small, abundant, widely distributed throughout body; uterus short, entirely anterior to ovary; parasites in liver, bile duct and small intestine of herbivorous mammals and human beings.

KEY TO GENERA

1a. Intestinal ceca without diverticula; ventral sucker much larger than oral sucker (Fig. 383). ....
....Genus *Fasciolopsis* Looss, 1899

Species of this genus do not occur in North America. In Asia *F. buski* is an important parasite in the small intestine of pigs and human beings. Three to seven weeks are required for development of the miracidium after the eggs are laid. They hatch in water and penetrate the planorbid snails, *Hippeutis cantori*, *Gyraulus saigonensis* and several species of *Segmentina*. One generation of sporocysts and two of rediae develop in the snails. Daughter rediae produce gymnocephalous cercariae (Fig. 46) which leave the snail and encyst on vegetation. In the native habitat the important cysts are those on the seed pods of the red ling, *Tropa natans;* or on the water chestnut, *Eliocharis tuberosa.* When human beings eat the enclosed nuts they customarily remove the outer covering with their teeth. Metacercariae are thus taken into the mouth and swallowed. Excystment occurs in the digestive tract and the trematode matures in the anterior part of the small intestine.

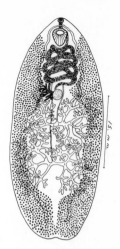

Fig. 383. *Fasciolopsis buski.*

1b. Intestinal ceca with many diverticula; suckers of nearly equal size. **2**

2a. Anterior end of body conical; body 2 to 3 cm. long; vitelline follicles located dorsal and ventral to intestinal ceca (Fig. 384). ....Genus *Fasciola* **Linnaeus, 1758**

Key to species in Skrjabin (1964).
Life cycle: *F. hepatica*—
The sheep liver fluke is a parasite of considerable economic importance in all parts of the world. Nonembryonated eggs pass in the feces of the host. About fifteen days are required for development and hatching of the miracidium which penetrates a variety of species of freshwater snails. Sporocysts and two generations of rediae develop in the snails and gymnocephalous cercariae develop in the daughter rediae. After leaving the snail, the cer-

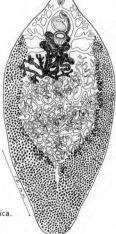

Fig. 384. *Fasciola hepatica.*

cariae encyst on aquatic vegetation. Definitive hosts such as sheep, goats, cattle, rabbits, deer, and human beings, become infected through accidental ingestion of metacercariae in their forage. Metacercariae encyst in the small intestine and migrate to the liver by way of the coelom, penetrating the outer surface of the liver. Human beings have been known to become infected by eating water cress, containing metacercariae (Leuckart, 1882; Thomas, 1883).

2b. **Anterior end of body rounded, not conical; body 3 to 10 cm. long; vitelline follicles only ventral to intestinal ceca (Fig. 385).** ....Genus *Fascioloides* **Ward, 1917**

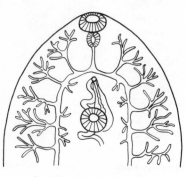

F. magna is the only known species. It is one of the largest known trematodes. The life cycle is similar to that of *Fasciola hepatica*, utilizing many of the same intermediate and definitive hosts.

Fig. 385. *Fascioloides magna.*

FAMILY PHILOPHTHALMIDAE Travassos, 1918

Body elongate, oval or fusiform, usually spinous; ventral sucker much larger than oral sucker; intestinal ceca long; testes opposite or tandem, lobed or oval and near posterior end of body; cirrus sac well developed; genital pore median and anterior to ventral sucker; ovary median, pretesticular; uterus entirely anterior to ovary; vitelline follicles few, forming a U- or V-shaped design anterior to testes; parasites in intestine, cloaca, bursa Fabricii or conjunctiva of birds.

KEY TO GENERA

1a. **Testes opposite; parasites in cloaca or bursa Fabricii of birds.** 2

1b. **Testes tandem; parasites in intestine or conjunctiva of birds....3**

2a. **Well developed spiny collar around oral sucker; testes lobed; genital pore just anterior to ventral sucker (Fig. 386).** ....Genus *Parorchis* **Nicoll, 1907**

Life cycle: *P. avitus—*

Miracidia hatch either before or soon after the eggs are laid. The miracidia already contain a mother redia. Echinostome-like cercariae develop in rediae in the marine molluscs, *Urosalpinx cinereus* and *Thais lapillus* and encyst in hemispherical cysts on vegetation. There is no second intermediate host needed for completion of the life cycle. The adult flukes develop in the cloaca of the common tern, *Sterna hirundo,* and the roseate tern, *S. dougalli,* which probably ingest the metacercariae. The cercariae resemble those of the echinostomes, having a spiny collar and the same type of excretory system (Stunkard and Cable, 1932).

Angel (1954) investigated the life cycle of *P. acanthus.* Cercariae of the megalura group (Fig. 45) develop in daughter rediae in the marine snail, *Nucella lapillus.* Cercariae penetrate mussels and cockles of the genera *Cardium* and *Mytilus* in which they probably encyst. The infected molluscs are eaten by gulls in which the mature trematode develops.

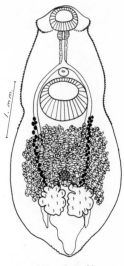

Fig. 386.   *Parorchis acanthus.*

2b. Spiny collar absent; testes oval; genital pore ventral to pharynx (Fig. 387). ....**Genus *Cloacitrema* Yamaguti, 1935**

Life cycle: *C. michiganense—*

Embryonated eggs hatch in the uterus of the adult fluke or shortly after oviposition. The miracidia penetrate the marine snail, *Cerithidea californica* in which megalurous cercariae (Fig. 45) develop in daughter rediae. After emergence from the snail, the cercariae encyst on snail shells and other solid objects. The mature fluke inhabits the cloaca of spotted sandpiper, black-necked stilt, western willet, and sea gull (Robinson, 1952).

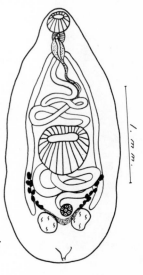

Fig. 387.   *Cloacitrema michiganense.*

3a. Vestigial spiny collar present around oral sucker; body spines large and dense; intestinal parasites of birds (Fig. 388). ....
....Genus *Echinostephilla* Lebour, 1909

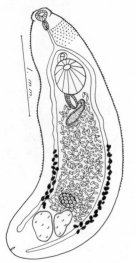

Fig. 388.   *Echinostephilla haematopi.*

3b. Body without a spiny collar; body spines of moderate size; parasites in the conjunctiva and beneath the nictitating membrane of birds (Fig. 389)..
....Genus *Philophthalmus* Looss, 1899

Two species have been reported as parasites in the human eye.

Life cycle: *P. gralli—*

Eggs are non-operculate and contain a miracidium when laid. The miracidium contains a mother redia. After hatching, the miracidium penetrates the epidermis of the freshwater operculate snails, *Pleurocera acuta* and *Goniobasis* spp., then releases the mother redia which migrates to the heart of the snail. Megalurous cercariae (Fig. 45) develop in daughter rediae and encyst in flask-shaped cyst (Fig. 48d) membranes on the exoskeleton of aquatic arthropods which are ingested by birds. The liberated metacercariae migrate

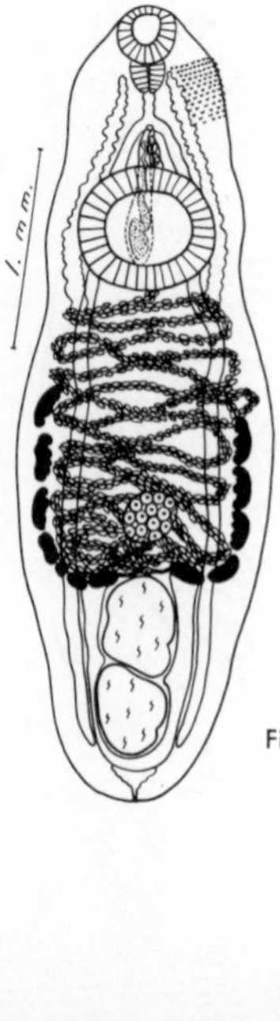

Fig. 389.   *Philophthalmus hegneri.*

from the mouth to the eye by way of the nasal cavities and naso-lacrimal ducts. The mature fluke develops beneath the nictitating membrane and around the upper end of the nasolacrimal duct (Ching, 1961; West, 1961).

Alicata (1962) found that eggs leave the definitive host by way of the mouth when the bird drinks water. He also observed that mother, daughter and granddaughter rediae are produced.

The life cycle of *P. hegneri* is similar to that of *P. gralli*. Mega-lurous cercariae develop in the marine snail, *Batillaria minima*, from the Gulf of Mexico. Experimental infections were estab-lished in chickens, pigeons, mute swan and western gull by ocular infection and by feeding metacercariae. Natural definitive hosts are royal tern, yellow-crowned night heron, laughing gull and willet (Penner and Fried, 1963).

FAMILY HAPLOSPLANCHNIDAE Poche, 1925

Body nonspinous, elongate; ventral sucker smaller than oral suck-er; one intestinal cecum; one testis; cirrus and cirrus sac absent; seminal vesicle long and sinuous, free in parenchyma; ovary an-terior to testis; seminal receptacle present; genital pore median, a short distance posterior to pharynx; vitelline follicles either few and antero-lateral to testis or abundant and distributed in lateral regions between level of pharynx and posterior end of body; uterine folds entirely anterior to ovary; excretory vesicle Y-shaped; intestinal parasites of marine fishes.

Only the genus *Schikhobalotrema* Skrjabin and Gus-chanskaja, 1955 is represented in North America (Fig. 390).

Life cycle: *S. acutum*—

Oculate cercariae with a single intestinal cecum and numerous finger-like lateral appendages on the tail (Fig. 31) develop in sporocysts in the marine snail, *Cerithium variabile*. The cercariae encyst on vegetation and solid objects in spherical cysts. The mature flukes develop in the intestine of halfbeaks, *Hyporhamphus unifasciatus*, and needlefish, *Strongy-lura* spp. (see Cable, 1954b).

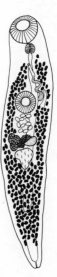

Fig. 390. *Schikhobalotrema kyphosi*. (Redrawn from Manter, 1947.)

FAMILY HAPLOPORIDAE Nicoll, 1914

Body small, spinous, pyriform, oval or elongate; suckers well developed, in anterior half of body, ventral sucker pedunculate in some genera; intestinal ceca usually half long, inflated in some genera; one or two testes, in posterior part of body; cirrus sac absent; hermaphroditic sac present, containing metraterm, internal seminal vesicle, genital sinus and prostate cells; external seminal vesicle also present; ovary pretesticular; genital pore median, anterior to ventral sucker; vitelline glands compact or follicular; uterus between ovary and genital pore or extending posterior to ovary in some genera; excretory vesicle saccular, I-shaped or Y-shaped; parasites of marine fishes.

KEY TO GENERA

1a. Ventral sucker pedunculate, retractile, with two pointed papillae; eggs have unipolar filament. 2
1b. Ventral sucker sessile, not retractile, papillae absent. 3
2a. Peduncle long; intestinal ceca united with excretory vesicle to form cloaca; one testis in posterior part of body; conspicuous dorso-ventral muscle bands in forebody (Fig. 391). ....Genus *Myodera* Montgomery, 1957
2b. Peduncle short; intestinal ceca end blindly; two unequal testes (one testis in immature forms); dorso-ventral muscle bands absent (Fig. 392). ....Genus *Scorpidicola* Montgomery, 1957

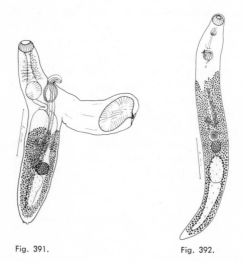

Fig. 391.   Fig. 392.

Fig. 391. *Myodera medialunae.* Fig. 392. *Scorpidicola californiensis.*

3a. Two testes; vitelline glands in form of thick dorso-ventral bands, one behind the other (Fig. 393). ....
....Genus *Vitellibaculum* Montgomery, 1957

3b. One testis; vitelline glands compact or follicular. 4

4a. Vitelline gland a single compact mass, dorsal to ovary and testis; intestinal ceca extend only to level of testis (Fig. 394). ....Genus *Dicrogaster* Looss, 1902

4b. Vitelline glands follicular. 5

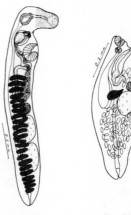

Fig. 393. *Vitellibaculum girella.* Fig. 394. *Dicrogaster fastigatus.*

Fig. 393.   Fig. 394.

5a. Vitelline follicles abundant, filling most of hindbody (Fig. 395). ....Genus *Hapladena* Linton, 1910

Key to species in Skrjabin (1964).

Life cycle: Cable (1962) described an oculate cercaria (*Cercaria caribbea* LII) having some echinostome-like anatomical features such as stenostomate excretory system, cystogenous glands, no penetration glands, no stylet, simple tail and spinous body. The cercariae develop in a redia in a marine snail, *Zebina browniana* and encyst on vegetation in thick ovoid cyst membranes. Experimental infections resulted in the production of very young adult specimens that bore some resemblance to *Hapladena varia.*

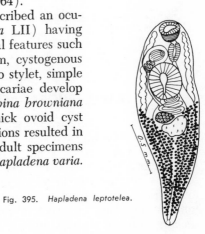

Fig. 395. *Hapladena leptotelea.*

5b. Vitelline follicles not as described above. 6
6a. Vitelline follicles in bilateral clusters, forming an H-shaped design at ends of ceca; eggs few and large (Fig. 396). ....
....Genus *Saccocoelium* Looss, 1902
6b. Vitelline follicles large, irregular in shape, distributed around testis and ends of ceca. 7
7a. Body pyriform; ceca half long; hermaphroditic sac nearly spherical, not extending posterior to ventral sucker (Fig. 397).
....Genus *Saccocoelioides* Szidat, 1954
7b. Body elongate or oval; ceca more than half long; hermaphroditic sac elongate, extending posterior to ventral sucker (Fig. 398). ....Genus *Carassotrema* Park, 1938

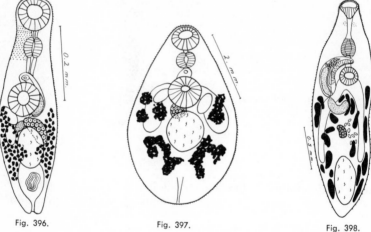

Fig. 396.   Fig. 397.   Fig. 398.

Fig. 396. *Saccocoelium beauforti.* Fig. 397. *Saccocoelioides sogandaresi.* Fig. 398. *Carassotrema mugilicola.*

FAMILY RHOPALIASIDAE Looss, 1899

Body oval to elongate, densely spinous; a retractile proboscis with large spines on each side of oral sucker; ventral sucker larger than oral sucker; ceca long; testes tandem, in middle third of body; cirrus sac very long, extending far posterior to ventral sucker; ovary anterior to testes; genital pore median and anterior to ventral sucker; uterus between ovary and genital pore; vitelline follicles abundant, filling lateral areas of body posterior to ventral sucker, confluent posterior to testes; intestinal parasites of opossum.

The family contains only the genus *Rhopalias* Stiles and Hassall, 1898 in which four species have been described. One species (Fig. 399) occurs in North America as a parasite of *Didelphis virginiana*. The trematodes in this family bear some resemblance to those of the families Echinostomatidae and Psilostomatidae. Key to species in Skrjabin (1964).

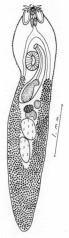

Fig. 399. *Rhopalias macracanthus.* (Redrawn from Chandler, 1932.)

SUPERFAMILY PARAMPHISTOMATOIDEA
Stiles and Goldberger, 1910

Miracidia have one pair of flame cells; cercariae of amphistome type with stenostomate excretory system, develop in rediae or in branched sporocysts (Heronimidae) in aquatic snails; life cycle involves two hosts; adults in digestive tract of vertebrates or in lungs of turtles.

FAMILY PARAMPHISTOMATIDAE Fischoeder, 1901

Body thick, muscular; ventral sucker large, located at posterior end of body; oral sucker usually treminal, containing one pair of diverticula in some genera; pharynx absent but esophagus has muscular bulb in some genera; intestinal ceca long, sometimes sinuous; testes tandem or oblique in middle third of body, smooth margins or lobed; ovary posterior to testes; vitelline follicles few or many, variable in distribution; uterus with ascending limb only, uterine folds entirely intercecal; in digestive tract of vertebrates.

KEY TO GENERA

1a. Oral sucker with a pair of pouch-like muscular diverticula (Fig. 400); primarily parasites of amphibians, reptiles and birds. 2

1b. Oral sucker without diverticula or with vestigial diverticula; parasites of fishes and mammals. 9

2a. Muscular esophageal bulb present (Fig. 400). 3
2b. Muscular esophageal bulb absent. 8
3a. Ventral sucker with a pair of muscular papillae on posterior margin; testes lobed; parasites in colon and cloaca of birds (Fig. 400). ....Genus *Zygocotyle* Stunkard, 1917

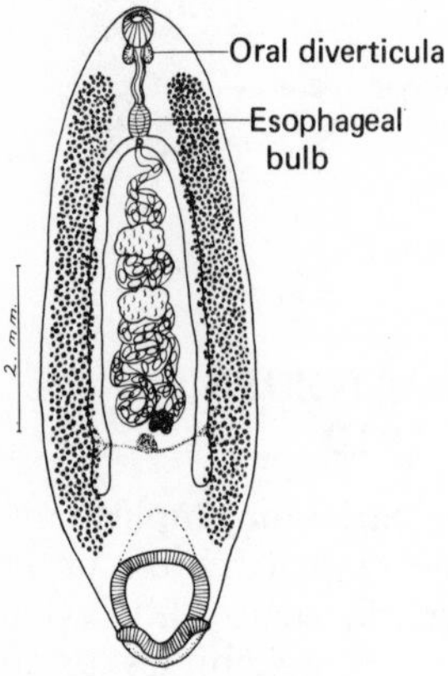

—Oral diverticula

—Esophageal bulb

2 m m

Fig. 400. *Zygocotyle lunata.*

Life cycle: *Z. lunata*—

Eggs passed in the feces of the host are in the one-celled stage. Twenty to 40 days are required for development of the miracidia which hatch and penetrate the fresh-water snail, *Helisoma antrosum.* Amphistome cercariae (= *Cercaria poconensis*) develop in rediae. Some rediae contain only cercariae while others contain both cercariae and daughter rediae. The cercariae leave the rediae while still immature and complete their development in the snail tissues. After emerging from the host snail they encyst on aquatic vegetation or any solid surface in brown, hemispherical membranes. Ducks probably serve as natural definitive host although geese, chickens and turkeys also harbor the parasite. Sexual maturity is attained in 41 to 44 days in the ceca and colon of ducks. Experimental infections were established in rats and sheep (Willey 1930, 1936, 1941).

3b. Ventral sucker without muscular papillae. 4

4a. Vitelline follicles few, located either ventral or medial to intestinal ceca; parasites of frogs, newts and snakes. 5

4b. Vitelline follicles abundant, located both medial and lateral to intestinal ceca; parasites of turtles. 7

5a. Ventral sucker twice as large as oral sucker; vitelline follicles medial to intestinal ceca; parasites of snakes (Fig. 401). ....
....Genus *Ophioxenos* Sumwalt, 1926

5b. Ventral sucker at least four times as large as oral sucker and having a navel-like papilla in center of sucker. 6

6a. Vitelline follicles entirely medial to posterior ends of ceca; parasites in colon of newts (Fig. 402). ....
.....................................Genus *Pseudopisthodiscus* Yamaguti, 1958
(= *Opisthodiscus* Holl, 1928)

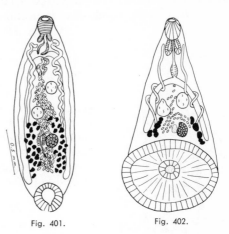

Fig. 401. *Ophioxenos dienteros.*
Fig. 402. *Pseudopisthodiscus americanus.* (Redrawn from Holl, 1928.)

Fig. 401.   Fig. 402.

6b. Vitelline follicles chiefly ventral to ceca; parasites in colon and cloaca of amphibians (Fig. 403). ....
....Genus *Megalodiscus* Chandler, 1923

Key to species in Skrjabin (1964).
Life cycle: *M. temperatus*—

Eggs are embryonated when laid. The miracidia hatch when eggs enter water and penetrate the freshwater snails of three species of *Helisoma* in which they metamorphose to sporocyst stage. Amphistome cercariae develop in daughter rediae and after leaving the snail, encyst on the darkly pigmented areas of skin of frogs and tadpoles. Frogs become infected when they eat pieces of molted epidermis or when eating tadpoles. The adult flukes inhabit the colon and cloaca of frogs. *Ferrissia fragilis* has also been reported as a possible host mollusc for the larval stages (Krull and Price, 1932; Herber, 1938, 1939; Smith, 1967).

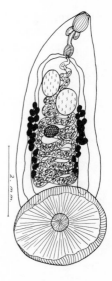

Fig. 403. *Megalodiscus temperatus.*

Macy (1960a) found the life cycle of *M. microphagus* to be similar to that of *M. temperatus* except for utilization of hosts. The host snails are *Menetus cooperi* and *Gyraulus* sp. The definitive hosts are *Hyla regilla, Rana aurora* and *Taricha granulosa.*

7a. **Vitelline follicles large; testes lobed, tandem; posterior end of body with corner-like projections (Fig. 404).** ....
....**Genus** *Allassostomoides* **Stunkard, 1925**

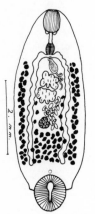

Life cycle: *A. parvum*—
The adult is a parasite in the colon, cloaca and urinary bladder of turtles. Amphistome cercariae (Fig. 33) develop in daughter rediae in *Helisoma trivolvis* and *H. antrosum.* Cercariae encyst on aquatic vegetation, crayfish and tadpoles. The definitive host becomes infected by ingesting these infected plants and animals (Beaver, 1929; Krull, 1933).

Fig. 404. *Allassostomoides chelydrae.*

7b. **Vitelline follicles small; testes oblique, small, oval or round; posterior end of body without corner-like projections (Fig. 405).**
....**Genus** *Allassostoma* **Stunkard, 1917**
8a. **Arms of excretory vesicle united dorsal to esophagus; vitelline follicles present only along posterior ends of intestinal ceca; parasites of freshwater and marine fishes (Fig. 406).** ....
....**Genus** *Cleptodiscus* **Linton, 1910**

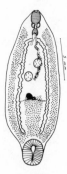

Fig. 405. *Allassostoma magnum.* Fig. 406. *Cleptodiscus reticulatus.*

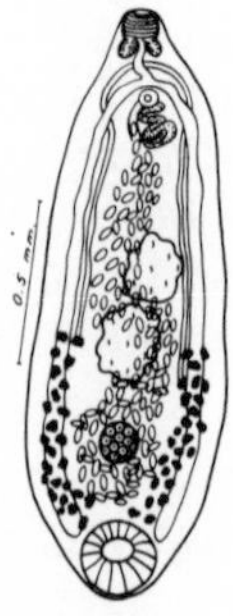

Fig. 405.   Fig. 406.

8b. Arms of excretory vesicle not united dorsal to esophagus; vitelline follicles distributed along full length of ceca; parasites in cecum and colon of muskrat (Fig. 407). ....
................................**Genus** *Wardius* **Barker and East, 1915**

Life cycle: *W. zibethicus*—

Amphistome cercariae develop in rediae in the freshwater snail, *Helisoma antrosum* and encyst on aquatic vegetation. When encysted metacercariae were fed to mice, hamsters, deer mouse and guinea pig, immature trematodes were recovered. It was thought that insufficient time had elapsed for complete development. The natural definitive host is the muskrat (Murrell, 1963, 1965).

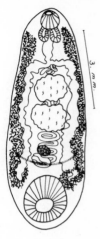

Fig. 407. *Wardius zibethicus.*

9a. Testes dendritic, tandem; oral sucker with vestigial divertticula; vitelline follicles restricted to area around posterior half of intestinal ceca; parasites in cecum and colon of beaver (Fig. 408). ....**Genus** *Stichorchis* **(Fischoeder, 1901)**

Life cycle: *S. subtriquetrus*—

Approximately three weeks are required for development of the miracidium which already contains a mother redia. The miracidium penetrates the freshwater snail, *Fossaria parva* and liberates the mother redia in the mantle cavity. The mother redia produces a generation of daughter rediae in which amphistome cercariae develop. After leaving the snail, the cercariae encyst on vegetation which is eventually eaten by the beaver, the natural definitive host (Bennett and Humes, 1939).

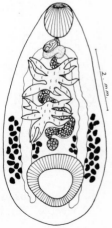

Fig. 408. *Stichorchis subtriquetrus.*

9b. Testes lobed or round, tandem or oblique; oral sucker without diverticula; vitelline follicles distributed along full length of intestinal ceca. **10**

10a. Muscular genital sucker enclosing genital pore (Fig. 409). .....
.................Genus *Cotylophoron* Stiles and Goldberger, 1910

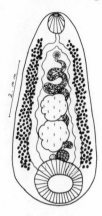

Life cycle: *C. cotylophorum*—

After eggs are laid, 11 to 29 days are required for development of the miracidium which hatches when eggs are placed in water. They penetrate the freshwater snails, *Fossaria parva* and *F. modicella* in which a sporocyst and a redial generation are produced. In one instance, two redial generations were observed. The rediae produce amphistome cercariae which encyst on vegetation which in turn is eaten by ruminant mammals. Five to eight months are required for completion of the entire life cycle. The mature trematode develops in the rumen of the host (many authors).

Fig. 409. *Cotylophoron cotylophorum*.

10b. Muscular genital sucker absent. **11**

11a. Esophagus with muscular bulb; testes round; intestinal parasites of fishes (Fig. 410). ....
.... Genus *Pisciamphistoma* Yamaguti, 1954

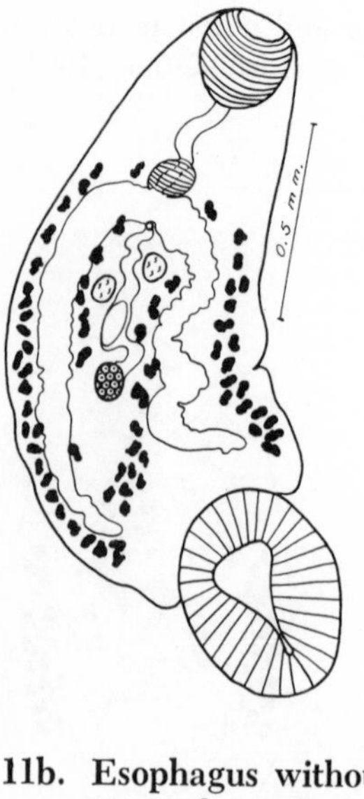

Fig. 410. *Pisciamphistoma stunkardi.*

11b. Esophagus without muscular bulb; testes lobed; in digestive tract of ruminant mammals (Fig. 411). ....
.................................Genus *Paramphistomum* Fischoeder, 1901

Life cycle: *P. cervi*—

The life cycle involves a generation of sporocysts, followed by mother and daughter rediae which develop in aquatic snails of the Genera *Physa, Bulinus, Galba* and *Pseudosuccinea*. The daughter rediae produce amphistome cercariae (= *Cercaria pigmentata*) which encyst on vegetation in hemispherical cyst membranes. Mammals such as sheep, goats and cattle ingest the encysted metacercariae with their forage. The metacercariae excyst in the duodenum then pass forward to the rumen where they develop to sexual maturity.

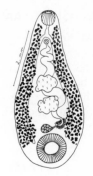

Fig. 411. *Paramphistomum cervi.*

FAMILY HERONIMIDAE Ward, 1917

Body elongate; ventral sucker absent; intestinal ceca long; testes tubular, 2/3 as long as body; cirrus sac absent; genital pore ventral to oral sucker; ovary ovoid, near anterior end of body; vitelline glands tubular, 3/4 as long as body; uterus with doubled descending and ascending limbs; excretory vesicle Y-shaped but inverted with the excretory pore dorsal to pharynx; parasites in lungs of turtle.

The family contains a single genus and species, *Heronimus chelydrae*, (Fig. 412) the life cycle of which was described by Crandall (1960) and by Ulmer (1960). The miracidia hatch while eggs are still in the uterus and penetrate the aquatic snails, *Physa gyrina, P. integra,* and *P. sayii,* in which amphistome-like cercariae develop in branched sporocysts. The cercariae remain in the sporocysts but do not encyst. Turtles become infected by eating infected snails. In the turtle the larvae migrate to the lungs by way of the esophagus, larynx and trachea. As the trematodes develop to the adult stage, the body expands ventrally and the ventral sucker disappears. This results in having the excretory pore on the dorsal surface at the anterior end of the body. Three months are required for development to sexual maturity in the turtle. The amphistome-like cercaria indicates relationship to trematodes of the family Paramphistomatidae.

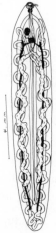

Fig. 412. *Heronimus chelydrae.*

SUPERFAMILY NOTOCOTYLOIDEA Larue, 1957

Miracidia have one pair of flame cell; cercariae of monostome type with stenostomate excretory system, having the main ducts fused in anterior part of body; adhesive glands at posterior end of body; develop in rediae in aquatic snails; two hosts involved in life cycle; ventral sucker and pharynx absent in cercariae, metacercariae and adults; eggs have bipolar filaments; parasites in intestine or urinary bladder of vertebrates.

FAMILY NOTOCOTYLIDAE Lühe, 1909

Body flat, either oval or elongate usually having longitudinal rows of glands on ventral body surface; ventral sucker and pharynx absent; intestinal ceca long; testes opposite, near posterior end of body; cirrus sac long; ovary median, between testes; vitelline follicles in lateral clusters, mostly anterior to testes; uterus consisting of many transverse folds which fill most of intercecal area between ovary and genital pore; eggs have long bipolar filaments; parasites in small intestine, colon and ceca of birds and mammals.

KEY TO GENERA

Note: Transverse sections through midbody region are useful for observation of ventral glands (Fig. 413).

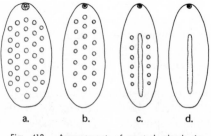

Fig. 413. Arrangement of ventral glands in Family Notocotylidae (a. *Quinqueserialis*, b. *Notocotylus*, c. *Catatropis*, d. *Hofmonostomum*).

Keys to species in Harwood (1939) and Skrjabin (1964).

1a. Vitelline follicles located anterior and lateral to testes; parasites of birds (Fig. 414). ....
....**Genus** *Hofmonostomum* **Harwood, 1939**

1b. Vitelline follicles entirely anterior to testes. 2

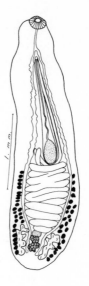

Fig. 414. *Hofmonostomum himantopodis.*
(Redrawn from Harwood, 1939.)

2a. Genital pore and cirrus sac in posterior part of body, posterior to uterus; parasites of mammals (Fig. 415). ....
....Genus *Nudacotyle* **Barker, 1916**

Life cycle: *N. novicia—*
Embryonated eggs in the feces of the host are ingested by the operculate snail, *Pomatiopsis lapidaria,* in which a sporocyst and two redial generations develop. Monostome cercariae (Fig. 32) with three pigmented eyespots develop in daughter rediae and after leaving the snail, encyst in hemispherical cyst membranes (Fig. 48c) on aquatic vegetation. The adult trematode develops in the bile duct of meadow mouse, *Microtus pennsylvanicus,* or in the small intestine of muskrat, *Ondatra zibethicus.* The metacercariae are ingested along with the aquatic vegetation (Ameel, 1944).

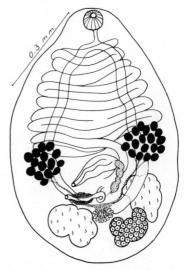

Fig. 415. *Nudacotyle novicia.*

2b. Genital pore and cirrus sac in anterior half of body, anterior
     to uterus. 3

3a. Body without ventral glands; parasites of birds and mammals
     (Fig. 416). ....Genus *Paramonostomum* Lühe, 1909

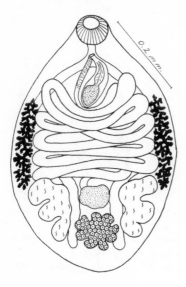

Fig. 416.   *Paramonostomum alveatum.*

3b. Body with three to five rows of ventral glands. 4

4a. Body with five rows of ventral glands (Fig. 417); parasites
     of mammals. ....Genus *Quinqueserialis* Skwortzow, 1935

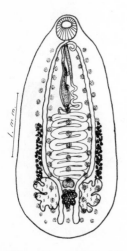

Fig. 417.   *Quinqueserialis
quinqueserialis.*

Life cycle: *Q. quinqueserialis*—

Embryonated eggs, passed in the feces of the host, are eaten by the freshwater snail, *Gyraulus parvus*. Miracidia hatch in the digestive tract of the snail and, after penetrating the intestinal wall, transform to a sporocyst. Mother and daughter rediae are produced, the latter finally giving rise to monostome cercariae (Fig. 32) which are released from the daughter redia before they are fully developed and complete their development in the tissues of the snail. Emerging cercariae encyst on vegetation in hemispherical cyst membranes. The trematode develops to sexual maturity in the cecum of muskrat, meadow mouse and jumping mouse in about 14 days after cysts are ingested (Herber, 1942).

4b. Body with three longitudinal rows of separate ventral glands or two lateral rows and a median ridge; parasites of birds and mammals. 5

5a. Body with three rows of separate ventral glands (Fig. 418). ....Genus *Notocotylus* **Diesing, 1839**

Life cycle: *N. stagnicolae—*

Embryonated eggs are eaten by the aquatic snail, *Stagnicola emarginata angulata,* in which miracidia hatch and metamorphose to the mother sporocyst after penetrating the wall of the digestive tract. Each sporocyst produces one mother redia which in turn produces a generation of daughter rediae. The latter produce monostome cercariae (Fig. 32) which after escaping from the snail encyst on vegetation in hemispherical cyst membranes. The adult fluke develops in several species of ducks and also in chickens (Herber, 1942).

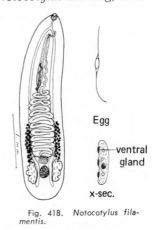

Egg

ventral gland

x-sec.

Fig. 418.   *Notocotylus filamentis.*

5b. Body with a median glandular ridge plus a row of separate glands on each side of the ridge (Figs. 413c and 419). ....Genus *Catatropis* **Odhner, 1905**

Life cycle: *C. johnstoni—*

Monostome cercariae (Fig. 32) develop in rediae in the marine snail, *Cerithidea californica* and encyst on vegetation. Metacercariae, fed to baby chicks, develop to maturity in nine to thirteen days (Martin 1956).

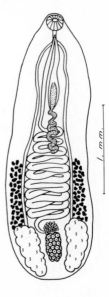

Fig. 419.   *Catatropis harwoodi.*

FAMILY PRONOCEPHALIDAE Looss, 1902

Body nonspinous, elongate with parallel sides and unarmed triangular head collar usually present around oral sucker; ventral sucker absent; intestinal ceca long, sometimes sinuous with lateral diverticula in some genera; testes two or follicular, near posterior end of body; cirrus sac present; external seminal vesicle present; ovary anterior to testes; genital pore to left of median line, in anterior third of body; vitelline follicles in lateral clusters, along ceca, anterior to testes; uterus long, numerous transverse folds between ovary and genital pore; eggs have polar filaments in some genera; excretory vesicle V- or Y-shaped with arms united in region of esophagus and having anastomosing branches throughout body; in intestine or urinary bladder of turtles.

KEY TO GENERA

1a. **Parasites of freshwater turtles; intestinal ceca straight, without diverticula; vestibular cavity at posterior end of body; eggs have bipolar filaments; cirrus sac large; folds of uterus entirely intercecal; vitelline follicles in grape-like clusters median to ceca (Fig. 420).** ....Genus *Macravestibulum* **Mackin, 1930**

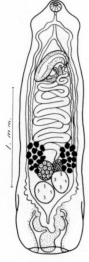

Life cycle: *M. eversum*—

Snails were not infected experimentally but it was assumed that embryonated eggs are ingested by the operculate snail, *Goniobasis livescens,* in which oculate monostomate cercariae develop in daughter rediae in the gills of the snail. The cercaria has a triangular head collar like that of the adult fluke. The cercariae encyst on the operculum of the snail. Turtles acquire the parasite by eating infected snails (Hsü 1937).

The life cycle of *M. obtusicaudum* is similar to that of *M. eversum* (see Horsfall, 1935).

Fig. 420.   *Macravestibulum obtusicaudum.*

1b. Vestibular cavity absent; intestinal ceca straight or sinuous, cecal diverticula present in some genera. 2

2a. Intestinal ceca straight with numerous short diverticula; head collar weakly developed or absent. 3

2b. Intestinal ceca sinuous, with or without diverticula; head collar well developed. 4

3a. Head collar weakly developed; two testes, opposite; metraterm as long as cirrus sac; esophagus long, about 1/4 as long as body (Fig. 421). ....Genus *Pleurogonius* Looss, 1901

3b. Head collar absent; testes follicular, the follicles arranged in a U-shaped group in posterior third of body; metraterm shorter than cirrus sac; esophagus very short, about 1/10 as long as body (Fig. 422). ....
....Genus *Diaschistorchis* Johnston, 1913

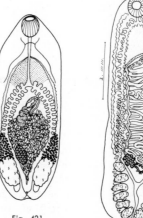

Fig. 421. *Pleurogonius malaclemmys.* Fig. 422. *Diaschistorchis ellipticus.* (Redrawn from Pratt, 1914.)

Fig. 421.

Fig. 422.

4a. Body large (15 to 20 mm.); Intestinal ceca without diverticula; vitelline follicles abundant, distributed along ceca and extending into anterior half of body (Fig. 423). ....
....Genus *Astrorchis* Poche, 1925

4b. Body moderately large (6 to 9 mm.); intestinal ceca with short diverticula or none; vitelline follicles in lateral clusters in posterior half of body, anterior to testes (Fig. 424). ....
....Genus *Pyelosomum* Looss, 1899

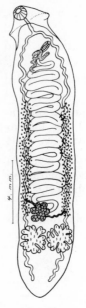

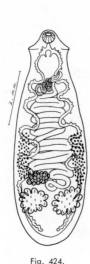

Fig. 423.   Astrorchis renicapite.
Fig. 424.   Pyelosomum longicaecum.

Fig. 424.

Fig. 423.

FAMILY MICROSCAPHIDIIDAE Travassos, 1922

Body elongate, nonspinous, ventral surface of body concave; ventral sucker absent; oral sucker large with triangular projections; pharynx absent but a muscular swelling is sometimes present at posterior end of esophagus; ceca long and sinuous; testes tandem, lobed or ovoid; cirrus sac absent; genital pore median, near intestinal bifurcation; ovary posterior to testes; seminal receptacle absent; vitelline follicles lateral to ceca; uterus looping between ovary and genital pore; excretory vesicle I-shaped or sac-shaped and also having a network of tubules; parasites in the large intestine of turtles.

Only the genus *Dictyangium* Stunkard, 1943 is known to occur in North America. The genus contains one species, *D. chelydrae* (Fig. 425); a parasite of the snapping turtle, *Chelydra serpentina*.

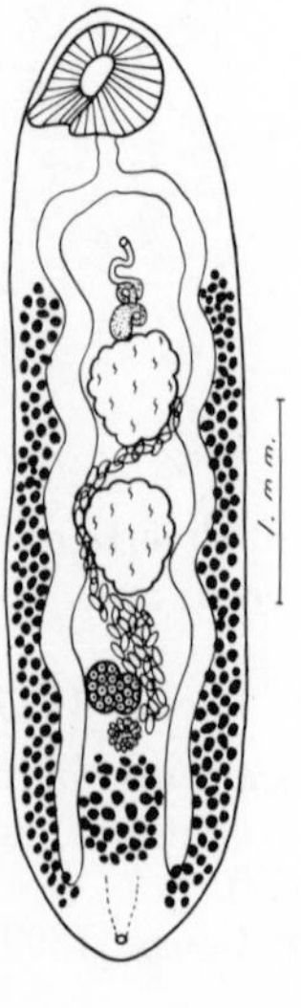

Fig. 425.   Dictyangium chelydrae

ORDER PLAGIORCHIIDA Larue, 1957
SUPERFAMILY PLAGIORCHIOIDEA Dollfus, 1930

Miracidia have one pair of flame cells; produce xiphidiocercariae (stylet) of the armatae, ubiquita, ornatae, virgulate, microcercous or tailless type, having mesostomate excretory system, develop in daughter sporocysts in aquatic or terrestrial snails; two or three hosts involved in life cycle; parasites in intestine, liver, lungs, ureters, esophagus, bursa Fabricii or cloaca of vertebrates.

FAMILY PLAGIORCHIIDAE Lühe, 1901,
emended Ward, 1917

Body spinous, oval, fusiform or elongate; suckers well developed, located in anterior half of body; intestinal ceca extending at least 2/3 of way through body; testes oblique or opposite, rarely tandem; cirrus sac present, usually dorsal to ventral sucker, sometimes extending posterior to ventral sucker; ovary anterior to testes; genital pore median or submedian, anterior to ventral sucker; vitelline follicles variable in number and distribution; uterus long, extending posterior to testes in most genera; eggs embryonated when laid; excretory vesicle Y-shaped; parasites in intestine, gall bladder, ureters or cloaca of all classes of vertebrates.

KEY TO GENERA

1a. Testes opposite. 2

1b. Testes oblique or tandem. 6

2a. Vitelline follicles in lateral clusters entirely anterior to level of ventral sucker; arms of excretory vesicle long, extending anterior to level of pharynx; in mouth and esophagus of snakes (Fig. 426). ....Genus *Stomatrema* Guberlet, 1928

2b. Vitelline follicles in lateral clusters anterior and posterior or only posterior to ventral sucker. 3

3a. Excretory vesicle Y-shaped with stem of the Y long and sinuous and having one pair of lateral diverticula near the posterior end, arms of Y embrace ventral sucker; parasites of turtles (Fig. 427). ....Genus *Styphlotrema* Odhner, 1911

3b. Excretory vesicle not as described above; parasites of newts and snakes or fishes. 4

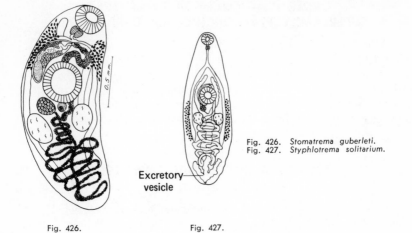

Fig. 426.   Stomatrema guberleti.
Fig. 427.   Styphlotrema solitarium.

Excretory
vesicle

Fig. 426.   Fig. 427.

4a. Metraterm well developed, surrounded by gland cells; vi-
     telline follicles few, in lateral clusters in region of ovary and
     testes; ventral sucker much larger than oral sucker; cirrus sac
     entirely anterior to ventral sucker; ovary close to testes (Fig.
     428); parasites of snakes. .... Genus *Leptophyllum* Cohn, 1902

4b. Metraterm not unusually prominent; vitelline follicles abun-
     dant, distributed anterior and posterior to ventral sucker;
     suckers nearly equal or ventral smaller than oral sucker. 5

5a. Testes median to intestinal ceca; ovary lobed; body broadly
     oval; intestinal parasites of freshwater fishes (Fig. 429). ....
     .... Genus *Vietosoma* Van Cleave and Mueller, 1932

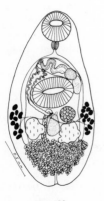 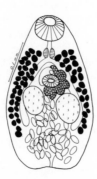

Fig. 428.   Leptophyllum tamia-
miense.   Fig. 429.   Vietosoma
parvum.   (Redrawn from Van-
Cleave and Mueller, 1932.)

Fig. 428.   Fig. 429.

5b. Testes posterior to ends of ceca; ovary oval; body elliptical; intestinal parasites of amphibians (Fig. 430). ....
....**Genus** *Plagitura* **Holl, 1928**

Some attempt has been made to make *Plagitura* a synonym of *Manodistomum* Stafford, 1905 but this synonymy is not observed here because of the uncertain status of the type and only species, *M. occultum,* which was described from immature specimens.

Life cycle: *P. parva*—

Eggs which contain miracidia when laid, are eaten by the planorbid snail, *Helisoma antrosa* in which xiphidiocercariae of the armatae group develop in daughter sporocysts. The cercariae encyst in Dobsonfly larvae (*Corydalis* sp.) and in the snails, *Physa heterostropha, Pseudosuccinea columella, Lymnaea stagnalis* and *Campeloma* sp. The definitive host is the newt, *Triturus viridescens* (Stunkard, 1936).

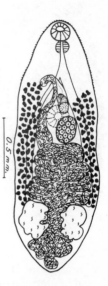

Fig. 430. *Plagitura parva.* (Redrawn from Stunkard, 1936.)

The life cycle of *P. salamandra* was studied by Owens (1946) who found that miracidia develop within one week after oviposition. The embryonated eggs are eaten by the snail, *Pseudosuccinea columella* in which xiphidiocercariae, with a finfold on the tail, develop in daughter sporocysts. They encyst in dragonfly nymphs, diving beetles and several species of snails. The newt, *Triturus viridescens* is definitive host.

6a. Testes tandem, near posterior end of body. 7

6b. Testes oblique, separated from posterior end of body by some distance. 8

7a. Parasites of mammals (shrews); body broadly oval; uterus not extending posterior to testes; vitelline follicles abundant, distributed in lateral zones from level of esophagus to posterior end of body (Fig. 431). ....
...............**Genus** *Neoglyphe* **(Shaldybin, 1954) Yamaguti, 1958**

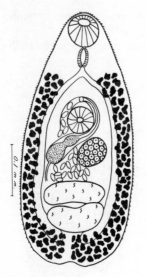

Life cycle: *N. locellus—*

Xiphidiocercariae of the armatae group develop in sporocysts in the freshwater snail, *Lymnaea bulimoides.* Cercariae either encyst in the sporocyst or emerge and encyst in water beetles, caddisfly larvae or in mayfly nymphs. Experimental infections with the adult fluke were established in hamsters. Natural infections are known to occur in shrews which probably ingest infected insects or snails (Macy and Moore, 1958).

Fig. 431. *Neoglyphe locellus.*

7b. **Parasites of freshwater fishes (catfish); body fusiform or elongate; uterus extends posterior to testes; vitelline follicles few, distributed in lateral rows between level of ventral sucker and testes (Fig. 432).** ....Genus *Parastiotrema* **Miller, 1940**

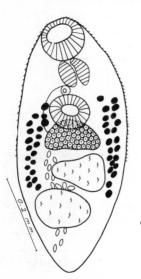

Fig. 432. *Parastiotrema ottawanense.* (Redrawn from Miller, 1940.)

8a. Oral sucker with one pair of lateral muscular papillae and twice as large as ventral sucker; excretory vesicle opens through funnel-shaped muscular chamber; intestinal parasites of turtles (Fig. 433). .... Genus *Eustomos* MacCallum, 1921

Life cycle: *E. chelydrae*—

Xiphidiocercariae of the armatae group develop in sporocysts in the freshwater snails, *Helisoma antrosa, Lymnaea stagnalis, Stagnicola emarginata angulata* and *Bulimoides megasoma*. The cercariae encyst in the branchial basket of dragonly nymphs and in the snails, *Helisoma trivolvis, H. antrosa, Lymnaea traskii* and *Pseudosuccinea columella*. Definitive hosts are the snapping turtle, *Chelydra serpentina*, and the painted turtle *Chrysemys picta*, six to ten weeks being required for development to sexual maturity after feeding metacercariae (Krull, 1934d, 1937; McMullen, 1935a).

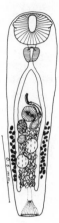

Fig. 433. *Eustomos chelydrae.*

8b. Oral sucker without muscular papillae; muscular excretory chamber absent. 9

9a. Intestinal parasites of vertebrates other than fishes; ovary immediately posterior to ventral sucker; testes located only a short distance from posterior end of body; excretory vesicle small, Y-shaped (Fig. 434). .... Genus *Plagiorchis* Lühe, 1899

Key to species in Olsen (1937a).

Life cycle: *P. muris*—

Embryonated eggs are ingested by the lymnaeid snail, *Stagnicola emarginata angulata* in which xiphidiocercariae of the armatae group develop in daughter sporocysts. Some cercariae encyst in the sporocyst and develop to infective metacercariae but most of the cercariae leave the sporocyst and the snail and encyst in dipterous larvae of the family Chironomidae. Natural definitive hosts are rat, dog, night hawk, robin, herring gull and spotted sandpiper. Experimental infections were established in mice, rats, pigeons and human beings (McMullen, 1937).

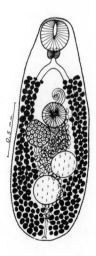

Fig. 434. *Plagiorchis proximus.*

Macy (1960b) published an account of the life cycle of *P. vespertilionis parorchis*. Larval stages develop in *Lymnaea stagnalis* which ingests embryonated eggs. The cercariae encyst in larvae of mosquitoes, caddisflies, mayflies and dragonflies. Bats serve as the natural definitive host. Experimental infections were established in white mice.

Najarian (1961) described the life cycle of *P. goodmani*.

9b. **Parasites in the gall bladder, kidneys or ureters of snakes; excretory vesicle not as described above; testes widely separated from posterior end of body by fold of uterus.** 10

10a. **Stem of excretory vesicle with numerous lateral diverticula; ovary immediately posterior to ventral sucker; testes in anterior half of body (Fig. 435).** ....
....**Genus *Styphlodora* Looss, 1899**
Key to species in Dawes (1942) and Skrjabin (1964).

10b. **Excretory vesicle voluminous, extending forward as far as ovary; ovary some distance posterior to ventral sucker; many folds of uterus between ovary and ventral sucker; testes in posterior half of body (Fig. 436).** ....
....**Genus *Allopharynx* Strom, 1928**
Key to species in Skrjabin (1964).

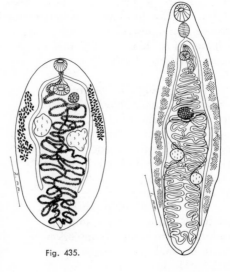

Fig. 435.

Fig. 436.

Fig. 435. *Styphlodora magna.* Fig. 436. *Allo-pharynx multispinosa.* (Redrawn from Bennett, 1935.)

FAMILY OCHETOSOMATIDAE Leão, 1944

Body spinous, oval, linguiform or elongate; suckers well developed; intestinal ceca variable in length, extending at least to midbody region; testes opposite or oblique; cirrus sac well developed; genital pore anterior to ventral sucker, median, sublateral, or lateral; ovary pretesticular; seminal receptacle absent; uterus with descending and ascending limbs and usually extending posterior to testes; eggs abundant, embryonated when laid; vitelline follicles variable in extent, usually lateral to ceca; excretory vesicle Y-shaped with the arms of the Y encircling ventral sucker; parasites in respiratory and upper digestive tract of snakes.

KEY TO GENERA

1a. **Genital pore lateral or sublateral (Fig. 437).** ....
....**Genus** *Ochetosoma* **Braun, 1901**

Life cycle: *O. aniarum* (= *Renifer aniarum*)—
Eggs passed in the feces of the host contain miracidia which hatch after the eggs are ingested by the aquatic snail, *Physa helei*. Xiphidiocercariae of the armatae group develop in daughter sporocysts. After leaving the snail, the cercariae penetrate and encyst in tadpoles of the Genera *Rana*, *Hyla* and *Pseudacris*. Infected tadpoles are eaten by snakes of the Genus *Natrix*. Mature trematodes were recovered from the mouth and esophagus 35 days after metacercariae were fed (Byrd, 1935; Walker, 1937, 1939).

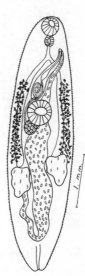

Fig. 437. *Ochetosoma ophiboli.*

1b. **Genital pore median.** 2
2a. **Ovary some distance posterior to ventral sucker; vitelline follicles few, in lateral areas posterior to level of ovary; body elongate (Fig. 438).** ....**Genus** *Natriodera* **Mehra, 1937**
2b. **Ovary immediately posterior to ventral sucker; some vitelline follicles anterior to level of ovary; body oval or slightly elongate.** 3

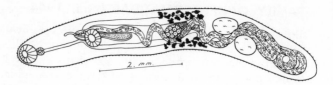

Fig. 438. *Natriodera verlata.*

3a. Ascending limb of uterus greatly inflated when gravid. 4
3b. Uterus with numerous transverse folds, ascending limb not inflated when gravid. 6

4a. Testes opposite, close to posterior end of body (Fig. 439). ....
...................Genus *Zeugorchis* Stafford, 1905

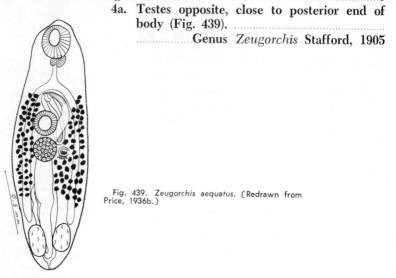

Fig. 439. *Zeugorchis aequatus.* (Redrawn from Price, 1936b.)

4b. Testes opposite or oblique, some distance from posterior end of body. 5
5a. Vitelline follicles in narrow bands, lateral to ceca which tend to pass between testes (Fig. 440). ....
....Genus *Lechriorchis* Stafford, 1905

Key to species in Byrd and Denton (1938) and in Skrjabin (1964). Life cycle: *L. primus—*

The adult trematodes inhabit the lungs of snakes of the Genus *Thamnophis.* Embryonated eggs that pass forward to the trachea are swallowed and leave the body in the feces. Eggs are eaten by several species of snails of the Genus *Physa* in which the miracidia hatch, penetrate the wall of the intestine and then metamorphose to the mother sporocyst stage. Xiphidiocercariae develop in daughter sporocysts and, after leaving the host snail,

penetrate the skin of tadpoles and frogs and encyst in the subcutaneous connective tissue. Snakes become infected by eating infected tadpoles and frogs (Talbot, 1933).

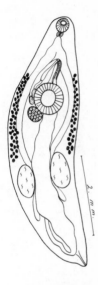

Fig. 440. *Lechriorchis primus.*

**5b. Vitelline follicles both lateral and medial to ceca which pass
      lateral to testes (Fig. 441).** .... **Genus** *Dasymetra* **Nicoll, 1911**

Key to species in Byrd and Denton (1938).
Byrd (1935) investigated the life cycle of
D. villicaeca and found it to be identical to
that of *Ochetosoma aniarum.*

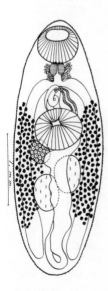

Fig. 441. *Dasymetra conferta.*

6a. Body pyriform, widest at level of testes; metraterm about two-thirds as long as cirrus sac (Fig. 442). ....
....Genus *Pneumatophilus* **Odhner, 1911**

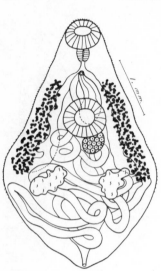

Key to species in Byrd and Denton (1938) and Skrjabin (1964).

Life cycle: *P. leidyi*—

The mature trematode inhabits the trachea of the island water snake, *Natrix sipedon insularum.* Embryonated eggs, in the feces of the host, are eaten by the aquatic snail, *Physa sayii* in which xiphidiocercariae of the armatae group (Fig. 38) develop in daughter sporocysts. The cercariae encyst in the subcutaneous connective tissue of tadpoles of the Genus *Rana,* in mudpuppies, *Necturus maculosus,* in cricket frogs, *Acris crepitans* and in the catfish, *Schilbeodes miurus.* Snakes become infected by eating the metacercariae in these hosts (Norris, 1945).

Fig. 442.   *Pneumatophilus leidyi.*

6b. Body linguiform; metraterm as long as cirrus sac (Fig. 443).
..........................Genus *Paralechriorchis* **Byrd and Denton, 1938**

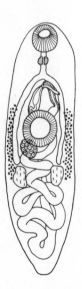

Key to species in Byrd and Denton (1938).

Life cycle: *P. syntomentera* (= *Zeugorchis syntomentera*)—

The adult trematode develops in the lungs and oro-nasal cavities of snakes. Embryonated eggs, passed by the host, are eaten by the freshwater snail, *Physa gyrina.* Xiphidiocercariae develop in what are probably daughter sporocysts. After leaving the snail, the cercariae penetrate the skin of tadpoles of *Hyla regilla, Rana aurora* and *Triturus torosus* in which they encyst. The definitive host ingests the infected tadpoles (Ingles, 1933).

Fig. 443.   *Paralechriorchis syntomentera.*

FAMILY PACHYPSOLIDAE Yamaguti, 1958

Body thick, oval, spinous anteriorly; suckers large, in anterior half of body; pharynx present; intestinal ceca long with diverticula in forebody region; two opposite testes; ovary pretesticular; cirrus sac present; genital pore submedian, anterior to ventral sucker; vitelline follicles small, arranged in stellate groups in middle third of body; most of uterus posterior to testes; excretory vesicle Y-shaped, the arms of the Y having diverticula and united dorsal to oral sucker; intestinal parasites of sea turtles.

The family contains only the Genus *Pachypsolus* Looss, 1901. One species, *P. ovalis* Linton, 1910 (= *P. tertius* Pratt, 1914) is known to occur in North America (Fig. 444).

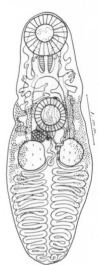

Fig. 444. *Pachypsolus tertius*. (Redrawn from Pratt, 1914.)

FAMILY TELORCHIIDAE Stunkard, 1924

Body elongate, spinous; ventral sucker smaller than oral sucker; intestinal ceca long; one or both testes near posterior end of body (testes widely separated in *Orchidasma*); cirrus sac long; genital pore median or submedian, ventral or dorsal; ovary pretesticular, usually widely separated from testes by uterine folds; uterus fills intercecal space between ovary and testes; eggs embryonated; vitelline follicles in narrow lateral bands; excretory vesicle Y-shaped with the stem of the Y long; intestinal parasites of amphibians and reptiles.

KEY TO GENERA

1a. Testes widely separated by uterine folds; parasites of marine turtles (Fig. 445). ....Genus *Orchidasma* Looss, 1900
1b. Both testes near posterior end of body. 2
2a. Cirrus sac entirely anterior to ventral sucker; genital pore dorsal, near left body margin; parasites of freshwater turtles (Fig. 446). ....Genus *Protenes* Barker and Covey, 1912
    Key to species in Bennett (1935).

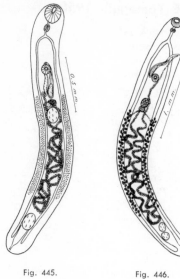

Fig. 445. *Orchidasma amphiorchis.*
Fig. 446. *Protenes angustus.*

Fig. 445.   Fig. 446.

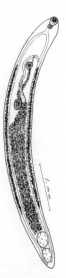

2b. Cirrus sac extending some distance posterior to ventral sucker; genital pore ventral, median; in intestine of amphibians and reptiles (Fig. 447).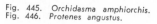
.................Genus *Telorchis* Lühe, 1899

Fig. 447. *Telorchis bonnerensis.*

Key to species in Wharton (1940).
Life cycle: *T. medius*—

Embryonated eggs from the feces of turtles are eaten by the freshwater snail, *Physa integra*. Xiphidiocercariae develop in daughter sporocysts and after leaving the snail, penetrate tadpoles in which they encyst. Turtles acquire the parasite by eating infected tadpoles (McMullen, 1934).

Schell (1962) investigated the life cycle of *T. bonnerensis*. Embryonated eggs are eaten by the physid snails, *Physa gyrina*, *P. ampullacea* and *P. propinqua*, in which the miracidia hatch. Mother and daughter sporocysts develop in the hemocoel of the snail. The daughter sporocysts produce xiphidiocercariae of the armatae group (Fig. 38). After leaving the snail, the cercariae encyst in other snails, fingernail clams, and in the tadpoles of frogs and salamanders. The adult fluke develops in tadpoles of the long-toed salamander, *Ambystoma macrodactylum*, which eat the infected intermediate hosts. Adult salamanders do not harbor the mature fluke.

FAMILY MACRODEROIDIDAE McMullen, 1937

Body spinous, elongate, oval or fusiform; ventral sucker smaller than oral sucker; ceca long; testes tandem, oblique or more rarely opposite and usually in midbody region; cirrus sac present; ovary pretesticular; genital pore median, immediately anterior to ventral sucker; uterus passing between testes to posterior end of body; vitelline follicles variable in number and distribution; excretory vesicle I-shaped; parasites in digestive tract of fishes and amphibians.

KEY TO GENERA

1a. Testes tandem to slightly oblique. 2
1b. Testes opposite to slightly oblique. 5
2a. Vitelline follicles distributed in fore- and hindbody; intestinal parasites of freshwater fishes (Fig. 448). ....
....Genus *Alloglossidium* Simer, 1929

Life cycle: *A. corti*—

Xiphidiocercariae develop in daughter sporocysts in the planorbid snails, *Helisoma trivolvis* and *H. campanulatum*. Cercariae encyst in the muscles and fatbody of mayfly and dragonfly nymphs and also in crayfish. The adult fluke develops in the madtom, *Schilbeodes gyrinas*, the brown bullhead, *Ictalurus nebulosus* and the yellow bullhead, *I. natalis* (see McMullen, 1936; Crawford, 1937).

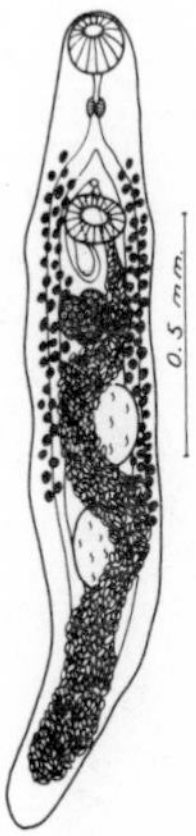

Fig. 448. *Alloglossidium corti.*

2b. Vitelline follicles confined to hindbody. 3

3a. Several circles of prominent spines on oral sucker; intestinal parasites of garfish (Fig. 449). ....
....**Genus** *Paramacroderoides* **Venard, 1941**

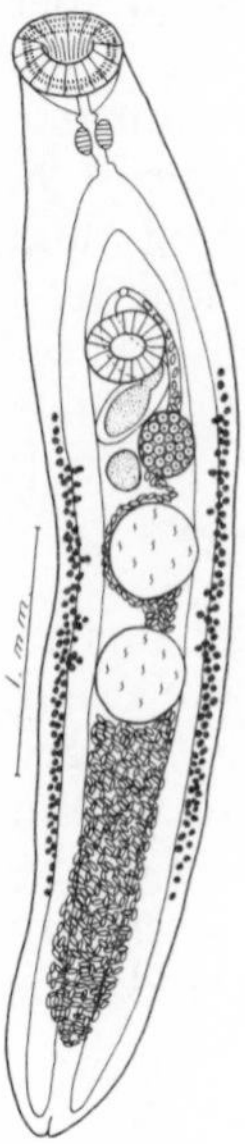

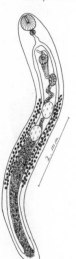

Life cycle: *P. echinus*—

Embryonated eggs, passed in the feces of the host, are eaten by the planorbid snail, *Helisoma duryi*, in which the miracidia hatch. Xiphidiocercariae of the ornatae group (Fig. 35) develop in daughter sporocysts and, after emerging from the snail, encyst in numerous small fishes of the Genera *Gambusia, Fundulus, Jordanella, Heterandria, Mollienesia* and also in the adults of *Rana sphenocephala* and tadpoles of *R. grylio*. Of these, *Gambusia affinis* is the most important intermediate host. The adult fluke develops in the intestine of the Florida gar, *Lepisosteus platyrhincus* (see Leigh and Holliman, 1956).

Fig. 449.   *Paramacroderoides echinus.*
(Redrawn from Venard, 1941.)

3b. Oral sucker without circles of spines. **4**

4a. Intestinal parasites of frogs; seminal receptacle present (Fig. 450). ....**Genus** *Haplometrana* **Lucker, 1931**

Life cycle: *H. intestinalis* (= *H. utahensis*)—

Embryonated eggs are ingested by several species of snails of the the Genus *Physa* in which xiphidiocercariae of the ornatae group develop in daughter sporocysts. The cercariae encyst in the epidermis of frogs which subsequently become infected by ingesting pieces of shed epidermis containing the cysts. *Rana pretiosa* is the definitive host (Olsen, 1937b).

Fig. 450.   *Haplometrana intestinalis.*

4b. Intestinal parasites of freshwater fishes; seminal receptacle absent (Fig. 451). .... **Genus** *Macroderoides* **Pearse, 1924**
Key to species in Van Cleave and Mueller (1934) and in Skrjabin (1964).
Life cycle: *M. spinifera—*
Embryonated eggs are eaten by the freshwater snail, *Helisoma duryi* in which xiphidiocercariae of the armatae group develop in daughter sporocysts. After leaving the snail, the cercariae encyst in the muscles of fishes of the Genera *Gambusia, Mollienesia, Heterandria* and *Fundulus* and also in tadpoles of several species of frogs. The adult trematode develops in the intestine of the garfish, *Lepisosteus platyrhincus,* attaining sexual maturity in 10 to 12 days (Leigh, 1958).

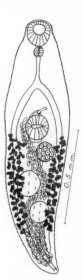

Fig. 451. *Macroderoides typica.*

5a. **Body linguiform; testes nearly opposite; vitelline follicles distributed along full length of ceca; uterus fills posterior 3/4 of body; intestinal parasites of chameleon (Fig. 452).** ....**Genus** *Alloglyptus* **Byrd, 1950**

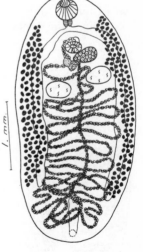

Fig. 452. *Alloglyptus crenshawi.*

5b. **Body fusiform; testes oblique; vitelline follicles largely restricted to middle third of body; intestinal parasites of frogs and toads.** **6**

6a. Uterine folds extend anterior to testes and overlap ceca laterally; cuticle thick with tubular spines; parenchymal cells present in area between oral and ventral suckers (Fig. 453). ....Genus *Choledocystus* Pereira and Cuocolo, 1941

Life cycle: *C. pennsylvaniensis* (= *Glypthelmins pennsylvaniensis*)—

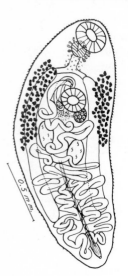

The results are not based entirely on experimental infections. Embryonated eggs are ingested by *Helisoma trivolvis* in which xiphidiocercariae develop in daughter sporocysts and encyst in the skin of frogs. Suitable definitive hosts are the spring peeper, *Hyla crucifer*, and the chorus frog, *Pseudacris nigrita*, which become infected by eating pieces of shed epidermis containing the encysted metacercariae (Cheng, 1961).

Fig. 453. *Choledocystus pennsylvaniensis.*
(Redrawn from Byrd and Maples, 1963.)

6b. Uterine folds entirely posttesticular and intercecal; cuticle thin; spines conical; parenchymal cells absent (Fig. 454). ....
....Genus *Glypthelmins* Stafford, 1905

Key to species in Skrjabin (1964).

Life cycle: *G. quieta*—

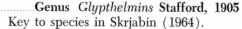

Embryonated eggs from frog feces are eaten by the freshwater snail, *Physa gyrina*. Xiphidiocercariae of the ornatae group (Fig. 35) develop in daughter sporocysts. After leaving the host snail, the cercariae penetrate the skin of frogs of the Genus *Rana* and encyst. Sheets of cast epidermis, containing metacercariae, are eaten by the frogs. The adult trematode develops in the small intestine (Rankin, 1944 and Leigh, 1946).

Fig. 454. *Glypthelmins quieta.*

FAMILY HAPLOMETRIDAE McMullen, 1937

Body elongate, spinous, flat, transparent; ventral sucker well developed or vestigial; intestinal ceca extend to posterior end of body; testes tandem, oblique or opposite, located in posterior half of body; cirrus sac present; ovary ovoid or lobed, pretesticular; seminal receptacle present; genital pore ventral to pharynx or esophagus; vitelline follicles arranged in many separate clusters throughout body; uterus very long, consisting of many folds which fill most of area around other internal organs; eggs small, abundant; excretory vesicle Y-shaped, the arms of the Y extending far forward in body; parasites in lungs of amphibians.

Only the Genus *Haematoloechus* Looss, 1899 (= *Pneumonoeces* Looss, 1902) (Figs. 455, 456) is represented in North America. The genus contains many species of which 17 have been reported from North America as parasites of amphibians of the Genera *Rana* and *Bufo*.

Life cycle: *H. parviplexus* and *H. medioplexus—*

Embryonated eggs of the former species are ingested by the planorbid snail, *Gyraulus parvus* in which the miracidia hatch, penetrate the intestinal wall and metamorphose to the sporocyst stage. Xiphidiocercariae of the ornatae group develop in sporocysts and after leaving the snail, are drawn into the branchial basket of dragonfly nymphs where they encyst. The infected insects are eaten by *Rana clamitans*. The mature flukes develop in the lungs.

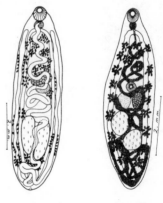

Fig. 455.   Fig. 456.

Fig. 455. *Haematoloechus longiplexus.*
Fig. 456. *H. similiplexus.*

The life cycle of *H. medioplexus* is similar except that the host snail is *Planorbula armigera* and the definitive host is *Rana pipiens* (Krull, 1931).

Schell (1965) described the life cycle of *H. breviplexus*. Mother and daughter sporocysts develop, the latter producing xiphidiocercariae of the ornatae group (Fig. 35). The host snail is *Gyraulis similaris*. Dragonfly nymphs of *Aeschna multicolor* serve as second intermediate host and the definitive host is *Rana pretiosa*.

FAMILY CEPHALOGONIMIDAE Nicoll, 1915

Body linguiform, spinous; suckers of about equal size; testes tandem to slightly oblique, in middle third of body; cirrus sac long, entirely anterior to ventral sucker; genital pore antero-dorsal to oral sucker; ovary pretesticular; seminal receptacle large; vitelline follicles lateral to ceca, in midde third of body; uterus has descending and ascending limbs, extends to posterior end of body; excretory vesicle Y-shaped with lateral diverticula; intestinal parasites of amphibians and reptiles.

The family is represented in North America by only the Genus *Cephalogonimus* Poirier, 1886, (Fig. 457). Key to species in Ogata (1934).

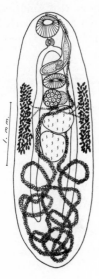

Life cycle: *C. americanus*—

Embryonated eggs are ingested by the planorbid snails, *Helisoma antrosa* and *H. trivolvis*. Xiphidiocercariae of the armatae group develop in daughter sporocysts in the snail hemocoel. After escaping from the snail, the cercariae penetrate tadpoles and encyst in the tissues. The adult fluke develops in the small intestine of frogs of the Genus *Rana* which acquire the infection by eating infected tadpoles. During development in the definitive host, the excretory vesicle develops prominent lateral diverticula (Lang, 1968).

Fig. 457. *Cephalogonimus amphiumae.*

FAMILY AURIDISTOMATIDAE Stunkard, 1924

Body elongate, spinous; oral sucker with one pair of lateral papillae and a dorsal transverse ridge; ventral sucker smaller than oral sucker and in anterior third of body; intestinal ceca extend to posterior end of body; testes tandem or oblique; cirrus sac present, anterior to ventral sucker; ovary just posterior to ventral sucker and pretesticular; seminal receptacle present; genital pore median, some distance anterior to ventral sucker; vitelline follicles abundant, all around ceca from level of ventral sucker to posterior end of body; uterus between anterior testis and genital pore; excretory vesicle Y-shaped with a long stem; intestinal parasites of turtles.

The family contains three genera but only the Genus *Auridistomum* Stafford, 1905 is represented in North America by the species *A. chelydrae* (Fig. 458).

Life cycle: *A. chelydrae—*

Xiphidiocercariae of the armatae group (= *Cercaria concavocorpa*) develop in sporocysts in the freshwater snail, *Helisoma trivolvis,* and encyst in the tissues of tadpoles of the bullfrog, *Rana catesbeiana.* Metacercariae were fed to young snapping turtles, *Chelydra serpentina* and young adults were recovered from the small intestine (Ralph, 1938).

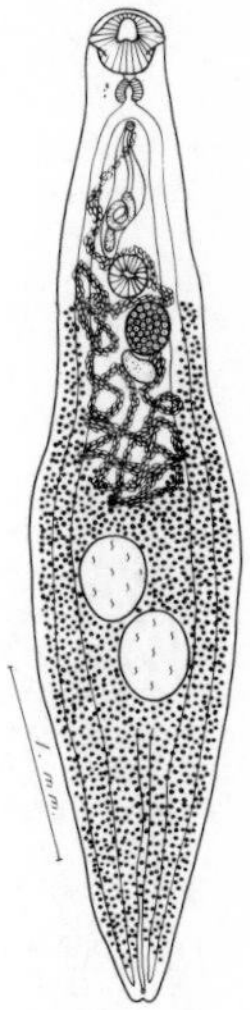

Fig. 458. *Auridistomum chelydrae.*

FAMILY LISSORCHIIDAE Poche, 1926

Body elongate, spinous, tapering toward posterior end; ceca long; ventral sucker larger than oral sucker; testes tandem; cirrus sac absent (?); ovary anterior to testes; genital pore on left margin of body at level of ventral sucker; uterus with descending and ascending limbs, extending posterior to testes; vitelline follicles in narrow rows along ceca between ventral sucker and testes; excretory vesicle Y-shaped; intestinal parasites of freshwater fishes.

The family contains only the Genus *Lissorchis* Magath, 1917. Life cycle investigations by Smith (1968) indicate that the Genus *Triganodistomum* Simer, 1929 is a synonym of *Lissorchis,* whereas the early work of Magath (1918) shows that the two genera might not be closely related. The adults of both genera are similar in their anatomy (Figs. 459, 460).

Life cycle: *Lissorchis mutabile* (= *Triganodistomum mutabile*)—

Tailless cercariae (= *Cercariaeum mutabile*) develop in rediae in the limpets, *Laevapex fuscus* and *Ferrissia rivularis,* and also in the planorbid snails, *Helisoma trivolvis* and *H. campanulatum.* Escaping cercariae are ingested by planarians, *Dugesia* sp., and by aquatic oligochaetes, *Chaetogaster limnaei,* in which metacercariae develop. The adult fluke develops in the chub and white suckers which probably ingest the infected planarians and oligochaetes (Wallace, 1941; Smith, 1968).

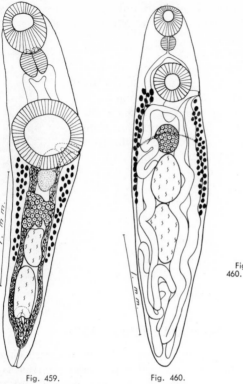

Fig. 459. *Lissorchis fairporti.* Fig. 460. *Triganodistomum attenuatum.*

Fig. 459.   Fig. 460.

The anatomy of the adults and the development of a tailless cercaria in the life cycle indicates possible relationship to the Family Zoogonidae.

The situation is confused by the work of Magath (1918) who reported tailed xiphidiocercariae which are produced in sporocysts in *Helisoma trivolvis* for *Lissorchis fairporti,* the type species. The cercariae penetrate the body wall of chironomid larvae and encyst in the hemocoel. The adult parasites develop in the intestine of buffalo fish, *Ictiobus bubalus* and *I. cyprinellus.*

FAMILY BRACHYCOELIIDAE Johnston, 1912

Body spinous, oval or elongate; intestinal ceca short; testes opposite or oblique, close to ventral sucker; cirrus sac present; genital pore median, anterior to ventral sucker; ovary either anterior or posterior to testes; uterus extends to posterior end of body; vitelline follicles restricted to anterior half of body; excretory vesicle I- or Y-shaped; intestinal parasites of amphibians and reptiles.

KEY TO GENERA

1a. Ovary posterior to testes; genital pore close to intestinal bifurcation (Fig. 461). .... Genus *Mesocoelium* Odhner, 1911

Life cycle: *M. brevicaecum*—
Only one intermediate host is involved in the life cycle. Cercariae develop in daughter sporocysts in the snail, *Euhadra quaesita* and encyst in the snail. Definitive hosts are *Bufo vulgaris, Rana nigromaculata, R. rugosa, R. catesbeiana, Elaphe quadrivirgata,* and *Eumeces latiscutatus* (see Ochi, 1930).

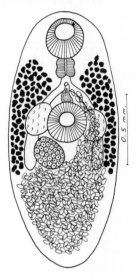

Fig. 461. *Mesocoelium waltoni.*

1b. Ovary anterior to testes; genital pore immediately anterior to ventral sucker. 2
2a. Testes oblique; cirrus sac large, extending posterior to ventral sucker; vitelline follicles in marginal bands; intestinal parasites of turtles (Fig. 462). ....
.... Genus *Cymatocarpus* Looss, 1899

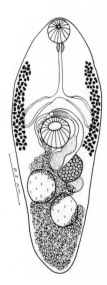

Fig. 462. *Cymatocarpus undulatus.*

2b. Testes opposite or nearly so; cirrus sac small, not extending posterior to ventral sucker; vitelline follicles in confluent clusters, largely anterior to ventral sucker; intestinal parasites of amphibians and reptiles (Fig. 463). ....

....Genus *Brachycoelium* (Dujardin, 1845)

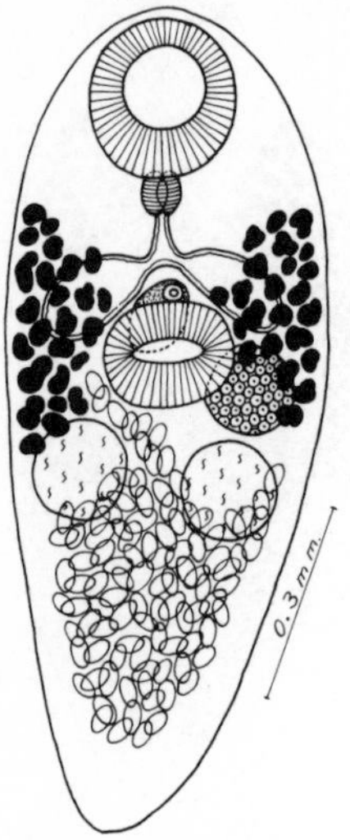

Life cycle: *B. mesorchium*—

Key to species in Byrd (1937).

Embryonated eggs are eaten by the terrestrial molluscs, *Triodopsis carolinensis, Mesodon inflectus, M. thyroidus* and *Agriolimax agrestis*. Miracidia hatch in the mollusc intestine, penetrate the intestinal wall and shed the ciliated epidermal plates. Tailless cercariae without a stylet develop in daughter sporocysts. The cercariae emerge from the mollusc and secrete a jelly-like capsule over themselves. The encapsulated cercariae are eaten by a variety of species of terrestrial molluscs in which they encyst. Encysted metacercariae were fed to the salamanders, *Desmognathus fuscus* and *Eurycea bislineata cirrigera*. Young trematodes were recovered after three weeks (Denton, 1962; Jordan, 1963; Jordan and Byrd, 1967).

Fig. 463. *Brachycoelium salamandrae.*

FAMILY DICROCOELIIDAE Odhner, 1911

Body translucent, lanceolate, filiform, fusiform or claviform; suckers well developed; intestinal ceca long; testes opposite, tandem or oblique; cirrus sac anterior to ventral sucker; genital pore median, between the suckers; ovary posterior to testes; uterus with descending and ascending limbs; parasites in the liver, gall bladder, bile duct or pancreatic duct of reptiles, birds and mammals. A taxonomic monograph of the family was published by Travassos (1944).

KEY TO GENERA

1a. Testes opposite. 2
1b. Testes tandem or oblique. 6
2a. Ventral sucker twice the diameter of oral sucker; body lanceolate, widest at level of testes (Fig. 464). ....
....Genus *Zonorchis* Travassos, 1944
2b. Ventral sucker only slightly larger than oral or of equal size; body fusiform widest at midbody region. 3

3a. Intestinal ceca inflated, sinuous; parasites of reptiles and birds (Fig. 465). ....Genus *Paradistomum* Kossack, 1910

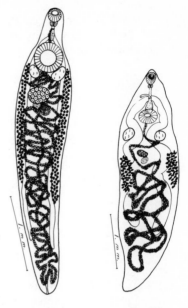

Fig. 464. *Zonorchis petiolatum.*
Fig. 465. *Paradistomum passerculum.*

Fig. 464.   Fig. 465.

3b. Intestinal ceca narrow and straight. 4
4a. Vitelline follicles large, few, restricted to lateral clusters in middle fifth of body; primarily parasites of mammals (Fig. 466) ....Genus *Concinnum* Bhalerao, 1936

Life cycle: *C. procyonis*—
Embryonated eggs are ingested by the land snail, *Mesodon thyroideus.* Cercariae, similar to the microcercous type, develop in daughter sporocysts. The cercariae remain in the daughter sporocysts which enter the mantle cavity and are then expelled through the spiracle and deposited on vegetation. Although a second intermediate host is not known for this species, some arthropod might be involved. The adult fluke develops in the pancreatic duct of raccoon (Denton, 1944).

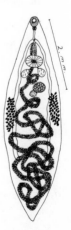

Fig. 466. *Concinnum burleighi.*

4b. Vitelline follicles small, abundant, distributed in lateral fields through at least the middle third of the body; parasites of birds. 5

5a. Ventral sucker larger than oral sucker and about one-third of body length from anterior end of body; body narrowly fusiform (Fig. 467). ....Genus *Conspicuum* Bhalerao, 1936

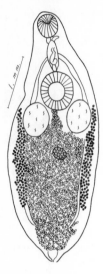

Life cycle: *C. icteridorum*—

Embryonated eggs, which pass in the feces of the host, are eaten by the land snails, *Zonitoides arboreus* and the slug, *Deroceras laeve*, in which microcercous cercariae are produced in daughter sporocysts. Entire daughter sporocysts, containing cercariae, are expelled through the spiracle of the snail. These sporocysts are ingested by the terrestrial isopods, *Oniscus asellus* and *Armadillium quadrifrons*, in the digestive tract of which the cercariae are liberated. They penetrate the gut wall and encyst. Adult flukes develop in the gall bladder of grackles, blackbirds and meadowlarks which feed on the infected isopods (Patten, 1952).

Fig. 467. *Conspicuum macrorchis.*

5b. Ventral and oral suckers of equal size; both in anterior fifth of body; body broadly fusiform (Fig. 468). ....
....Genus *Lubens* Travassos, 1920

6a. Vitelline follicles unilateral; testes distinctly lobed; parasites of birds and mammals (Fig. 469). ....
....Genus *Athesmia* Looss, 1899

Key to species in McIntosh (1937) and Skrjabin (1964).

6b. Vitelline follicles bilateral; testes usually not lobed. 7

7a. One intestinal cecum present; parasites of birds (Fig. 470). ....Genus *Lutztrema* Travassos, 1941

7b. Two intestinal ceca present. 8

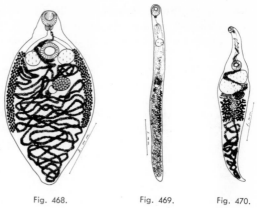

Fig. 468. *Lubens lubens.*
Fig. 469. *Athesmia jolliei.*
Fig. 470. *Lutztrema monenteron.*

Fig. 468.   Fig. 469.   Fig. 470.

8a. Body narrowly fusiform, widest at the middle; testes with irregular margins; vitelline follicles few, restricted to area posterior to level of ovary; parasites of birds and mammals (Fig. 471). .... Genus *Dicrocoelium* **Dujardin, 1845**

Key to species in Macy (1931) and in Skrjabin (1964).

Life cycle: *D. dendriticum—*

Embryonated eggs in the feces of the host are eaten by the land snail, *Cionella lubrica*. Miracidia hatch in the snail intestine and penetrate the gut wall. Xiphidiocercariae with a long tail (= *Cercaria vitrina*) develop in daughter sporocysts. As the cercariae leave the sporocysts, the snail secretes mucus around masses of several hundred cercariae to form so-called "slime balls" which are expelled through the spiracle of the snail. The slime balls are eaten by the ant, *Formica fusca,* in which the cercariae encyst. Infected ants are ingested by the definitive host along with their forage. Metacercariae excyst in the host intestine and migrate to the liver by way of the common bile duct. Sexually mature adults develop within six to seven weeks. Sheep, goats, cattle, pigs, deer, marmot and rabbit are the normal hosts (Krull and Mapes, 1952, 1953; Mapes, 1951; Mapes and Krull, 1951).

8b. Body lanceolate or filiform; testes have smooth margins. 9

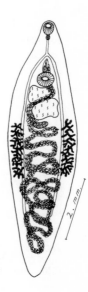

Fig. 471. *Dicrocoelium dendriticum.*

9a. **Body filiform, delicate; vitelline follicles small, abundant, some follicles anterior to level of ovary; genital pore ventral to pharynx; parasites of birds and mammals (Fig. 472).** ....
....Genus *Lyperosomum* Looss, 1899

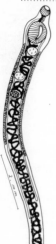

Life cycle: *Lyperosomum* spp.—

Embryonated eggs from the feces of the host are eaten by the land snails, *Polygyra texasiana* and *Practicollela berlandieriana.* Xiphidiocercariae of the armatae group develop in daughter sporocysts. Cercariae leave the sporocysts and accumulate in the mantle cavity of the snail where mucus is secreted around masses of 150 to 300 cercariae. The masses are expelled periodically and deposited on vegetation. Development to this stage requires 100 or more days. Metacercariae develop in the chrysomelid beetle, *Gastroidia cyanea,* which probably feed on the mucus-cercaria masses. Normal definitive hosts are meadowlarks and bronzed grackles which feed upon the infected beetles (Denton, 1941).

Fig. 472. *Lyperosomum oswaldoi.*

9b. **Body lanceolate; vitelline follicles large, few, distributed in a limited area posterior to level of ovary; genital pore ventral to intestinal bifurcation (Fig. 473).** ....
....Genus *Brachylecithum* Strom, 1940

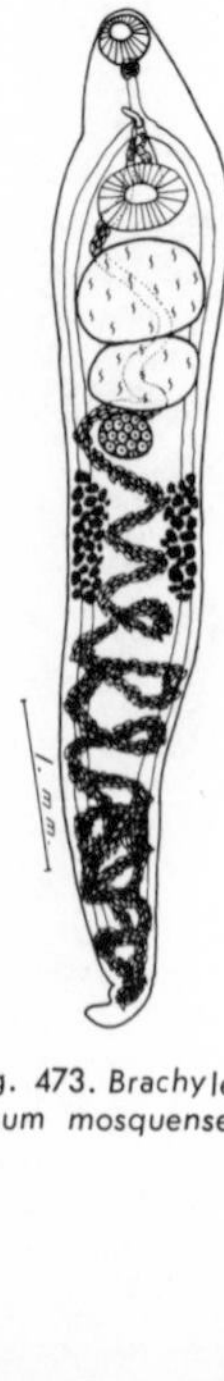

Life cycle: *B. mosquense*—

The adult flukes occupy the bile passages of the robin. Embryonated eggs, passed in the feces of robins, are eaten by the terrestrial polygyrid snail, *Allogona ptychophora,* in which the miracidia hatch, penetrate the intestinal wall and migrate to the digestive gland. Mother and daughter sporocysts develop there. Xiphidiocercariae with a long tail develop in daughter sporocysts. The cercariae leave the sporocysts, migrate to the mantle cavity, then emerge from the snail in a mass of mucus secreted by the snail. These "slime balls" are eaten by carpenter ants of the Genus *Camponotus.* The cercariae encyst in the hemocoel of ants and robins become infected by eating infected ants. The parasites migrate to the bird's liver by way of the common bile duct. Over one hundred days are required to attain maturity in the robin (Carney, 1967).

Fig. 473. *Brachylecithum mosquense.*

Denton (1945) studied the life cycle of *B. americanum.*

FAMILY EUCOTYLIDAE Skrjabin, 1924

Triangular unarmed head collar present or absent; intestinal ceca end blindly or are fused at posterior end; ventral sucker absent or vestigial; testes opposite or oblique, oval or lobed, in middle of body; cirrus sac absent; genital pore median; ovary pretesticular, lobed; uterus with descending and ascending limbs; eggs abundant; vitelline follicles distributed along lateral margins of ceca; parasites in the urinary tract of birds.

KEY TO GENERA

1a. **Triangular unarmed head collar around oral sucker; ceca end blindly; testes opposite (Fig. 474).** ....
....**Genus** *Eucotyle* **Cohn, 1904**
Key to species in Schell (1967b).

1b. **Without triangular head collar; ceca fused at posterior end; testes opposite, tandem or oblique (Fig. 475).** ....
....**Genus** *Tanaisia* **Skrjabin, 1924**
Key to species in Byrd and
Denton (1950).

Life cycle: *T. bragai—*
Embryonated eggs are eaten by the land snails, *Subulina octona,* in which microcercous cercariae develop in daughter sporocysts. The cercariae encyst in the daughter sporocysts. The definitive host probably acquires the parasite by ingesting infected snails. Development to sexual maturity takes place in the kidneys of pigeon, chickens, turkeys, grackles and oven bird. The encysted metacercariae migrate there by way of the cloaca and ureters. The cercariae have fused ceca like the adults. A ventral sucker is present in the cercaria, metacercaria and young adult but it gradually atrophies by the time the mature adult develops (Maldonado, 1945).

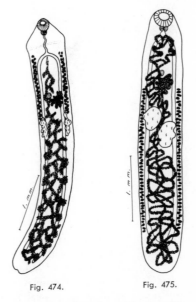

Fig. 474.   Fig. 475.

Fig. 474. *Eucotyle wehri.* Fig. 475. *Tanaisia fedtschenkoi.*

FAMILY LECITHODENDRIIDAE Odhner, 1910

Body small, spinous or nonspinous, round, pyriform or oval; suckers about equal; intestinal ceca short in most genera; testes opposite, usually lateral to ventral sucker; cirrus sac present or absent; genital pore median, sublateral or lateral; genital atrium rarely present; ovary submedian, anterior to testes or between testes and either anterior or posterior to ventral sucker; vitelline follicles in lateral clusters in anterior part of body; uterus confined to posterior part of body; eggs numerous; primarily parasites of bats, a few species in birds and amphibians.

KEY TO GENERA

1a. Vitelline follicles posterior to ventral sucker. 2
1b. Vitelline follicles anterior to ventral sucker. 3

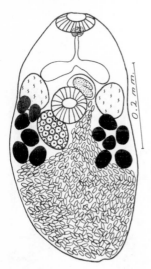

2a. Vitelline follicles entirely posterior to testes; genital pore ventral and median, anterior to ventral sucker; intestinal parasites of bats (Fig. 476). ....Genus *Lecithodendrium* Looss, 1896

Fig. 476. *Lecithodendrium breckenridgei.*

2b. Some vitelline follicles lateral to testes; genital pore dorsal and to left of oral sucker; uterus restricted to forebody; intestinal parasites of salamanders (Fig. 477). ....
...........................Genus *Cephalouterina* Senger and Macy, 1953
3a. Genital pore at lateral margin of body. 4
3b. Genital pore median or sublateral. 8

Life cycle: *C. dicamptodoni*—

The first intermediate host is the operculate hydrobiid snail, *Bythinella hemphilli*, in which xiphidiocercariae develop
in daughter sporocysts. Following emergence from the snail, the cercariae penetrate and encyst in the nymph of the
stonefly, *Acroneuria californica*. The natural definitive host is the Pacific giant
salamander, *Dicamptodon ensatus* and the
tailed frog, *Ascaphus truei*. Experimental
infections were established in *Rana aurora*
(see Anderson, Martin and Pratt, 1966).

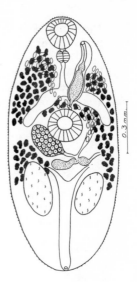

Fig. 477. *Cephalouterina dicamptodoni.*

4a. Intestinal ceca long, extending beyond testes. 5
4b. Intestinal ceca short, not extending beyond testes. 6
5a. Intestinal ceca extending to posterior end of body; body
broadly pyriform, nonspinous; intestinal parasites of muskrat
and bats (Fig. 478). ....Genus *Allassogonoporus* Olivier, 1938

Life cycle: *A. vespertilionis*—

Virgulate xiphidiocercariae
(Fig. 36) develop in sporocysts in the river snail, *Fluminicola virens*. The cercariae
are weak swimmers, usually
creep on the substrate. Upon
coming in contact with caddisfly larvae, the cercaria
loses the tail, secretes a mucous covering over itself,
penetrates the gills and encysts inside the gill. The
metacercariae are infective in
about one week. Adult trematodes develop in the in-
testine of bats which devour
the infected insects (Knight
and Pratt, 1955; Burns, 1961
b).

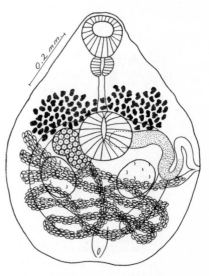

Fig. 478. *Allassogonoporus marginalis.*

5b. Intestinal ceca extend to middle of body; body oval, spinous;
     parasites of bats (Fig. 479). ....
     ....Genus *Myotitrema* **Macy, 1939**
6a. Genital pore marginal and posterior to level of ventral sucker;
     parasites of birds (Fig. 480). ....Genus *Macyella* **Neiland, 1951**
6b. Genital pore marginal and anterior to level of ventral sucker.
    7

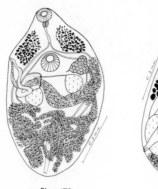

Fig. 479. *Myotitrema asymmetricum.*
Fig. 480. *Macyella postgonoporus.*

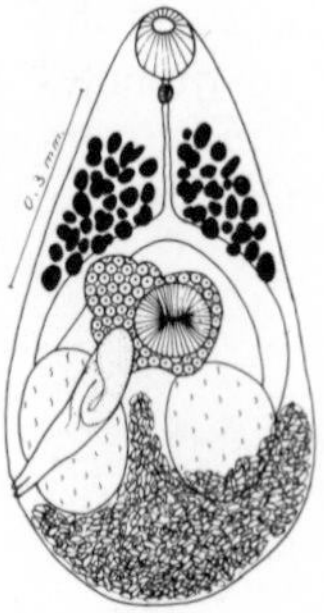

Fig. 479.   Fig. 480.

7a. Cirrus sac present, well developed; vitelline follicles in a
     cluster on each side of esophagus; parasites of reptiles and
     amphibians (Fig. 481). ....
     ....Genus *Pleurogenoides* **Travassos, 1921**

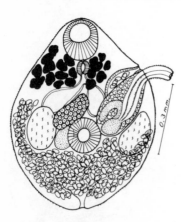

Fig. 481. *Pleurogenoides stromi.*

Life cycle: *P. tener—*
    Virgulate xiphidiocercariae develop in sporocysts in the snail,
Bithynia subdiella and after leaving the snail, enter the rectum of
several species of dragonfly nymphs and encyst in the rectal wall.
Adult flukes were recovered from the intestine of the lizard,

Chalcides ocellatus, 22 days after metacercariae were fed. Some development toward maturity also occurred in the frog, *Rana mascareniensis.* This work was done in Egypt (Macy, 1964).

7b. **Cirrus sac absent; seminal vesicle long, free in parenchyma; vitelline follicles lateral to ventral sucker; parasites of mink (Fig. 482).** ....Genus *Cephalophallus* Macy and Moore, 1954

Life cycle: *C. obscurus*—
Virgulate xiphidiocercariae (Fig. 36) develop in sporocysts in the river snail, *Fluminicola virens* and encyst in the muscles of the crayfish, *Astacus trowbridgii.* The adult fluke develops in the small intestine of mink in the Pacific Northwest (Macy and Moore, 1954).

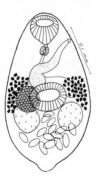

Fig. 482. *Cephalophallus obscurus.*

8a. Intestinal ceca long, extending beyond middle of body. 9
8b. Intestinal ceca short, not extending beyond middle of body. 10
9a. Intestinal ceca dilated, extending to posterior end of body; body broadly oval; testes some distance posterior to ventral sucker; ovary lobed, dorsal to ventral sucker; in bile duct of frogs (Fig. 483). ....Genus *Loxogenoides* Kaw, 1945
9b. Intestinal ceca narrow, extending through 3/4 of body; body oval or fusiform; testes lateral to ventral sucker; ovary follicular, some distance anterior to ventral sucker; in intestine of birds (Fig. 484). ....
....Genus *Metoliophilus* Macy and Bell, 1968

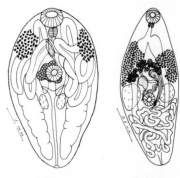

Fig. 483. *Loxogenoides bicolor.*
Fig. 484. *Metoliophilus uvaticus.*

Fig. 483.   Fig. 484.

Life cycle: *M. uvaticus*—

Adults were recovered from baby chicks five days after feeding metacercariae found in the nymphs of stonefly, *Acroneuria pacifica*. The water ouzel, *Cinclus mexicanus unicolor*, is the natural definitive host (Macy and Bell, 1968).

10a. Intestinal ceca extend to level of testes; parasites of birds.....11

10b. Intestinal ceca entirely anterior to ventral sucker; parasites of amphibians or bats. 12

11a. Vitelline follicles in clusters on each side of esophagus; genital pore median, posterior to ventral sucker; excretory vesicle I-shaped (Fig. 485). ....
....................Genus *Echinuscodendrium* Skarbilovich, 1943

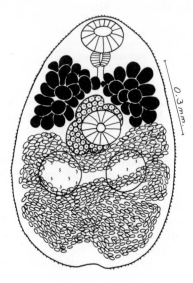

Fig. 485. *Echinuscodendrium echinus.*

11b. Vitelline follicles distributed along lateral margins of intestinal ceca; excretory vesicle V-shaped (Fig. 486). ....
....................................Genus *Mosesia* Travassos, 1921

Life cycle: *M. chordeilesia*—

Virgulate xiphidiocercariae develop in sporocysts in the freshwater operculate snails, *Goniobasis livescens* and *Pleurocera acuta*. The cercariae encyst in the hemocoel of mayfly nymphs. The adult fluke develops in the intestine of night hawks (Hall, 1959).

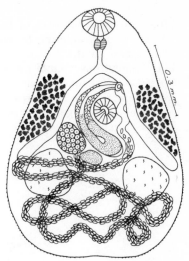

Fig. 486. *Mosesia chordeilesia.*

12a. Encysted in wall of duodenum or pyloric end of stomach of frogs; ovary lobed; genital pore dorsal, sinistral, and anterior to level of ventral sucker (Fig. 487). ....
....Genus *Loxogenes* Stafford, 1905

Life cycle: *L. arcanum*—

Metacercariae of this species occur encysted in the muscles of the abdomen of nine species of dragonfly nymphs which might be eaten by frogs. The adult parasites are usually encysted in the duodenal wall or in the pyloric area of the stomach (Crawford, 1938).

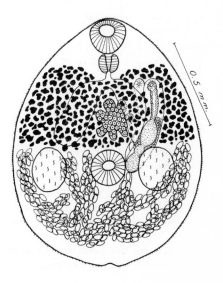

Fig. 487. *Loxogenes arcanum.*

12b. Intestinal parasites of bats; genital pore and cirrus sac me-
     dian and anterior to ventral sucker or lateral or postero-
     lateral to it. 13
13a. Genital pore and cirrus sac median, anterior to ventral sucker;
     genital atrium present. 14
13b. Genital pore and cirrus sac lateral or postero-lateral to ven-
     tral sucker; genital atrium absent. 15
14a. Genital atrium spinous (Fig. 488). ....
     ....Genus *Acanthatrium* Faust, 1919

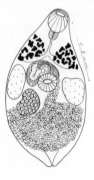 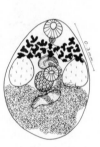

Fig. 488. *Acanthatrium micra-
canthum.* Fig. 489. *Prosthodendrium
naviculum.*

Fig. 488.   Fig. 489.

Key to species in Williams (1960).
Life cycle: *A. oregonense—*
Virgulate xiphidiocercariae develop in sporocysts in the snail,
Oxytrema silicula. The cercariae penetrate caddisfly larvae, enter
the hemocoel but do not encyst. Bats, which serve as definitive
host, probably acquire the parasite by eating infected caddisflies
(Knight and Pratt, 1955; Burns, 1961b).
14b. Genital atrium nonspinous (Fig. 489). ....
     ....Genus *Prosthodendrium* Dollfus, 1931
Life cycle: *P. pyramidum* (= *Lecithodendrium pyramidum*)—
Virgulate xiphidiocercariae develop in sporocysts in the snail,
Melania tuberculata. The cercariae are thought to be eaten by
anopheline mosquito larvae in which they encyst. The adult trematode develops in the intestine of bats (Abdel-Azim, 1936).
15a. Cirrus sac lateral to ventral sucker with base of sac directed
     toward anterior end of body (Fig. 490). ....
     ....Genus *Limatulum* Travassos, 1921
15b. Cirrus sac posterior to ventral sucker with base of sac di-
     rected toward posterior end of body (Fig. 491). ....
     ....Genus *Gyrabascus* Macy, 1935

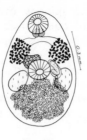
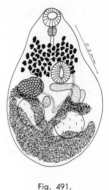

Fig. 490. *Limatulum gastroides.*
Fig. 491. *Gyrabascus brevigastrus.*

Fig. 490.

Fig. 491.

FAMILY UROTREMATIDAE Poche, 1926

Body elongate, spinous; suckers small, close to anterior end of body; intestinal ceca long; testes tandem, in posterior part of body; genital pore and cirrus sac near posterior end of body; ovary pretesticular, separated from testes by uterine folds; vitelline follicles variable in extent; uterus long, folded between ovary and genital pore; excretory vesicle V-shaped; primarily intestinal parasites of bats.

KEY TO GENERA

1a. Testes and ovary lobed; ventral sucker far anterior to ovary. (Fig. 492). ....Genus *Urotrematulum* Macy, 1933
1b. Testes and ovary with smooth margins; ventral sucker only a short distance anterior to ovary (Fig. 493). ....
....Genus *Urotrema* Braun, 1900
Key to species in Macy (1933) and Skrjabin (1964).

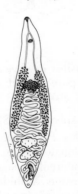
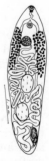

Fig. 492. *Urotrematulum attenuatum.* Fig. 493. *Urotrema lasiurensis.*

Fig. 492.

Fig. 493.

FAMILY PROSTHOGONIMIDAE Nicoll, 1924

Body flat, translucent, spinous, oval or pyriform; suckers in anterior third of body, of equal size; intestinal ceca extend nearly to posterior end of body; testes opposite, in hindbody; cirrus sac long, between the suckers; genital pore ventral to pharynx or lateral to oral sucker; ovary lobed, pretesticular; vitelline follicles occupy lateral zones in middle third of body; uterus long, folds fill most of body posterior to ventral sucker; excretory vesicle Y-shaped; parasites in cloaca, bursa Fabricii and oviducts of birds or in the liver of mammals.

KEY TO GENERA

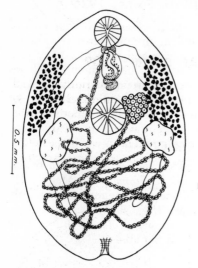

1a. Parasites in liver of mammals; genital pore ventral to pharynx; cirrus sac thick, ovoid (Fig. 494). .... Genus *Mediogonimus* Woodhead and Malewitz, 1936

Fig. 494.　*Mediogonimus ovilacus.*

1b. Parasites in cloaca, bursa Fabricii and oviducts of birds; genital pore lateral to oral sucker; cirrus sac slender, sinuous (Fig. 495). ....Genus *Prosthogonimus* Lühe, 1899

Key to species in Skrjabin (1964).

Life cycle: *P. macroorchis*—

Embryonated eggs, passed in the feces of the host, are eaten by the operculate snail, *Amnicola limosa*. Miracidia hatch in the snail intestine. Xiphidiocercariae with a short tail develop in sporocysts. After leaving the snail, they are drawn into the branchial basket (rectum) of dragonfly nymphs, enter the hemocoel and

encyst in the abdominal muscles. Definitive hosts such as
ducks, chickens, crows and
pheasants eat the infected
nymphs or the adult dragonflies. Infected birds seem to
lay fewer eggs (Macy, 1934,
1939, 1940b).

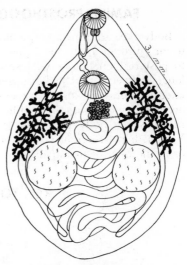

Fig. 495. *Prosthogonimus macrorchis.*

FAMILY RENICOLIDAE Dollfus, 1939

Body spinous, rounded anteriorly and tapered posteriorly; ventral
sucker rudimentary, in posterior half of body; intestinal ceca extend about to midbody region; testes opposite, in hindbody; cirrus
sac absent?; genital pore anterior to ventral sucker; ovary submedian, pretesticular; vitelline follicles in lateral areas of posterior
half of body; uterus fills most of body, anterior to ovary; excretory
vesicle Y-shaped; in kidneys of aquatic birds.

The Genus *Renicola* Cohn, 1904 is represented in North America
by at least two species (Fig. 496).

Life cycle: *R. thaidus—*

Eggs are embryonated when laid.
The early larval stages have been
observed only from natural infections in the marine snail, *Thais lapillus,* in which xiphidiocercariae
develop in daughter sporocysts. The
cercariae encyst in the marine lamellibranchs, *Mytilus edulis, Pecten
irradians* and *Gemma gemma.* The
adult develops in the herring gull,
Larus argentatus, when metacercariae are ingested (Stunkard, 1964b)

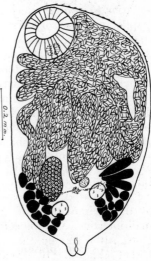

Fig. 496. *Renicola thaidus.* (Redrawn
from Stunkard, 1964b.)

FAMILY STOMYLOTREMATIDAE Poche, 1926

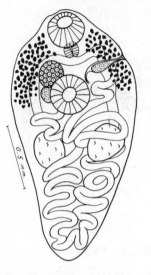

Body small (1-2 mm.), nonspinous; suckers large, the ventral sucker near center of body; ceca half long to long; testes opposite, anterior or posterior to ventral sucker; cirrus sac anterior to ventral sucker near right or left margin of body; ovary anterior to testes and on side opposite cirrus sac; genital pore on right or left margin of body at level of pharynx; seminal receptacle present; vitelline follicles in lateral rows in anterior half of body; uterus long, the folds filling posterior half of body; excretory vesicle Y-shaped; parasites in bursa Fabricii and cloaca of birds.

Only the Genus *Laterotrema* Semenow, 1928 occurs in North America. *L. americanum* has been reported as a

Fig. 497. *Laterotrema americanum.*   parasite of songbirds (Fig. 497).

FAMILY MICROPHALLIDAE Travassos, 1920

Body small, pyriform or oval, usually spinous; suckers of equal size or the ventral sucker smaller than the oral; intestinal ceca short, divergent; testes opposite, posterior to ventral sucker; cirrus sac present or absent; seminal vesicle and cirrus sac transverse, anterior to ventral sucker; genital atrium present, containing male papilla or accessory suckers in some genera and receiving male and female sex ducts; ovary usually anterior to right or left testis; seminal receptacle absent; vitelline follicles in small lateral clusters, variable in location; uterus extends posterior to ovary; excretory vesicle V-shaped; primarily intestinal parasites of birds, a few species in fishes and mammals.

Adult trematodes of this family bear some resemblance to those of the family Heterophyidae. Microphallid life cycles resemble those of the plagiorchioid trematodes in that xiphidiocercariae, usually of the ubiquita type (Fig. 37), develop in sporocysts and encyst in crustaceans. In some genera, tailless cercariae are produced.

KEY TO GENERA

1a. **Cirrus sac present, enclosing seminal vesicle and prostatic complex.** **2**

1b. Cirrus sac absent, seminal vesicle and prostatic complex free in parenchyma. 6

2a. Vitelline follicles entirely anterior and lateral to intestinal ceca; part of uterus extending anterior to ventral sucker; eggs large; genital pore a longitudinal slit; intestinal parasites of birds (Fig. 498). ....

........Genus *Plenosoma* Ching, 1960

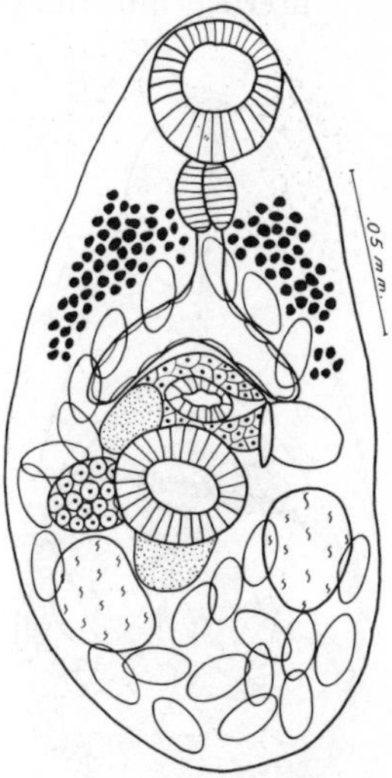

Fig. 498. *Plenosoma minimum.* (Redrawn from Ching, 1960.)

2b. Vitelline follicles posterior to intestinal ceca; uterus entirely posterior to ventral sucker. 3

3a. Two ventral suckers side by side (one probably encloses uterine pore); coiled muscular cirrus to right of ventral sucker; intestinal parasites of birds (Fig. 499). ....
...........Genus *Gynaecotyla* Yamaguti, 1939

Key to species in Dery (1958).

Life cycle: *G. nassicola*—

Miracidia hatch and penetrate the marine snail, *Nassa obsoleta* in which xiphidiocercariae of the ubiquita group (Fig. 37) develop in daughter sporocysts. The cercariae penetrate the gill lamellae of the sand flea, *Talorchestia longicornis* and encyst in the pericardial cavity. The adult fluke develops in the intestine of shore birds, such as plovers and sandpipers which eat the infected sandfleas (Rankin, 1940).

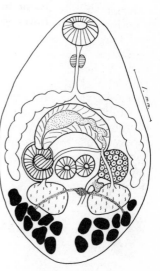

Fig. 499. *Gynaecotyla sippiwissettensis.* (Redrawn from Rankin, 1939b.)

3b. One ventral sucker present. **4**

4a. Vitelline follicles form a complete ring encircling testes and uterus; intestinal parasites of birds and mammals (Fig. 500).
....**Genus *Maritrema* Nicoll, 1907**

Key to species in Deblock and Combes (1965).

Life cycle: *M. caridiniae*—

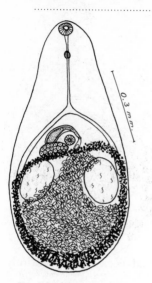

Xiphidiocercariae, resembling those of the ubiquita group, develop in daughter sporocysts in the snail, *Oncomelania nosophora*. The cercariae encyst in the freshwater shrimp, *Neocaridina denticulata*, and in dragonfly nymphs, *Anax parthenope julius*. In the shrimp, the older metacercariae tend to be precocial as numerous eggs develop in the uterus. The painted snipe, *Rostratula benghalensis* is a natural definitive host for this parasite. Experimental infections can be established in rats by feeding metacercariae (Shibue, 1951).

Fig. 500. *Maritrema ovatum.*

4b. Vitelline follicles not forming a ring; intestinal parasites of birds. **5**

5a. Vitelline follicles in lateral bands, primarily anterior to testes; uterus between and posterior to testes (Fig. 501). ....
....**Genus *Odhneria* Travassos, 1921**

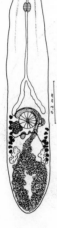

Fig. 501. *Odhneria limnodromi.*

5b. Vitelline follicles in irregular clusters around testes sometimes in form of an inverted U; uterus between, posterior and lateral to testes (Fig. 502). ....Genus *Maritreminoides* Rankin, 1939

Life cycle: *M. obstipus*—

Approximately 35 days are required for development of the miracidium after the eggs pass in the feces of the host. Miracidia did not hatch in water so it was assumed that the eggs are eaten by the freshwater snail, *Amnicola pilsburyi,* in which xiphidiocercariae (not the ubiquita type) develop in sporocysts. The cercariae encyst in the hemocoel of the aquatic freshwater isopod, *Asellus communis,* which are eaten by ducks (Etges, 1953).

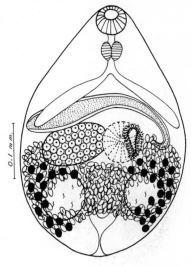

Fig. 502.   *Maritreminoides nettae.*

6a. Genital atrium large, containing a fleshy trilobed male copulatory organ; parasites of birds (Fig. 503). ....
.............................Genus *Carneophallus* Cable and Kuns, 1951

6b. Genital atrium large or small but not containing a trilobed copulatory organ; parasites of fishes, birds or mammals. 7

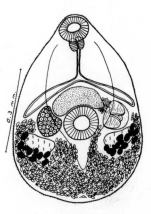

Fig. 503.   *Carneophallus trilobatus.*

7a. Genital atrium small, without muscular suckers or alveoli .....
(Fig. 504). ....Genus *Microphallus* Ward, 1901

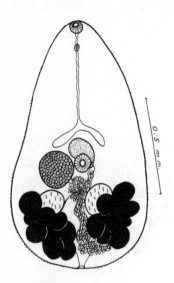

Fig. 504. *Microphallus opacus.*

Life cycle: *M. nicolli* (= *Spelotrema nicolli*)—

Miracidia develop slowly after eggs are passed by the host. Xiphidiocercariae of the ubiquita group develop in sporocysts in the marine snail, *Bittium alternatum* and after leaving the snail, penetrate the gills of the blue crab, *Callinectes sapidus* in which they encyst. The host produces a thick capsule around the cyst membrane. Metacercariae from crabs were fed to young herring gulls, *Larus argentatus,* in which the adult trematodes developed. A natural definitive host is the seaside sparrow, *Ammospiza maritima macgillivraii* (Cable and Hunninen, 1940).

7b. Genital atrium contains accessory suckers, muscular papilla, several small alveoli or denticles. 8

8a. Genital atrium contains several accessory suckers or alveoli or sometimes denticles; parasites of birds (Fig. 505). ....
............................Genus *Levinseniella* Stiles and Hassall, 1901

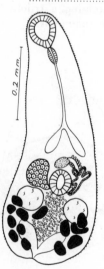

Etges (1953) investigated the life cycle of *L. amnicolae* and found it to be similar to that of *Maritreminoides obstipus* except that the cercaria is of the ubiquita type in *L. amnicolae.* Both species utilize the same host animals. Experimental infections were established in chicks and mice. Natural infections occur in ducks.

Stunkard (1958) described the life cycle of *L. minuta,* a parasite of the scaup duck, *Nyroca affinis.* Embryonated eggs were fed

Fig. 505. *Levinseniella amnicolae.*

to *Hydrobia minuta* in which mother and daughter sporocysts developed. The latter produced monostomate tailless cercariae which encysted in the host snail. The adult flukes developed in one to three days in mice that were fed metacercariae.

8b. Genital atrium contains one muscular papilla; parasites of birds and mammals (Fig. 506). ....
....**Genus** *Spelotrema* **Jägerskiold, 1901**

Life cycle: *S. pirum*—

Embryonated eggs are eaten by the snail, *Thais emarginata,* in which xiphidiocercariae resembling the armatae group develop in daughter sporocysts. Natural infections of the metacercaria occur in the hermit crab, *Pagurus hirsutiusculus.* Metacercariae were fed to hamsters, red fox, arctic fox, and glaucus-winged gull and the adult fluke developed in all of them. The sea otter is a natural definitive host (Schiller, 1959).

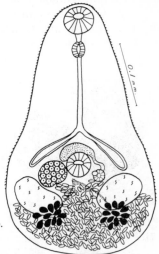

Fig. 506. *Spelotrema pygmaeum.*

SUPERFAMILY ALLOCREADIOIDEA Nicoll, 1934

Miracidia have one pair of flame cells; a variety of cercariae such as microcercous and macrocercous, which develop in sporocysts, or oculate trichocercous and ophthalmoxiphidiocercariae which develop in rediae are produced in snails or lamellibranch molluscs; excretory system of cercariae usually of mesostomate type; cercariae usually encyst in arthropods; three hosts involved in life cycle.

FAMILY ALLOCREADIIDAE Stossich, 1903

Body nonspinous, suckers well developed, oral sucker with muscular papillae in some genera; intestinal ceca end blindly, usually long, more rarely half long; testes tandem, opposite or oblique; cirrus sac present; seminal vesicle internal; ovary pretesticular; uterus extending posterior to ovary; vitelline follicles abundant, filling most of lateral regions of body; excretory vesicle I-shaped or saccular; parasites of freshwater fishes, one genus in amphibians.

It has been proposed that this family be reserved for those trematodes that produce ophthalmoxiphidiocercariae (Fig. 34) in rediae as part of their life cycle.

KEY TO GENERA

1a. Oral sucker with two or more muscular papillae. 2
1b. Oral sucker without muscular papillae. 7
2a. One pair of lateral muscular papillae present; parasites of freshwater fishes. 3
2b. Two or more pairs of muscular papillae present. 4
3a. Two testes, tandem; uterus entirely anterior to testes (Fig. 507).
........Genus *Creptotrema* Travassos, Artigas and Pereira, 1928
3b. Four testes, arranged in two opposite pairs; part of uterus between testes (Fig. 508). ....Genus *Megalogonia* Surber, 1928

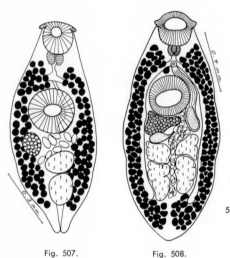

Fig. 507. *Creptotrema funduli.* Fig. 508. *Megalogonia ictaluri.*

Fig. 507.   Fig. 508.

Life cycle: *M. ictaluri*—
Ophthalmoxiphidiocercariae (Fig. 34) develop in rediae in the gill lamellae of fingernail clams (Sphaeriidae) and encyst in the gills of mayfly nymphs. The mature trematode develops in the intestine of freshwater fishes of the Genera *Ictalurus, Micropterus* and *Noturus* (see Hopkins, 1934a).

4a. One pair of ventro-lateral and one pair of transverse dorsal papillae on oral sucker; intestinal parasites of frogs (Fig. 509).
....Genus *Bunoderella* Schell, 1964

Life cycle: *B. metteri*—

About 35 days are required for development of the miracidium after eggs are laid. Ophthalmoxiphidiocercariae develop in rediae in the fingernail clam, *Pisidium idahoense.* The cercariae penetrate and encyst in the hemocoel of caddisfly and chironomid larvae. The adult fluke develops in the intestine of the tailed-frog, *Ascaphus truei,* which eats the infected insects (Anderson, Schell and Pratt, 1965).

oral sucker, dorsal view

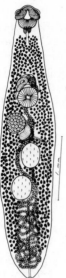

Fig. 509. *Bunoderella metteri.*

4b. One pair of ventro-lateral and two pairs of dorsal muscular papillae on oral sucker; intestinal parasites freshwater fishes.
....**5**

5a. Uterus entirely anterior to testes (Fig. 510). ....
....**Genus *Crepidostomum* Braun, 1900**

Key to species in Hopkins (1931).

Life cycle: *C. cooperi*—

Miracidia develop within seven days and hatch within 10 days after eggs are laid. They penetrate fingernail clams of the Genus *Musculium* in which ophthalmoxiphidiocercariae develop in daughter rediae. Some rediae are known to contain daughter rediae and cercariae simultaneously. The cercariae encyst in the abdominal hemocoel of mayfly nymphs. The adult flukes develop in the pyloric ceca of several species of freshwater fishes (Hopkins, 1934a).

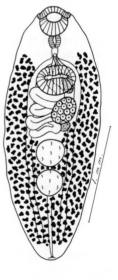

oral sucker, dorsal view

Fig. 510. *Crepidostomum farionis.*

Ameel (1937) described the life cycle of *C. cornutum*. The rediae and cercariae develop in clams of the Genera *Musculium* and *Sphaerium*. Cercariae encyst around the heart of the crayfish, *Cambarus immunis*.

5b. Uterus extends posterior to testes. 6

6a. Intestinal ceca extend only to level of testes which are nearly opposite; vitelline follicles in lateral areas of body between pharynx and cecal ends (Fig. 511). ....
....**Genus *Bunoderina* Miller, 1936**

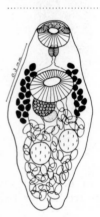

Life cycle: *B. eucaliae*—
    The work was not based on experimental infections. The eggs are embryonated at time of oviposition but do not hatch in water. Ophthalmoxiphidiocercariae develop in the fingernail clam, *Pisidium novebracense*. The second intermediate host is unknown. The adult trematode develops in the stickleback, *Eucalia inconstans* and in the mudminnow, *Umbra limi* (see Hoffman, 1955).

Fig. 511.   *Bunoderina eucaliae.*

6b. Intestinal ceca extend to posterior end of body; testes tandem or nearly so; vitelline follicles distributed all along lateral areas of body (Fig. 512). .... **Genus *Bunodera* Railliet, 1896**

Life cycle: *B. luciopercae*—
    Ophthalmoxiphidiocercariae develop in rediae in the fingernail clams, *Sphaerium rivicola* and *S. corneum*. The cercariae encyst in the hemocoel of several genera and species of cladocerans, ostracods and copepods. The adult fluke develops in numerous species of freshwater fishes that ingest the infected crustaceans (Wisniewski, 1958).

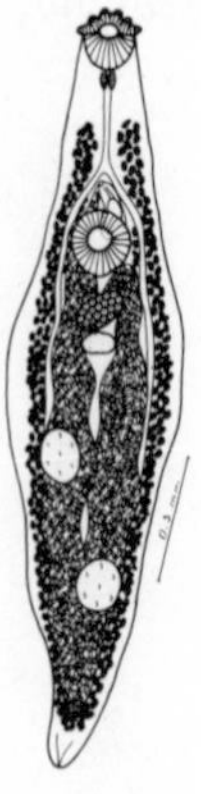

Fig. 512.   *Bunodera luciopercae.*

7a. Vitelline follicles few, in lateral rows between level of ventral sucker and ovary;
uterus extending posterior to testes; genital pore near left body margin (Fig. 513).
....................Genus *Plagiocirrus* Van Cleave
and Mueller, 1932

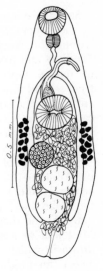

Fig. 513. *Plagiocirrus primus.*

7b. Vitelline follicles abundant, distributed along ceca; genital
pore median (Figs. 514, 515). ....
....Genus *Allocreadium* Looss, 1900

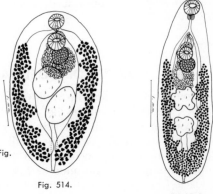

Fig. 514. *Allocreadium neotenicum.* Fig.
515. *A. lobatum.*

Fig. 514.

Fig. 515.

There is a tendency for species in this genus to be neotenic by
retaining such larval structures as the stylet and eyespots, and
progenetic by attaining sexual maturity in an arthropod which
might normally be utilized only as a second intermediate host.
Life cycle: *A. neotenicum—*

Sexually mature adults develop in the hemocoel of diving beetles of the genera *Dytiscus* and *Acilius*. Miracidia develop and hatch within two weeks and penetrate fingernail clams of the Genera *Pisidium* and *Sphaerium* in which sporocysts produce a generation of rediae. Ophthalmoxiphidiocercariae develop in the latter. A true second intermediate host is not utilized as cercariae apparently penetrate the dytiscid larvae in which developmental stages can be found. The adults retain the stylet and eyespots of the cercaria. Eggs are trapped until the beetle dies and decays (Crawford, 1940; Peters, 1955).

An account of the life cycle of *A. alloneotenicum* was published by Wootton (1957). The adult occurs in the hemocoel of caddisfly larvae of the Genus *Limnephilus*. Miracidia hatch from eggs in the debris left by decaying larvae and also from eggs that are ingested and then passed in the feces of the snail, *Aplexa hypnorum*. Miracidia penetrate the gills of the fingernail clam *Pisidium abditum* in which sporocysts develop and give rise to mother rediae. The latter produce a generation of daughter rediae in which ophthalmoxiphidiocercariae develop. Some rediae produce cercariae and rediae simultaneously. The cercariae penetrate caddisfly larvae in which the adult trematode develops.

DeGiusti (1962) described the development of *A. lobatum* to the adult stage in the digestive tract of the chub, *Semotilus atromaculatus* and the sucker, *Catostomus commersonii*. This species is also progenetic in the hemocoel of amphipods. The eggs remain trapped in the amphipod until it dies and decays. The host mollusc is *Pisidium* sp.

FAMILY OPECOELIDAE Ozaki, 1925

Body oval or elongate, nonspinous (minute spines in *Manteriella*); ventral sucker sessile or pedunculate, usually larger than oral sucker and having marginal papillae in some genera; pharynx present; intestinal ceca long (half long in *Eurycreadium*), end blindly, form a cyclocoel, open through separate ani, fuse and open through a single anus or fuse to excretory vesicle to form a cloaca (= uroproct); two testes, usually tandem, rarely opposite or oblique (nine testes in *Helicometrina*); cirrus sac usually present, rarely weakly developed or absent; genital pore ventral (dorsal in *Neonotoporus*), median or submedian; ovary pretesticular, smooth or lobed; vitelline follicles large, distributed along ceca; uterus entirely anterior to ovary; excretory vesicle I-shaped; chiefly intestinal parasites of marine fishes, a few in freshwater fishes.

KEY TO GENERA

1a. Intestinal ceca end blindly. 2
1b. Intestinal ceca open through one or two ani or unite with excretory vesicle to form a cloaca (= uroproct). 16
2a. Genital pore located on dorsal body surface, near left margin; testes oblique (Fig. 516).
............Genus *Neonotoporus* Srivastava, 1942
2b. Genital pore on ventral body surface. 3

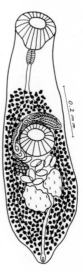

Fig. 516. *Neonotoporus yamagutii.*

3a. Eggs have unipolar filaments. 4
3b. Eggs oval, polar filaments absent. 6
4a. Nine testes present, in two longitudinal rows (Fig. 517). ....
....Genus *Helicometrina* Linton, 1910
Life cycle: *H. nimia—*
Metacercariae were found encysted in the thoracic muscles of two species of shrimp, *Lysmata intermedia* and *Crangon formosum.* A microcercous cercaria (Cercaria J of Miller, 1925), which develops in the marine snail, *Columbella mercatoria,* is thought to be the cercaria of *H. nimia.* In a laboratory experiment these cercariae encysted in the shrimp, *L. intermedia* which died later from over exposure (Manter, 1934a).

4b. One or two testes present. 5
5a. Cirrus sac long, extending far posterior to ventral sucker; vitelline follicles confined to hindbody; intestinal parasites of squirrelfish (Fig. 518). ....Genus *Stenopera* Manter, 1933

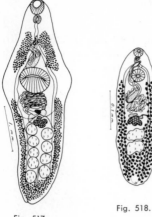

Fig. 517. *Helicometrina elongata.* (Redrawn from Noble and Park, 1937.) Fig. 518. *Stenopera equilata.*

Fig. 518.

Fig. 517.

5b. Cirrus sac short, not extending posterior to ventral sucker; vitelline follicles distributed in fore- and hindbody (one testis in H. execta) (Fig. 519). ....
....Genus *Helicometra* Odhner, 1902
Key to species in Manter (1934a) and in Skrjabin (1964).

6a. Intestinal ceca half long, extending to anterior margins of opposite testes; vitelline follicles mostly anterior to testes (Fig. 520). ....Genus *Eurycreadium* Manter, 1934

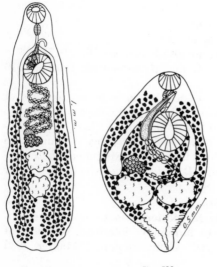

Fig. 519. *Helicometra torta.* Fig. 520. *Eurycreadium vitellosum.*

Fig. 519.   Fig. 520.

6b. Intestinal ceca long; testes tandem or oblique; many vitelline follicles posterior to testes. 7

7a. Accessory sucker between ventral sucker and genital pore; ventral sucker in fold of body wall (Fig. 521). ....
....**Genus** *Genitocotyle* **Park, 1937**

7b. Accessory sucker absent. 8

8a. Body with minute spines; posterior margin of body wavy; genital pore to left of pharynx; testes oblique or nearly opposite (Fig. 522). ....**Genus** *Manteriella* **Yamaguti, 1958** (Note: Because of the body spines there is some doubt about placing this genus in the Family Opecoelidae)

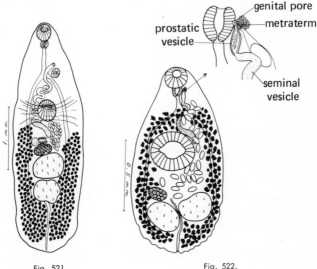

Fig. 521.   Fig. 522.

Fig. 521. *Genitocotyle acirrus.* Fig. 522. *Manteriella crassum.* (Redrawn from Manter, 1947.)

8b. Body nonspinous; posterior margin smooth; testes tandem or oblique. 9

9a. Cirrus sac absent; seminal vesicle free in parenchyma, extending posterior to ventral sucker; genital pore to left of pharynx; vitelline follicles mostly in hindbody (Fig. 523). ....
..............................**Genus** *Pseudopecoelus* **von Wicklen, 1946**

9b. Cirrus sac present, enclosing seminal vesicle; genital pore posterior to pharynx. 10

10a. Cirrus sac long, extending some distance posterior to ventral sucker; genital pore median or sinistral; ovary lobed (Fig. 524). ....**Genus** *Cainocreadium* **Nicoll, 1909**

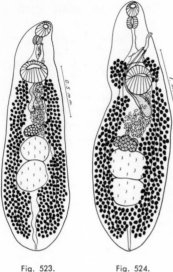

Fig. 523. *Pseudopecoelus barkeri*. Fig. 524. *Cainocreadium shawi*.

Fig. 523.   Fig. 524.

10b. Cirrus sac short, not extending posterior to ventral sucker.....11
11a. Vitelline follicles restricted to hindbody. 12
11b. Vitelline follicles distributed in fore- and hindbody; genital
      pore sinistral. 15
12a. Genital pore median, at level of cecal bifurcation or slightly
      posterior to this; ovary lobed; cirrus sac short, anterior to
      ventral sucker (Fig. 525). ....
      ....**Genus** *Apopodocotyle* **Pritchard, 1966**
12b. Genital pore sinistral, at level of cecal bifurcation or to left
      of esophagus. 13
13a. Ovary smooth; ventral sucker sessile; genital pore to left of
      cecal bifurcation (Fig. 526). ....
      .... **Genus** *Allopodocotyle* **Pritchard, 1966**
Life cycle: *A. lepomis* (= *Plagioporus lepomis*)—
   Cotylomicrocercous cercariae (Fig. 18) develop in daughter
sporocysts in the freshwater operculate snail, *Goniobasis livescens.*
They penetrate the integument of the amphipod, *Hyalella knicker-
bockeri* and encyst in the hemocoel. The adult flukes develop in
several species of freshwater fishes of the Genus *Lepomis* which
ingest infected amphipods (Dobrovolny, 1939b).
13b. Ovary lobed; genital pore sinistral. 14
14a. Ventral sucker pedunculate; genital pore to left of cecal bi-
      furcation (Fig. 527). ....
      ....**Genus** *Neopodocotyloides* **Pritchard, 1966**

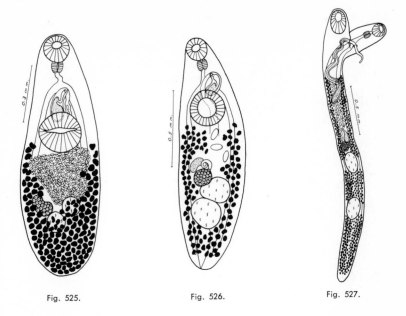

Fig. 525.   Fig. 526.   Fig. 527.

Fig. 525. *Apopodocotyle oscitans.* Fig. 526. *Allopodocotyle lepomis.* Fig. 527. *Neopodocotyloides sinusaccus.*

14b. Ventral sucker sessile; genital pore to left of esophagus (Fig. 528). ....Genus *Podocotyle* (Dujardin, 1845)

Life cycle: *P. atomon*—

Cotylomicrocercous cercariae develop in daughter sporocysts in the marine snail, *Littorina rudis* and encyst in the hemocoel of marine amphipods of the genera *Gammarus, Amphithoe* and *Carinogammarus.* From here the cycle can follow two possible courses. The metacercaria can develop to sexual maturity in the amphipods, or the infected amphipods can be eaten by the common eel, *Anguilla rostrata* or by the four-spine stickleback, *Apeltes quadracus,* in which the adult fluke then develops (Hunninen and Cable, 1943a).

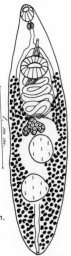

Fig. 528. *Podocotyle atomon.*

15a. Testes oblique; ovary lobed (Fig. 529). ....
....**Genus** *Hamacreadium* **Linton, 1910**

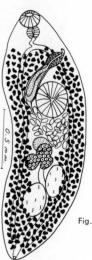

Life cycle: *H. mutabile* and *H. gulella*—

The life cycles of these species are similar. Cotylomicrocercous cercariae develop in sporocysts in the marine snail, *Astraea americana*. They encyst in marine fishes of the genera *Sparisoma, Halichoeres, Haemulon* and *Neomaenus*. The metacercariae are known to be infective for the definitive host within three days after encystment. The adult trematode develops in the intestine of a variety of marine fishes (McCoy, 1929, 1930).

Fig. 529. *Hamacreadium mutabile.*

15b. Testes tandem, ovary lobed or smooth; or testes oblique, ovary smooth (Fig. 530, 531). ....
....**Genus** *Plagioporus* **Stafford, 1904**

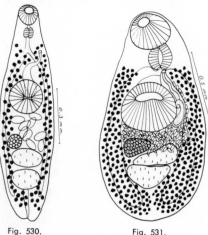

Fig. 530. *Plagioporus serotinus.* (Redrawn from Miller, 1940.) Fig. 531. *P. crassigulus.*

Fig. 530.   Fig. 531.

Key to species in Manter (1954) and in Skrjabin (1964). Life cycle: *P. sinitsini*—

Miracidia develop and hatch within 12 to 20 days after oviposition. Cotylomicrocercous cercariae develop in daughter sporocysts in the freshwater operculate snail, *Goniobasis livescens*. The cercariae lose their tails and encyst in the sporocysts which eventually escape from the snail and fall into the water. These sporocysts are ingested by cyprinid and catostomatid fishes in the gall bladder of which the adult trematodes develop within 15 to 30 days (Dobrovolny, 1939a).

The life cycle of *P. siliculus* differs from the above cycle in that the cercariae leave the sporocyst and the snail and finally encyst in the muscles of the crayfish, *Potamobius* sp. The adult fluke develops in the intestine of cutthroat trout (Sinitsin, 1931).

16a. **Ventral sucker distinctly pedunculate; intestinal ceca united with excretory vesicle to form a cloaca.** 17

16b. **Ventral sucker sessile or on a very short peduncle; intestinal ceca open through one or two ani.** 18

17a. **Accessory sucker at base of peduncle; papillae present on ventral sucker; genital pore near base of peduncle (Fig. 532).** ....**Genus *Opecoeloides* Odhner, 1928**

Life cycle: *O. vitellosus* (= *Anisoporus manteri*)—

Cotylomicrocercous cercariae develop in sporocysts in the marine snail, *Mitrella lunata* and encyst in the marine amphipods, *Carinogammarus mucronatus* and *Amphithoe longimana*. Several species of marine fishes serve as definitive host (Hunninen and Cable, 1941).

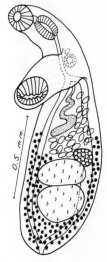

Fig. 532. *Opecoeloides brachyteleus.* (Redrawn from Manter, 1947.)

17b. **Accessory sucker absent; no papillae on ventral sucker; genital pore at level of pharynx (Fig. 533).** ....
...................**Genus *Pseudopecoeloides* Yamaguti, 1940**

18a. **Papillae present on ventral sucker; intestinal ceca fused and open through a single anus; external seminal vesicle present.** 19

18b. Papillae absent on ventral sucker; intestinal ceca open through one or two ani; external seminal vesicle present or absent. 20

19a. Seminal vesicle does not extend posterior to ventral sucker; vitelline follicles present in fore- and hindbody (Fig. 534). ....Genus *Opegaster* Ozaki, 1928

19b. Seminal vesicle extends posterior to ventral sucker; vitelline follicles restricted to hindbody (Fig. 535). ....Genus *Opecoelus* Ozaki, 1925

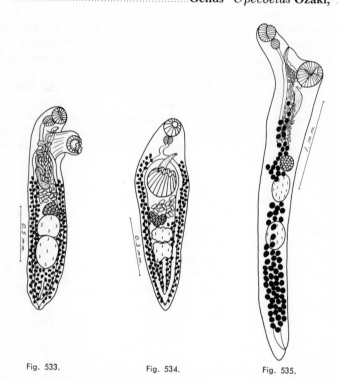

Fig. 533.   Fig. 534.   Fig. 535.

Fig. 533. *Pseudopecoeloides equesi.* Fig. 534. *Opegaster synodi.* Fig. 535. *Opecoelus adsphaericus.* (Redrawn from Manter and Van Cleave, 1951.)

20a. Genital pore to left of esophagus; cirrus sac and external seminal vesicle present; ceca fused and open through a single anus (Fig. 536). ....Genus *Opecoelina* Manter, 1934

20b. Genital pore to left of pharynx; cirrus sac present or absent, but if present, no external seminal vesicle; intestinal ceca open through separate ani. 21

21a. Cirrus sac present; ventral sucker large and conical (Fig. 537).
....Genus *Pellamyzon* Montgomery, 1957

21b. Cirrus sac absent; seminal vesicle and prostate cells free in parenchyma; ventral sucker spherical (Fig. 538). ....
....Genus *Neopecoelus* Manter, 1947

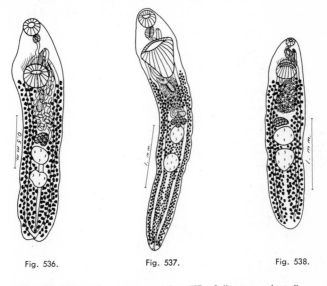

Fig. 536.   Fig. 537.   Fig. 538.

Fig. 536. *Opecoelina scorpaenae.* Fig. 537. *Pellamyzon sebastodis.*
Fig. 538. *Neopecoelus scorpaenae.*

FAMILY LEPOCREADIIDAE Nicoll, 1934

Body spinous, elongate, oval or round; pigmented eyespots present in younger specimens; intestinal ceca usually long, end blindly (open through separate ani in *Bianium* and *Diploproctodaeum*); testes tandem, opposite or oblique, usually two (10 to 11 in *Multitestis* and *Rhagorchis*); cirrus sac usually present (absent in *Barbulostomum, Homalometron* and *Crassicutis*); internal and external seminal vesicles present; genital pore usually anterior to ventral sucker (posterior to ventral sucker in *Postporus*); ovary pretesticular; seminal receptacle present; vitelline follicles numerous; uterus entirely anterior to ovary; excretory vesicle I-shaped; primarily intestinal parasites of marine fishes, a few species in freshwater fishes. At present it is assumed that trematodes in this family produce oculate trichocercous or homalometronine cercariae in rediae in snails.

KEY TO GENERA

1a. Body round, flat, margins curved ventrally; testes opposite, lobed; intestinal ceca arcuate; parasites of trunkfish. 2
1b. Body elongate or oval, plump; testes tandem or oblique, not lobed. 3
2a. Ventral surface of body with numerous glands (Fig. 539). ....
....Genus *Dermadena* Manter, 1946

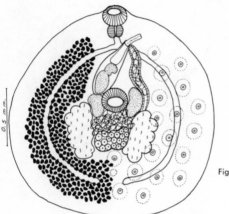

Fig. 539. *Dermadena lactophrysi.*

2b. Ventral surface of body without glands (Fig. 540). ....
....Genus *Pseudocreadium* Layman, 1930

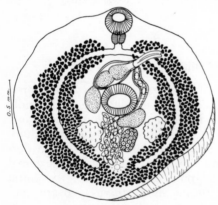

Fig. 540. *Pseudocreadium lamelli-forme.*

3a. Ten to 11 testes present. 4
3b. One or two testes present. 5
4a. Testes arranged in two opposite clusters with the ovary between them; some vitelline follicles anterior to ventral sucker (Fig. 541). ....Genus *Multitestis* Manter, 1931

Key to species in Skrjabin (1964).

4b. **Testes in a single median group; ovary pretesticular; vitelline follicles restricted to area posterior to ventral sucker (Fig. 542); parasite of filefishes.** ....Genus *Rhagorchis* **Manter, 1931**

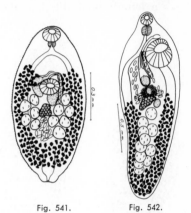

Fig. 541.   *Multitestis inconstans.*
Fig. 542.   *Rhagorchis odhneri.*

Fig. 541.   Fig. 542.

5a. **Intestinal ceca opening through separate ani at posterior end of body; anterior part of body flattened and wider than posterior part.** **6**

5b. **Intestinal ceca and body not as described above.** **7**

6a. **Vitelline follicles extend from level of ventral sucker to posterior end of body; ovary lobed (Fig. 543).** ....
....Genus *Bianium* **Stunkard, 1930**

6b. **Vitelline follicles some distance posterior to ventral sucker; ovary ovoid (Fig. 544); parasite of filefishes.** ....
....Genus *Diploproctodaeum* **LaRue, 1926**

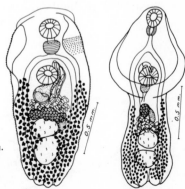

Fig. 543.   *Bianium plicitum.* Fig.
544. *Diploproctodaeum haustrum.*

Fig. 543.   Fig. 544.

7a. Genital pore posterior to ventral sucker; pigment granules in forebody (Fig. 545). ....Genus *Postporus* Manter, 1949
7b. Genital pore anterior to ventral sucker. 8
8a. Posterior margin of body crenulate; cavity of ventral sucker a longitudinal slit; bounded by semicircular striae (Fig. 546). ....Genus *Myzoxenus* Manter, 1934

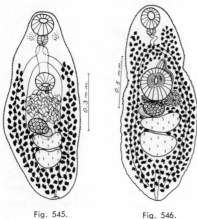

Fig. 545. *Postporus epinepheli.* Fig. 546. *Myzoxenus vitellosus.*

Fig. 545.   Fig. 546.

Key to species in Skrjabin (1964).
8b. Body not crenulate; ventral sucker not as described above. 9
9a. Oral sucker with two or more muscular papillae. 10
9b. Oral sucker without muscular papillae. 12
10a. Oral sucker with one pair of ventro-lateral muscular papillae; cirrus sac absent; body linguiform; vitelline follicles restricted to hindbody (Fig. 547). ....
..............................Genus *Barbulostomum* Ramsey, 1965

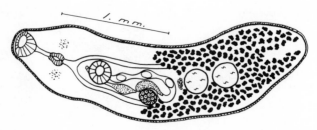

Fig. 547. *Barbulostomum cupuloris.*

10b. Eight to 10 muscular papillae on anterior margin of oral sucker. 11

11a. One testis; small accessory sucker anterior to ventral sucker; ceca fused with excretory vesicle to form cloaca (Fig. 548). ....Genus *Cadenatella* Dollfus, 1946

11b. Two testes; accessory sucker absent; ceca fused at posterior end, opening through an anus (Fig. 549). ....
....Genus *Enenterum* Linton, 1910

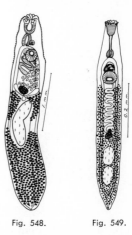

Fig. 548. *Cadenatella americana.* (Redrawn from Manter, 1949.) Fig. 549. *Enenterum aureum.*

Fig. 548.   Fig. 549.

12a. Terminal portions of male and female reproductive ducts fused to form long hermaphroditic duct (Fig. 550). ....
....Genus *Apocreadium* Manter, 1937

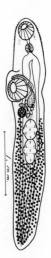

Fig. 550. *Apocreadium balistis.* (Redrawn from Manter, 1947.)

12b. Hermaphroditic duct absent. 13

13a. Testes opposite; vitelline follicles entirely posterior to testes; body less than 1 mm. long (Fig. 551). ....
....**Genus** *Microcreadium* **Simer, 1929**

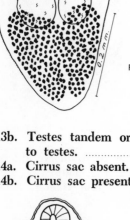

Life cycle: *M. parvum—*

The life cycle is similar to that of *Homalometron armatum.* Cercariae of the homalometronine type develop in rediae in the operculate freshwater snail, *Amnicola peracuta* and encyst in the fingernail clam, *Musculium ferrissi* (see Hopkins, 1937).

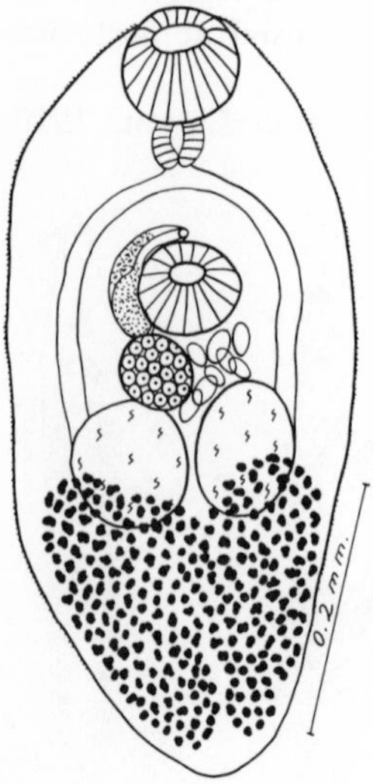

Fig. 551.　*Microcreadium parvum.*

13b. Testes tandem or oblique; most vitelline follicles anterior to testes. 14

14a. Cirrus sac absent. 15

14b. Cirrus sac present. 16

15a. Vitelline follicles confluent anterior to ventral sucker; body spines absent; cuticle thick (Fig. 552). ....
.... **Genus** *Crassicutis* **Manter, 1936**

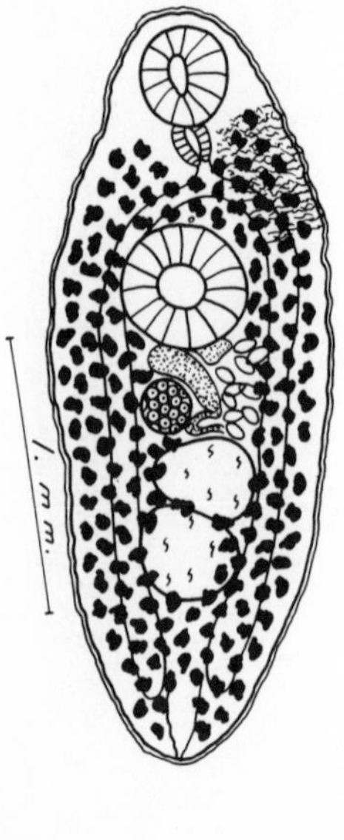

Fig. 552.　*Crassicutis marina.*

15b. Vitelline follicles confined to hindbody; body spines present; cuticle thin (Fig. 553). .... Genus *Homalometron* **Stafford, 1904** (= *Anallocreadium* **Simer, 1929**)

Key to species in Skrjabin (1964).
Life cycle: *H. pallidum—*

Eggs, which are nonembryonated when laid, were incubated in seawater and after miracidia developed, were fed to the marine snail, *Hydrobia minuta*, in which homalometronine cercariae developed in daughter rediae. The cercariae encysted in *H. minuta, Gemma gemma* and in small polychaete annelids. The natural definitive host is *Fundulus heteroclitus* (see Stunkard, 1964a).

Hopkins (1934b, 1937) described the life cycle of *H. armatum*. Homalometronine cercariae develop in rediae in the operculate freshwater snail, *Amnicola peracuta*, and encyst in clams of the Families Unionidae and Sphaeriidae.

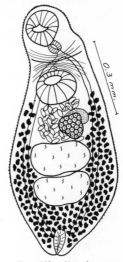

Fig. 553. *Homalometron pallidum.*

16a. Cirrus sac short, not extending posterior to ventral sucker; testes tandem; body plump; vitelline follicles in fore- and hindbody (Fig. 554). .... Genus *Lepidauchen* **Nicoll, 1913**

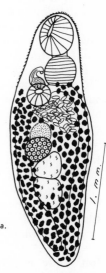

Fig. 554. *Lepidauchen hysterospina.*

16b. Cirrus sac long, extending posterior to ventral sucker. 17

17a. External seminal vesicle not surrounded by prostate cells or a membranous sac. 18

17b. External seminal vesicle surrounded at least in part by prostate cells; membranous sac present or absent. 19

18a. Esophagus short; external seminal vesicle elongate; vitelline follicles in fore- and hindbody or only in hindbody (Figs. 555, 556). ....Genus *Lepocreadium* Stossich, 1904

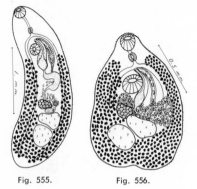

Fig. 555. *Lepocreadium retrusum.* Fig. 556. *L. trulla.*

Fig. 555.   Fig. 556.

Key to species in Edwards and Nahhas (1968).

Life cycle: *L. setiferoides*—Oculate trichocercous cercariae (Fig. 41) develop in rediae in the marine snail, *Nassa obsoleta.* They encyst in the turbellarian, *Procerodes warreni* and in the annelid, *Spio* sp. The adult fluke develops in the flounder and the sand dab (Martin, 1938).

Palombi (1931, 1937) described the life cycle of *L. album.* Miracidia hatch and penetrate the marine snails, *Nassa mutabilis* and *N. corniculum,* in which trichocercous cercariae are produced in rediae. The cercariae encyst in nudibranchs. Marine fishes of several species serve as definitive host, but experimental infections were established only in the blenny, *Blennius gattorugine.*

18b. Esophagus long and partly glandular; external seminal vesicle ovoid; vitelline follicles usually confined to hindbody (Fig. 557). .... Genus *Opechona* Looss, 1907
Key to species in Skrjabin (1964).

19a. External seminal vesicle surrounded by prostate cells and a membranous sac (Fig. 558). ....
....Genus *Lepidapedon* Stafford, 1904

19b. Only anterior portion of external seminal vesicle surrounded by prostate cells; membranous sac absent (Fig. 559). ....
....Genus *Neolepidapedon* Manter, 1954

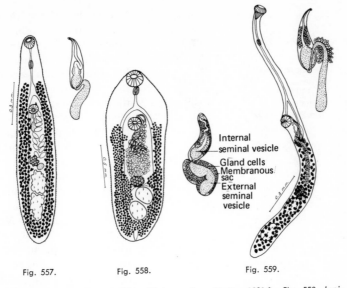

Fig. 557.   Fig. 558.   Fig. 559.

Fig. 557. *Opechona menidiae.* (Redrawn from Manter, 1931.) Fig. 558. *Lepidapedon nicolli.* (Redrawn from Manter, 1934b.) Fig. 559. *Neolepidapedon medialunae.*

FAMILY DEROPRISTIIDAE Skrjabin, 1958
emended Peters, 1961

Body elongate, densely spinous, spines sometimes locally enlarged to form spiny collar or spiny patches; eyespots present in young adult; ceca long; testes tandem or slightly oblique; cirrus sac contains spiny cirrus and usually a bipartite seminal vesicle; hermaphroditic duct present; genital pore median or submedian, anterior to ventral sucker; ovary pretesticular; seminal receptacle present; vitelline follicles restricted to hindbody; uterus extends posterior to ovary, sometimes posterior to testes; metraterm well developed, sometimes spiny; excretory vesicle saccular; intestinal parasites of freshwater and marine fishes.

KEY TO GENERA

1a. Anterior end of body inflated (widened). 2
1b. Anterior end of body not inflated; parasites of sturgeon. 3
2a. Anterior end of body with distinct patches of enlarged spines; ovary separated from seminal vesicle by some folds of uterus; ceca extend to posterior end of body; uterus extends posterior to testes; parasites of common eel and sturgeon (Fig. 560). ....Genus *Deropristis* Odhner, 1902

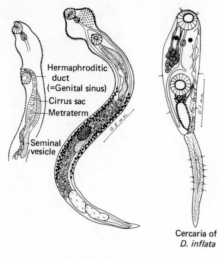

Fig. 560.   Deropristis inflata.

Cercaria of
D. inflata

Life cycle: *D. inflata*—

Eggs in the terminal portion of the uterus are embryonated but do not hatch in water. It is assumed that eggs are ingested by the first intermediate host. Oculate cercariae, resembling the homalometronine type, develop in daughter rediae in the marine snail, *Bittium alternatum* and encyst in the parapodia and body tissues of the polychaete annelid, *Nereis virens*. The adult trematode develops in the intestine of the common eel, *Anguilla rostrata* (Cable and Hunninen, 1942a).

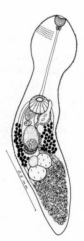

2b.   Body without patches of enlarged spines, anterior end of body just uniformly spinous; ovary close to seminal vesicle, not separated from it by folds of uterus; ceca extend only to testes; uterus extends posterior to testes (Fig. 561). ......
..................Genus *Cestrahelmins* Fischthal, 1957

Fig. 561.   Cestrahelmins laruei.

3a.   Anterior end of body with a ventrally-interrupted collar of large spines; cirrus sac, metraterm and hermaphroditic duct long (Fig. 562). ....Genus *Pristicola* Cable, 1952

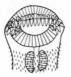

Circumoral spines, dorsal view

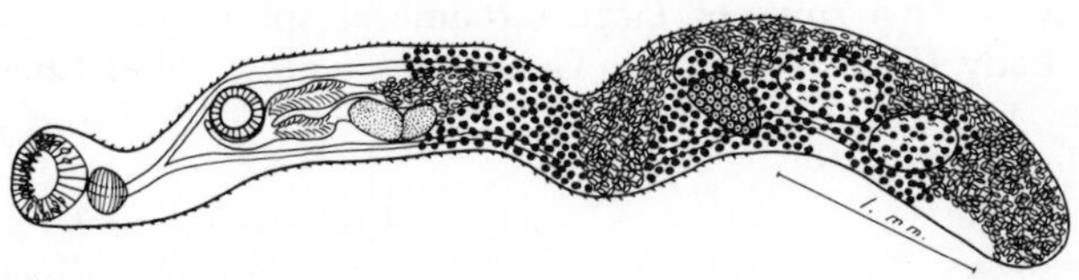

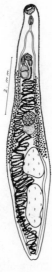

Fig. 562. *Pristicola sturionis.* (Redrawn from Little, 1930.)

3b. Anterior end of body without collar of large spines, body just uniformly spinous; cirrus sac, metraterm and hermaphroditic duct short (Fig. 563). ....
....**Genus** *Skrjabinopsolus* **Ivanov, 1935**

Life cycle: *S. manteri*—
Peters (1961) proposed a possible life cycle for this species, based on circumstantial evidence obtained through observation of natural infections and some experimental infections. He maintains that the oculate trichocercous cercaria reported by Seitner (1951) for *Allocreadium ictaluri* is really the cercaria of *S. manteri*. This cercaria develops in a redia in an operculate freshwater snail, *Pleurocera acuta*. It has an epithelial excretory vesicle, pigmented eyespots and single setae on body and tail, thus resembling the homalometronine type of cercaria. The metacercariae occur in freshwater oligochaetes upon which sturgeon feed.

Fig. 563. *Skrjabinopsolus manteri.*

FAMILY ACANTHOCOLPIDAE Lühe, 1902

Body elongate, densely spinous, large circumoral spines present in some genera; eyespots present in young adults; intestinal ceca end blindly or fuse with excretory vesicle; testes tandem, in posterior third of body; ovary pretesticular; seminal receptacle absent; hermaphroditic duct present; genital pore anterior to ventral sucker; vitelline follicles abundant, restricted to hindbody; uterus entirely anterior to ovary; excretory vesicle Y-shaped; parasites of fishes.

KEY TO GENERA

1a. **One or two rows of large circumoral spines at anterior end of body (Fig. 564).** ....Genus *Stephanostomum* Looss, 1899
Key to species in Manter and Van Cleave (1951) and in Caballero (1952).

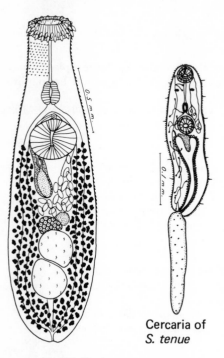

Fig. 564. *Stephanostomum casum.*

Cercaria of
S. tenue

Life cycle: *S. tenue*—
Oculate xiphidiocercariae with a spiny body and epithelial excretory vesicle develop in rediae in the marine snail, *Nassa obsoleta*. After leaving the snail, the cercariae are probably ingested by the silverside, *Menidia notata*, in which they encyst. Metacercariae were fed to the Northern puffer, *Sphaeroides maculatus* and the adult flukes recovered. The natural definitive host is the striped bass, *Roccus saxatilis* (see Martin 1939a).

Wolfgang (1955) described the life cycle of *S. baccatum*. Oculate cercariae, without a stylet, develop in rediae in the marine snails, *Buccinum undatum* and *Neptunea decumcostatum*. Cercariae encyst in the subcutaneous connective tissue, muscles and gills of flounder. The adult fluke develops in the rectum of several species of marine fishes.

Stunkard (1961) investigated the life cycle of *S. dentatum*. The cercaria is probably *C. dipterocerca* which differs from other cercariae reported for species of *Stephanostomum* in having lateral and ventral finfolds on the tail.

1b. Large circumoral spines absent (Fig. 565). ....
.............................Genus *Tormopsolus* **Poche, 1926**
Key to species in Skrjabin (1964).

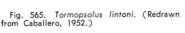

Fig. 565. *Tormopsolus lintoni.* (Redrawn
from Caballero, 1952.)

FAMILY MEGAPERIDAE Manter, 1934

Body round, oval or elongate, spinous anteriorly; oral sucker
larger than ventral sucker; pharynx wide, anterior margin lobed;
intestinal ceca wide, opening through separate ani; testes opposite, anterior to ventral sucker; cirrus sac absent; genital pore anterior to ventral sucker; ovary in hindbody; vitelline follicles fill
most of hindbody; uterus entirely anterior to ovary; excretory
vesicle I-shaped; intestinal parasites of trunk-, cow- and filefishes.

KEY TO GENERA

1a. Oral sucker without plasmic regions between muscle bands;
oral sucker enclosed in fold of body wall (Fig. 566). ....
....Genus *Thysanopharynx* **Manter, 1933**
1b. Oral sucker has plasmic regions separating radial muscle bands;
oral sucker not in cuticular fold of body wall (Fig. 567). ....
....Genus *Megapera* **Manter, 1934**

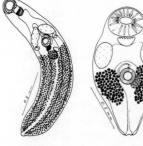

Fig. 566. *Thysanopharynx elongatus.* Fig.
567. *Megapera pseudura.*

Fig. 566.   Fig. 567.

Life cycle: *M. gyrina*—Oculate cercariae with ventral and lateral finfolds on the tail, develop in rediae in the gastropod, *Crepidula convexa*. This cercaria cannot now be assigned to a specific group. They encyst in the open (Cable, 1954c).

FAMILY OPISTHOLEBETIDAE Fukui, 1929

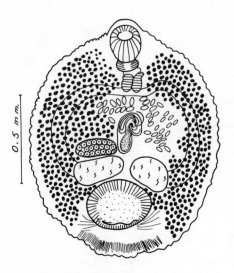

Fig. 568. *Opistholebes adcotylophorus.* (Redrawn from Manter, 1947.)

Body flat, round, margins crenulate; ventral sucker near posterior end of body and larger than oral sucker; muscular ring between oral sucker and pharynx; intestinal ceca long, arcuate; testes opposite, anterior to ventral sucker; cirrus sac present; genital pore median, in middle of body; ovary anterior to testes; vitelline follicles in wide zone along ceca; uterus fills intercecal space anterior to testes; intestinal parasites of marine fishes.

Two species of the Genus *Opistholebes* Nicoll, 1915 (Fig. 568) occur in North America as parasites of porcupine fishes. Key to species in Cable (1956).

FAMILY ORCHIPEDIDAE Skrjabin, 1924

Body elongate, nonspinous; ventral sucker larger than oral sucker; ceca long, end blindly; testes follicular (15 to 300); cirrus sac absent; ovary pretesticular; genital pore median, anterior to ventral sucker; vitelline follicles abundant, distributed along ceca; uterus entirely anterior to ovary; excretory vesicle tubular; parasites in trachea, nasal cavities and esophagus of birds.

Although two genera have been described in the family, only the Genus *Orchipedum* Braun, 1901 (Fig. 569) is regarded as valid for the following reason. Metacercariae, supposedly of *O. isostomum*, from the muscles of crayfishes were fed to several different carnivorous mammals and the adult trematodes recovered from their nasal cavities. For these specimens Skrjabin (1947) proposed the generic name *Mammorchipedum*. The latter genus is not here regarded as valid because of the lack of satisfactory diagnostic features.

Key to species in Schell (1967b).

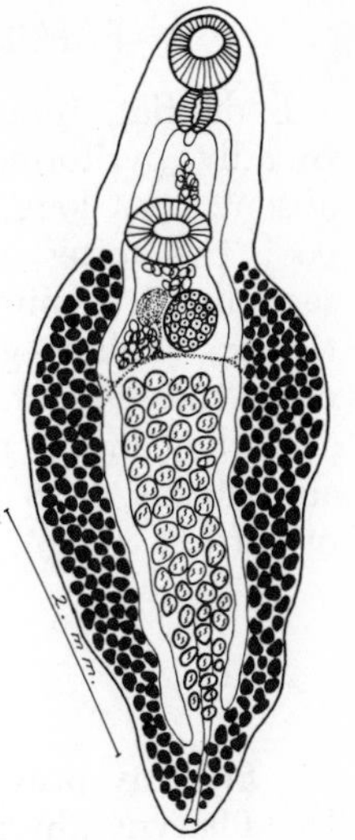

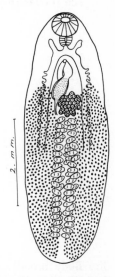

Fig. 569.   *Orchipedum tracheicola.*

FAMILY PLEORCHIIDAE Poche, 1926

Body linguiform to elongate, spinous; pigmented eyespots present; suckers well developed, in anterior third of body; intestinal ceca long, each with an anterior diverticulum; testes numerous (follicular) arranged in several longitudinal rows between ceca; cirrus sac present; ovary lobed, anterior to testes; genital pore median, anterior to ventral sucker; vitelline follicles small, fill lateral areas of hindbody; uterus entirely anterior to ovary; intestinal parasites of marine fishes.

The family contains one genus, *Pleorchis* Railliet, 1896 (Fig. 570). Two species have been reported from North America as parasites of sea trout and sea bass. Key to species in Skrjabin (1964).

Fig. 570.   *Pleorchis californiensis.*

FAMILY GORGODERIDAE Looss, 1901

Body flat, translucent, nonspinous, lanceolate, banjo-shaped or broadly pyriform; suckers well developed; pharynx present or absent; ceca long, sinuous, ending blindly or fused to form cyclocoel; two testes, usually opposite (9 to 11 in *Gorgodera*); cirrus sac absent; genital pore median; ovary pretesticular or intertesticular; vitelline glands in form of two opposite compact or dendritic masses, anterior to testes; uterus long with descending and ascending limbs; parasites in the urinary bladder of teleost fishes, amphibians or in the coelom of elasmobranchs, or in gall bladder of turtles.

KEY TO GENERA

1a. Pharynx present. 2
1b. Pharynx absent. 5
2a. Body with parallel sides, truncate at posterior end with two posterior papillae; two compact vitelline glands; in gall bladder of turtles (Fig. 571). ....
....Genus *Bicornuata* Pearse, 1949
2b. Body pyriform or nearly banjo-shaped; vitelline glands dendritic. 3
3a. Body nearly banjo-shaped; in urinary bladder and cloaca of sea turtles (Fig. 572). ....Genus *Plesiochorus* Looss, 1901

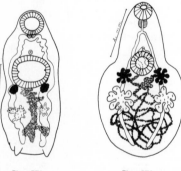

Fig. 571. *Bicornuata caretta.* (Redrawn from Pearse, 1949.) Fig. 572. *Plesiochorus cymbiformis.*

Fig. 571.   Fig. 572.

3b. Body broadly pyriform; in coelom of elasmobranchs. 4
4a. Vitelline glands lateral to intestinal ceca; ceca without diverticula (Fig. 573). ....Genus *Probolitrema* Looss, 1902

4b. Vitelline glands median to intestinal ceca; ceca with short diverticula (Fig. 574). ....Genus *Nagmia* Nagaty, 1930

5a. Body banjo-shaped; parasites of fishes and amphibians. 6

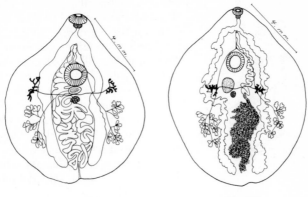

Fig. 573.   Fig. 574.

Fig. 573. *Probolitrema californiense*. (Redrawn from Stunkard, 1935.) Fig. 574. *Nagmia floridensis*. (Redrawn from Markell, 1953.)

5b. Body lanceolate; parasites of amphibians. 7

6a. Intestinal ceca fused posteriorly to form a cyclocoel; in urinary bladder of marine fishes (Fig. 575). .... Genus *Xystretum* Linton, 1910

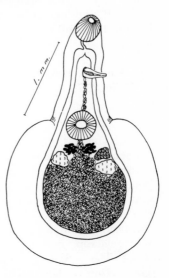

Fig. 575. *Xystretum solidum*.

6b. Intestinal ceca end blindly; in urinary bladder of marine and freshwater fishes and amphibians (Fig. 576). ....
....Genus *Phyllodistomum* Braun, 1899
Key to species in Skrjabin (1964).

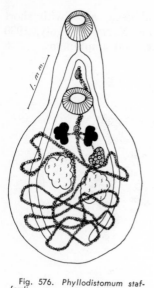

Fig. 576. *Phyllodistomum staffordi.*

Life cycle: *P. solidum—*

Embryonated eggs pass in the urine and miracidia hatch as soon as the eggs enter water. The miracidia are drawn into the incurrent siphon of fingernail clams of the Genus *Pisidium* in which cystocercous cercariae (Fig. 22) are produced in daughter sporocysts which develop in the gill lamellae of the clam. After leaving the clam, the cercariae encyst in the thoracic haemocoel of dragonfly nymphs. The mature trematode develops in the urinary bladder of the dusky salamander, *Desmognathus fuscus* and in the two-lined salamander, *Eurycea bislineata* which eat the infected insects (Goodchild, 1943; Groves, 1945).

Schell (1967a) described the life cycle of *P. staffordi,* a parasite in the urinary bladder of brown bullhead, *Ameiurus nebulosus.* Cystocercous cercariae develop in daughter sporocysts in the fingernail clam, *Musculium ryckholti* and encyst in naiads of damselflies and trichopterous larvae. The bullheads acquire the parasite by ingesting infected insects.

7a. **Nine to eleven testes, arranged in two longitudinal rows (Fig. 577).** ....**Genus** *Gorgodera* **Looss, 1899**

Life cycle: *G. amplicava—*

Embryonated, nonoperculate eggs pass in the urine of the host. Miracidia hatch when eggs enter water and are swept into the incurrent siphon of the fingernail clam, *Musculium partumeium.* They penetrate the gill lamellae and metamorphose to the mother sporocyst stage. Cystocercous cercariae (Fig. 22) develop in daughter sporocysts and leave the snail by way of the excurrent siphon. The cercariae are eaten by snails, *Physa, Lymnaea, Pseudosuccinea* and *Helisoma* spp., by tadpoles of frogs and salamanders, and by crayfishes. The cercariae encyst in the intestinal wall of these hosts. The definitive hosts which might be frogs (*Rana* spp.), toads (*Bufo* spp.) or salamanders (*Ambystoma maculatum*) acquire their parasites by eating the infected intermediate hosts. The trematodes undergo their final development in the urinary bladder (Krull, 1935d; Goodchild, 1948).

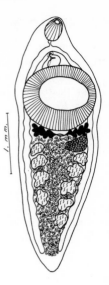

Fig. 577. Gorgodera sp.

7b. Two testes (Fig. 578). ....Genus *Gorgoderina* Looss, 1902

Key to species in Skrjabin (1964).
Life cycle: *G. attenuata*—
Embryonated eggs from the feces of the host hatch
when they enter water. The miracidia enter the fingernail clam, *Sphaerium occidentalis* by way of the incurrent siphon. Cystocercous cercariae (Fig. 22) develop in daughter sporocysts in the gill chamber of
the clam. After leaving the clam, the cercariae are
eaten by tadpoles in which they encyst around the
heart and liver. Frogs become infected by eating infected tadpoles. The developmental stages remain for
a time in the Wolffian ducts and kidneys of the frogs
then finally enter the urinary bladder where they mature. Natural infections by the adult fluke have been
found in frogs of the Genus *Rana* and in the newt,
Triturus viridescens.

The metacercariae have nine testes like trematodes
in the Genus *Gorgodera,* but by the time the adult
stage develops, only two testes are present (Rankin,
1939a).

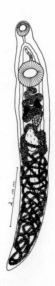

Fig. 578. Gorgoderina sp.

FAMILY TROGLOTREMATIDAE Odhner, 1914

Body spinous, large or small, fusiform, oval or pyriform; intestinal ceca variable in length; suckers well developed (ventral sucker absent in *Collyriclum*); testes opposite, oval or lobed, located in middle or posterior part of body; cirrus sac present; genital pore posterior to ventral sucker; ovary pretesticular; uterus extends posterior to ovary; excretory vesicle V-, Y- or I-shaped; parasites in lungs or intestine of mammals or encysted in the skin of birds (*Collyriclum*).

As presented here, the family contains an odd assortment of genera. The adult trematodes all have the genital pore located posterior to the ventral sucker (*Collyriclum* excepted) and opposite testes. Life cycles are known for species in three genera. Microcercous cercariae develop in rediae in operculate snails. With more knowledge of life cycles, better disposition of genera will be possible.

KEY TO GENERA

1a. Ventral sucker absent; ovary deeply lobed; vitelline follicles in lateral clusters in anterior half of body; encysted in the skin of birds (Fig. 579). ....Genus *Collyriclum* Kossack, 1911

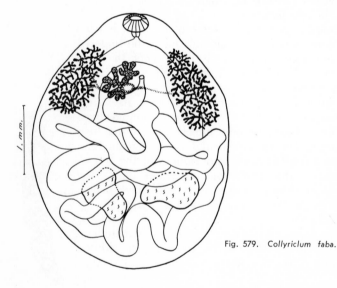

Fig. 579. *Collyriclum faba.*

1b. Ventral sucker present; parasites in intestine or lungs of mammals. 2

2a. **Body large (4 mm. or more), muscular, densely spinous; ovary and testes lobed; encysted in the lungs of mammals (Fig. 580).**
....Genus *Paragonimus* Braun, 1899

Life cycle: *P. kellicotti—*
The adult is a lung parasite of mink in North America. Eggs are swept up the trachea to the pharynx, then swallowed and leave the host in the feces. Miracidia develop and hatch in about two weeks. They penetrate the freshwater operculate snail, *Pomatiopsis lapidaria,* in which sporocysts and mother and daughter rediae develop. The latter give rise to chaetomicrocercous cercariae (Fig. 19) which leave the snail and encyst around the heart of crayfishes of the Genus *Cambarus.* The definitive host acquires the parasite by eating infected crayfish. The excysted metacercariae penetrate the intestinal wall and the diaphragm and enter the outer surface of the lungs in which they become loosely encysted in pairs (Ameel, 1934).

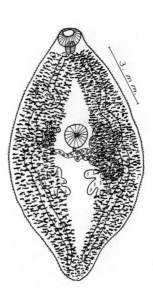

Fig. 580. *Paragonimus kellicotti.*

P. westermani is restricted to the Far East where it parasitizes human beings as well as species of feline, canine and porcine mammals. In its life cycle it utilizes the snail, *Semisulcospira libertina* as first intermediate host and edible crabs and crayfishes as second intermediate hosts. The adults are known to survive up to 20 years in the lungs of human beings. Eggs pass in human sputum and feces.

/

2b. **Body small (2 mm. or less); ovary and testes ovoid; intestinal parasites of mammals.** 3
3a. **Oral sucker with a small stylet; testes anterior to ventral sucker; vitelline follicles large, few, restricted to lateral regions posterior to level of ventral suckers; parasites of Insectivora (shrews) (Fig. 581).** ....Genus *Xiphidiotrema* Senger, 1953

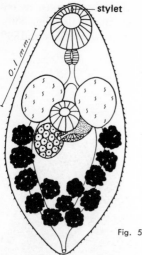

Fig. 581. *Xiphidiotrema lockerae.*

3b. Stylet absent; testes posterior to ventral sucker; vitelline follicles small, abundant, some follicles anterior to ventral sucker; intestinal parasites of Carnivora. 4

4a. Body ovoid; cirrus sac present, dorsal to ventral sucker; intestinal ceca long; vitelline follicles in lateral areas from level of pharynx to posterior end of body (Fig. 582). ....
....Genus *Nanophyetus* Chapin, 1927

Life cycle: *N. salmincola—*

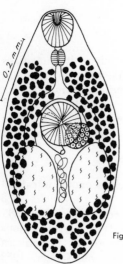

The eggs, passed in the feces of the host, are nonembryonated. About three months are required for development of the miracidium and considerably more time for hatching. The miracidia penetrate the freshwater snail, *Oxytrema silicula* in which chaetomicrocercous cercariae develop in rediae. The cercariae, discharged in mucous secretions, penetrate the skin of salmonid and other fishes, enter the blood vessels and finally encyst in the muscles, gills, kidneys and subcutaneous connective tissues. Penetration by numerous cercariae causes extensive

Fig. 582. *Nanophyetus salmincola.*

injury to the fins and gills of fishes. The adult fluke develops in the intestine of mammals such as dog, cat, fox, coyote, mink, bear and raccoon which are likely to eat infected fish (Bennington and Pratt, 1960).

The parasite is of economic importance in the Pacific Northwest because of its role in the transmission of *Neorickettsia helmintheca*, the organism that causes Salmon-poisoning disease in dogs and other members of the family Canidae.

4b. **Body pyriform; cirrus sac absent; intestinal ceca short, extending only to level of ventral sucker; vitelline follicles mostly anterior to ventral sucker (Fig. 583).** ....
....**Genus** *Sellacotyle* **Wallace, 1935**

Life cycle: *S. mustelae*—
Sulcatomicrocercous cercariae (Fig. 20) develop in rediae in the operculate freshwater snail, *Campeloma rufum*. After losing the stubby tail, the cercariae penetrate the skin of a variety of freshwater fishes such as Northern pike, yellow perch, black bullhead, mudminnow, shiners and white sucker and finally encyst in the muscles and connective tissue. Mink, the natural definitive host, acquire the parasite by eating the infected fish. Experimental infections were established in dog, cat, rat, ferret, fox, raccoon and skunk (Wallace, 1935).

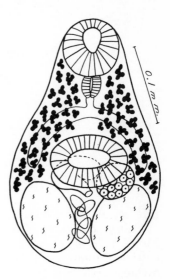

Fig. 583. *Sellacotyle mustelae.*

FAMILY ZOOGONIDAE Odhner, 1911

Body small, spinous, elongate, fusiform or linguiform; ventral sucker usually larger than oral sucker; intestinal ceca usually short; testes opposite; cirrus sac large, clubshaped, oriented transversely; ovary between, anterior, or posterior to testes; genital pore marginal or submarginal; accessory seminal receptacle sometimes present; vitelline glands exist as clusters of follicles or as one or two compact masses; uterus long, filling most of posterior half of body; excretory vesicle tubular or sac shaped; primarily parasites of marine fishes.

KEY TO GENERA

1a. Vitelline glands in the form of one or two compact masses. 2
1b. Vitelline glands follicular. 5
2a. Vitelline glands compact, bilobed, between testes; ovary between or slightly anterior to testes (Fig. 584). ....
....Genus *Diphtherostomum* Stossich, 1904

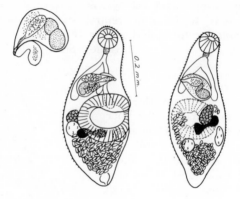

Fig. 584. *Diphtherostomum americanum.* (Redrawn from Manter, 1947.)

Life cycle: *D. brusinae*—
Tailless cercariae develop in sporocysts in the marine snails, *Natica poliana*, *Nassa mutabilis* and *N. reticulata*. Cercariae encyst and transform to metacercariae directly in the sporocysts. Metacercariae are later emitted by the snail, fall to the ocean floor and are ingested from there by marine fishes (Palombi, 1930; Prevot, 1966).

2b. Vitelline gland a single compact mass, located posterior to testes; ovary posterior to testes. 3

3a. Well developed genital atrium at right margin of body with an accessory seminal receptacle attached to it; cirrus sac sharply curved; intestinal ceca inflated and extend to posterior end of body (Fig. 585); parasite of black perch. ....
.... Genus *Neozoogonus* Arai, 1954

3b. Genital atrium absent; no accessory seminal receptacle; cirrus sac straight; intestinal ceca half long, extending to ventral sucker. 4

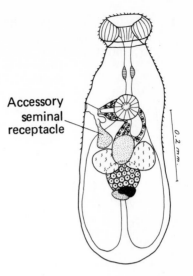

Accessory
seminal
receptacle

Fig. 585. *Neozoogonus californicus.*
(Redrawn from Arai, 1954.)

**4a. Intestinal bifurcation and cirrus sac far anterior to ventral
sucker; testes level with ventral sucker (Fig. 586).** ....
....Genus *Zoogonoides* **Odhner, 1902**

Life cycle: *Z. laevis—*

Embryonated eggs pass in the feces of
the host. The miracidium is covered by a
very thin membrane but no rigid shell as
in other trematodes. They hatch in sea
water and penetrate the marine snail, *Columbella lunata* (= *Mitrella lunata*) in
which tailless cercariae develop in daughter sporocysts. The cercariae leave the
sporocyst prematurely and complete their
development in the tissues of the snail.
After leaving the snail, the cercariae encyst in the parapodia and body wall of
the marine polychaete, *Nereis virens*. The
adut fluke develops in the tautog, *Tautoga
onitis*, and the Atlantic round herring,
Etrumeus sadina (see Stunkard, 1943).

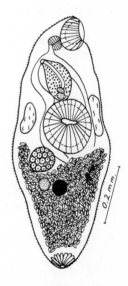

Fig. 586. *Zoogonoides laevis.*
(Redrawn from Linton, 1940.)

4b. Intestinal bifurcation dorsal or posterior to ventral sucker; cirrus sac lateral and close to ventral sucker; testes posterior to ventral sucker (Fig. 587). .... Genus *Zoogonus* Looss, 1901

Life cycle: *Z. rubellus* (= *Z. mirus*)—

Miracidia are enclosed only in the vitelline membrane. They hatch in seawater and penetrate the marine snail, *Nassa obsoleta*. Tailless cercariae develop in daughter sporocysts and encyst in the parapodia of *Nereis virens*. The adult fluke develops in the eel, *Anguilla chrysypa*, and in the toadfish, *Opsanus tau*.

Metacercariae of an unidentified species of *Zoogonus* have been found in several genera and species of sea urchins (Stunkard, 1938b, 1940).

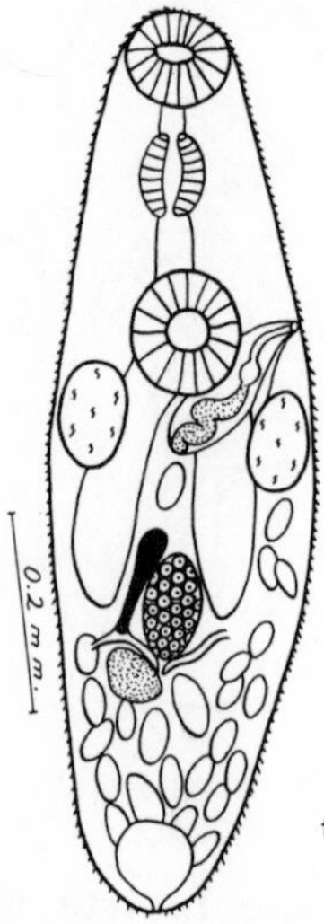

Fig. 587. *Zoogonus rubellus.* (Redrawn from Odhner, 1902.)

5a. Intestinal ceca very short, terminating anterior to ventral sucker; excretory vesicle tubular (Fig. 588). ....
.... Genus *Brachyenteron* Manter, 1934

5b. Intestinal ceca at least half long, extending some distance posterior to ventral sucker; excretory vesicle sac shaped. 6

6a. Ventral sucker near middle of body; some folds of uterus anterior to ventral sucker (Fig. 589). ....
.... Genus *Deretrema* Linton, 1910

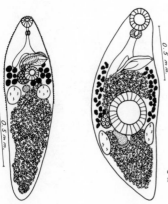

Fig. 588. *Brachyenteron peristedioni.* (Redrawn from Manter, 1934b.) Fig. 589. *Deretrema fusillus.* (Redrawn from Linton, 1910.)

Fig. 588.   Fig. 589.

6b. Ventral sucker in anterior third of body; uterus mostly posterior to ventral sucker. 7

7a. Vitelline follicles in small clusters antero-medial to testes; genital pore dorsal and sublateral (Fig. 590). ....
....Genus *Lepidophyllum* Odhner, 1902

7b. Vitelline follicles in elongate clusters anterior to testes; genital pore ventral and sublateral (Fig. 591). ....
....Genus *Steganoderma* Stafford, 1904

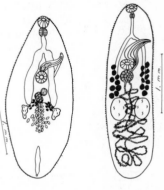

Fig. 590. *Lepidophyllum steenstrupi.* (Redrawn from Odhner, 1902.) Fig. 591. *Steganoderma formosum.* (Redrawn from Manter, 1925.)

Fig. 590.   Fig. 591.

The genus has been subdivided into two subgenera on the basis of length of intestinal ceca.

Subgenus *Steganoderma*: ceca not extending beyond testes.

Subgenus *Lecithostaphylus*: ceca extend posterior beyond testes.

FAMILY MONORCHIIDAE Odhner, 1911

Body small, spinous; suckers well developed; one or two testes; cirrus sac present; ovary pretesticular; genital atrium usually present; uterus fills posterior part of body, metraterm in the form of a spinous terminal organ enclosed in a metraterm sac; vitelline follicles usually in small compact lateral clusters; excretory vesicle tubular, saccular or V-shaped; parasites of marine and freshwater fishes.

The peculiar terminal organ (Fig. 234) is the most useful diagnostic feature for the family. The life cycles, as known for three genera, involve three kinds of cercariae some of which develop in sporocysts and some in rediae.

KEY TO GENERA

1a. Two testes, opposite. 2
1b. One testis. 3
2a. Excretory vesicle Y-shaped; uterus opens into base of terminal organ; vitelline follicles mostly anterior to testes (Fig. 592). ....**Genus** *Monorcheides* **Odhner, 1905**

Key to species in Skrjabin (1964).

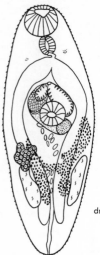

Life cycle: *M. cumingiae—*

Oculate cercariae, with lappets on the tail, develop in sporocysts in the marine clams, *Cumingia tellinoides* and *Tellina tenera.* The cercariae are swept out through the excurrent siphon and may reenter the same or a different clam and encyst in the foot, gill, mantle or wall of the incurrent siphon. The adult fluke develops in the intestine of eels and flounders which ingest infected clams (Martin, 1939b, 1940).

Fig. 592. *Monorcheides cumingiae.* (Re - drawn from Martin, 1940.)

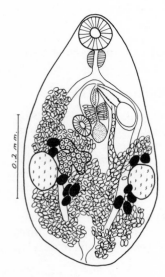

2b. Excretory vesicle tubular; uterus opens into anterior end of terminal organ; vitelline follicles medial and posterior to testes (Fig. 593). ....

.... **Genus** *Diplomonorchis* **Hopkins, 1941**

Fig. 593. *Diplomonorchis leiostomi.* (Re- drawn from Hopkins, 1941.)

3a. Parasites of freshwater fishes; genital pore marginal or submarginal, at level of ventral sucker (Fig. 594). ....
....Genus *Asymphylodora* Looss, 1899

Key to species in Skrjabin (1964).
Life cycle: *A. amnicolae—*
Embryonated eggs, passed in the feces of the host, are eaten by the operculate snail, *Amnicola limosa,* in which the miracidia hatch and transform to a sporocyst which in turn produces a generation of rediae. The latter produce tailless cercariae of the cercariaeum group. The cercariae leave the snail and enter another uninfected snail in which they either encyst and transform to metacercariae or develop directly to sexually mature adults. If they encyst, the cysts must be ingested by a fish in which they develop to the adult stage. Suitable fish are perch, killifish, small-mouthed bass or pumpkinseed (Stunkard, 1959).

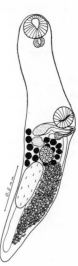

Fig. 594. *Asymphylodora atherinopsidis.*

3b. Parasites of marine fish; genital pore median or nearly median.
....**4**

4a. Vitelline follicles posterior to testis (Fig. 595). ....
........................Genus *Telolecithus* Lloyd and Guberlet, 1932

Life cycle: *T. pugetensis—*
Eggs do not contain fully developed miracidium at time of oviposition. Miracidia complete their development only after eggs are ingested by the clam, *Transennella tantilla.* Only one generation of sporocysts was observed but those were of two sizes, possibly the result of transverse fission. The cercariae have short furcae but no tail stem. The furcae are oriented in a dorso-ventral plane. They leave the clam through the excurrent siphon and upon coming into contact with any one of five species of bivalve molluscs, they penetrate and encyst. The clams that

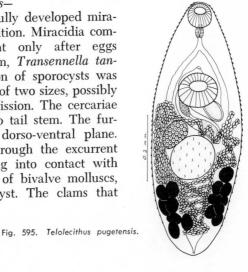

Fig. 595. *Telolecithus pugetensis.*

serve most commonly as second intermediate host are *Tellina salmonea* and *Mocona nasuta*. The definitive hosts are shiner perch, *Cymatogaster aggregata*, striped seaperch, *Embiotoca lateralis*, and the white seaperch, *Phanerodon furcatus* (see DeMartini and Pratt, 1964).

4b. Vitelline follicles anterior to testis. 5
5a. Eggs with monopolar filament. 6
5b. Eggs without monopolar filament. 7
6a. Ceca half long; eyespots present; vitelline follicles in two lateral groups (Fig. 596). ....
    ....Genus *Pseudohurleytrema* Yamaguti, 1954
6b. Ceca long; no eyespots; vitelline follicles in a single confluent mass between ovary and cirrus sac (Fig. 597). ....

    ....Genus *Hurleytrematoides* Yamaguti, 1954

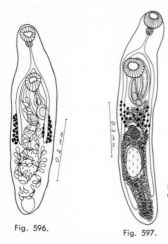

Fig. 596. *Pseudohurleytrema eucinostomi.*
Fig. 597. *Hurleytrematoides chaetodoni.* (Redrawn from Manter, 1942.)

Fig. 596.   Fig. 597.

7a. Vitelline follicles anterior or lateral to ventral sucker; body small and broadly oval (Fig. 598). ....
    ....Genus *Monorchis* Looss, 1902

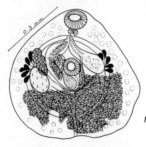

Fig. 598. *Monorchis latus.* (Redrawn from Manter, 1942.)

7b. Vitelline follicles posterior to ventral sucker. 8
8a. Uterus not extending posterior to testis (Fig. 599). ....
....Genus *Pristisomum* Looss, 1907

Life cycle: *P. donacis* (= *Post-monorchis donacis*)—

Spinous oculate cercariae (Fig. 599) develop in sporocysts in the bean clam, *Donax gouldii*, which can apparently serve as first and second intermediate host. Encysted metacercariae were fed to shiner perch, black perch, California corbina and spotfin croaker and later adult flukes were recovered (Young, 1953).

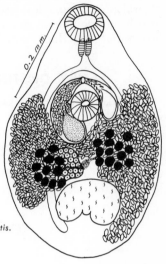

Fig. 599. *Pristisomum orthopristis*.

8b. Some folds of uterus extending posterior to testis. 9
9a. Uterus joins base of terminal organ (Fig. 600). ....
....Genus *Lasiotocus* Looss, 1907
9b. Uterus joins distal end of terminal organ (Fig. 601). ....
....Genus *Genolopa* Linton, 1910
Key to species in Skrjabin (1964).

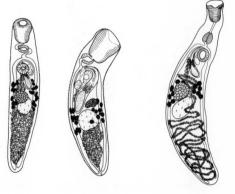

Fig. 600. *Lasiotocus longicaecum*. (Redrawn from Manter, 1940.) Fig. 601. *Genolopa beauforti*.

Fig. 600.   Fig. 601.

ORDER OPISTHORCHIIDA Larue, 1957
SUPERFAMILY OPISTHORCHIOIDEA Faust, 1929

Miracidia have one pair of flame cells; cercariae pleuro- or para-pleurolophocercous, develop in rediae in aquatic snails and encyst in fish or amphibians; three hosts involved in life cycles; parasites in intestine, bile ducts, gall bladder, or liver of vertebrates.

FAMILY OPISTHORCHIIDAE Braun, 1901

Body flat, translucent, elongate, fusiform or oval; suckers weakly developed or absent; testes usually tandem, rarely opposite or oblique, located in posterior part of body; cirrus sac usually absent; tubular seminal vesicle free in parenchyma; ovary usually pre-testicular, lobed; vitelline follicles in narrow bands lateral to ceca; uterus with ascending limb only; excretory vesicle Y-shaped; in liver, gall bladder or bile duct of reptiles, birds and mammals.

KEY TO GENERA

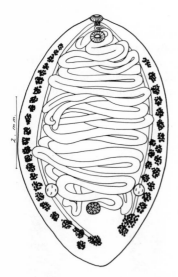

1a. Body broadly oval; suckers close together; testes opposite; ovary between or posterior to testes; parasites of birds (Fig. 602). .... **Genus** *Pachytrema* **Looss, 1907**
Key to species in Skrjabin (1964).

Fig. 602. *Pachytrema sanguineum.* (Redrawn from Linton, 1928.)

1b. Body fusiform or elongate; suckers separated by a distance equal to at least four times their diameter; testes tandem or oblique; ovary pretesticular. 2

Life cycle: *M. conjunctus*—

Embryonated eggs, passed in the feces of the host, are ingested by the operculate snail, *Amnicola limosa* in which a generation of sporocysts is followed by a generation of rediae. Pleurolophocercous cercariae develop in the rediae. After emerging from the snail, the cercariae penetrate the common sucker, *Catostomus commersoni*, and encyst in the muscles. The definitive host, which can be any one of a variety of fish-eating mammals including man, becomes infected by eating infected fish. Excysted metacercariae migrate to the liver and gall bladder by way of the bile duct (Cameron, 1944).

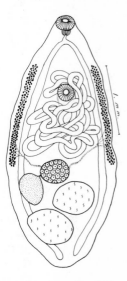

Fig. 603. *Metorchis albidus.*

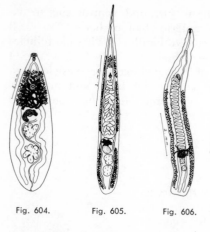

Fig. 604. *Parametorchis complexus.*
Fig. 605. *Pseudamphimerus sterni.*
(Redrawn from Gower, 1940.) Fig.
606. *Plotnikovia podilymbae.*

Fig. 604.   Fig. 605.   Fig. 606.

6a. **Testes dendritic, overlapping ceca laterally; vitelline follicles restricted to lateral areas between level of ovary and ventral sucker; parasites of mammals (Fig. 607).** ....
....**Genus** *Clonorchis* **Looss, 1907**

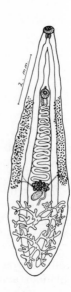

C. *sinensis,* the Chinese liver fluke, does not occur in North America but it is included here because of its importance as a parasite of cat, dog and human beings in Asia. The mature fluke inhabits the liver and bile duct. Embryonated eggs, from the feces of the host, are eaten by the operculate snails, *Parafossarulus manchouricus* and *Bulimus japonicus.* A generation of sporocysts and one of rediae develop in the snails. Pleurolophocercous cercariae develop in the rediae. Following emergence from the snail, the cercariae encyst in the muscles and connective tissues of numerous freshwater fishes. The definitive host acquires the parasite by eating infected fish. Defecation by human beings in exposed places and the custom of eating raw fish are important in the epidemiology associated with this parasite in the Orient.

Fig. 607. *Clonorchis sinensis.*

6b. **Testes lobed or with smooth margins, not overlapping ceca laterally; vitelline follicles usually extending posterior to level of ovary.** **7**

7a. Body very elongate, slender; ventral sucker distinctly smaller than oral sucker; vitelline follicles distributed in lateral areas along most of length of body but interrupted at level of ovary; parasites of reptiles, birds and mammals (Fig. 608). ....
....Genus *Amphimerus* Barker, 1911

Life cycle: *Amphimerus* sp.—
Miracidia developed in eggs kept in water but did not hatch until eggs were ingested by the aquatic snail, *Goniobasis semicarinata*. Pleurolophocercous cercariae develop in daughter rediae. Ninety days were required for development of the cercariae. The second intermediate host is unkown. The mature fluke develops in the bile duct and gall bladder of the snapping turtle, *Chelydra serpentina* (see Cable, 1939).

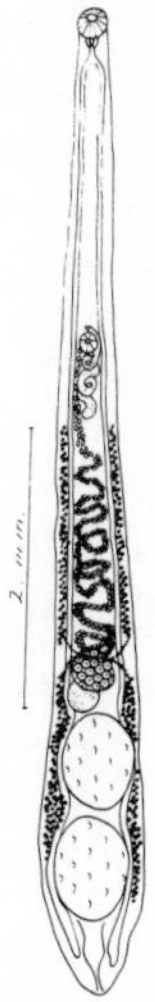

Fig. 608. *Amphimerus* sp.

7b. Body moderately elongate; suckers of equal size; vitelline follicles not interrupted at level of ovary; parasites of birds and mammals (Fig. 609). ....Genus *Opisthorchis* Blanchard, 1895

Life cycle: *O. tonkae*—
Embryonated eggs from the feces of the host are ingested by the operculate snail, *Amnicola limosa* in which pleurolophocercous cercariae develop in rediae. Cercariae encyst in the sand shiner, pumpkinseed and the bluntnosed minnow. Natural definitive hosts for this species are the muskrat and the Eastern meadow mouse. Experimental infections were established in dog, cat, rat and guinea pig (Wallace and Penner, 1939; Wallace, 1940; Sillman, 1953).

The life cycle of *O. tenuicollis* differs slightly from that of *O. tonkae*. The host snail is *Bithynia tentaculata* in which sporocysts and rediae develop. Metacercariae occur in the tissues of carp, bream and roach. The adult fluke develops in the bile and pancreatic ducts and in the small intestine of cat, dog, fox, pig and human being.

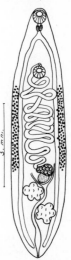

Fig. 609. *Opisthorchis tenuicollis.*

FAMILY HETEROPHYIDAE Odhner, 1914

Body small, spinous; ceca usually long; ventro-genital sac present, containing ventral sucker, one or more gonotyls and genital pore; male and female ducts fused to form hermaphroditic duct; one or two testes (six in *Larelmintha*), opposite or oblique; cirrus sac absent; seminal vesicle free in parenchyma; ovary pretesticular; vitelline follicles variable in extent; uterus extends posterior to ovary, posterior to testes in some genera; excretory vesicle Y-, V- or T-shaped, the arms extend anterior as far as the ovary; intestinal parasites of birds and mammals.

KEY TO GENERA

1a. **One testis.** 2

1b. **Two or more testes.** 4

2a. **One row of spines encircling oral opening; muscular genital ejector between ventral sucker and prostatic organ (Fig. 610).** .... Genus *Pygidiopsoides* Martin, 1951

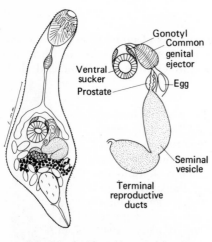

Fig. 610. *Pygidiopsoides spindalis*. (Redrawn from Martin, 1951.)

Life cycle: *P. spindalis*—
Metacercariae from the gills of the California killifish, *Fundulus parvipinnis*, were fed to cats and chicks and mature trematodes were recovered four to six days later. The natural definitive host is unknown. The early larval stages develop in the marine snail, *Cerithidea californica*. Cercariae, resembling the pleurolophocercous type except for absence of finfold on the tail, develop in rediae (Martin, 1951, 1964).

2b. **Spines absent around oral sucker.** 3

3a. **Body covered with numerous transverse rows of broad, scale-like spines; ceca long; ventro-genital sac large (Fig. 611).** .... Genus *Phocitremoides* Martin, 1950

Life cycle: *P. ovale*—

Pleurolophocercous cercariae develop in rediae in the marine snail, *Cerithidea californica* and encyst beneath the scales of the jack smelt, *Atherinopsis californica* and the California killifish, *Fundulus parvipinnis*. The natural definitive host is unknown but experimental infections were established in cats and chicks after feeding metacercariae (Martin, 1950a).

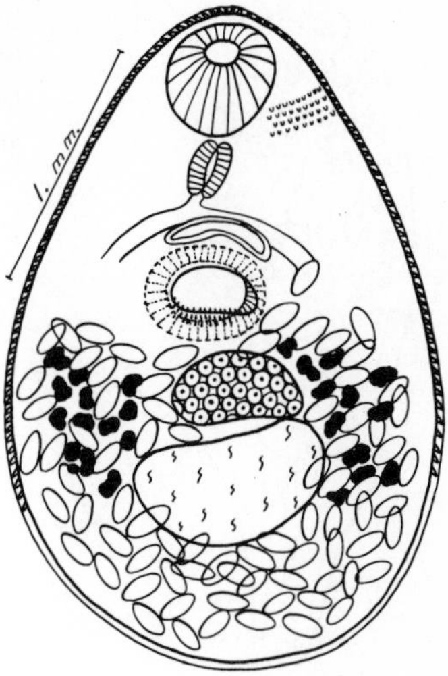

Fig. 611. *Phocitremoides ovale.*

3b. Body covered with conical spines; ceca short, dilated, not surpassing ventral sucker; genital atrium small (Fig. 612). ....Genus *Euhaplorchis* **Martin, 1950**

Life cycle: *E. californiensis*—

Parapleurolophocercous cercariae (Fig. 43) develop in rediae in the marine snail, *Cerithidea californica* and encyst around the brain of the California killifish, *Fundulus parvipinnis*. The natural definitive host is the California gull, *Larus californicus*. Experimental infections were established in chicks (Martin, 1950b).

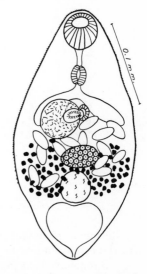

Fig. 612. *Euhaplorchis californiensis.*

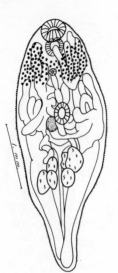

4a. Six testes, arranged in two groups; vitelline follicles near anterior end of body; most of uterus anterior to ventral sucker (Fig. 613). ....
.... **Genus** *Larelmintha*
Lautenschlager and Cheng, 1958

Fig. 613. *Larelmintha polyorchis.* (Redrawn from Lautenschlager and Cheng, 1958.)

4b. Two testes. 5
5a. Oral sucker conical; body pyriform, very small; one or two rows of spines around oral opening (Fig. 614). ....
....**Genus** *Ascocotyle* **Looss, 1899**

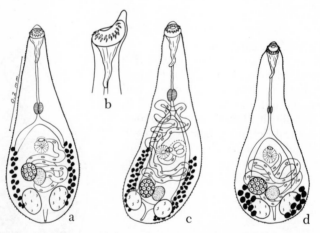

Fig. 614. Subgenera of *Ascocotyle* (a. *Ascocotyle;* b. oral sucker, lateral view; c. *Leighia;* d. *Phagicola.*)

Recent work by Sogandares-Bernal and Lumsden (1963) resulted in the establishment of three subgenera.

Subgenus *Ascocotyle* Looss, 1899: Vitelline follicles in lateral rows extending forward to level of ventral sucker; two rows of spines around oral opening; uterus confined to hindbody; cercaria parapleurolophocercous.

Subgenus *Phagicola* Faust, 1920: Vitelline follicles confined to region of ovary and testes; one, two or no rows of spines around oral opening; uterus confined to hindbody; cercaria pleurolophocercous.

Subgenus *Leighia* Sogandares-Bernal and Lumsden, 1963: Vitelline follicles in lateral rows, extending forward to level of ventral sucker; two rows of spines around oral opening; uterus extending forward to level of pharynx; cercaria ophthalmogymnocephalous.

Life cycle: *A. pachycystis*—

Parapleurolophocercous cercariae (Fig. 43) develop in rediae in the amnicolid snail, *Littoradinops tenuipes*. After leaving the snail, the cercariae attach to the gills of the killifish, *Cyprinodon variegatus*. They penetrate the gill arteries and migrate to the bulbus arteriosus in which they encyst and develop to infective metacercariae within 25 days. The infected bulbus enlarges to 20 times its normal size. The sexually mature trematode develops in the small intestine of raccoon (Schroeder and Leigh, 1965).

5b. Oral sucker not funnel-shaped; spines absent around mouth....6
6a. Testes and ovary lobed, or irregular in shape. 7
6b. Testes and ovary round or oval. 9

7a. **Vitelline follicles confined to ovarian and testicular area of hindbody; body pyriform (Fig. 615).** ....
.... **Genus** *Pygidiopsis*
Looss, 1907
Key to species in Skrjabin (1964).

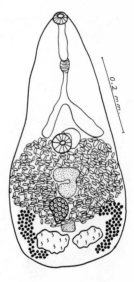

Fig. 615. *Pygidiopsis plana.* (Redrawn from Linton, 1928.)

7b. **Vitelline follicles distributed in fore- and hindbody.** 8

8a. Body oval or linguiform; primarily parasites of birds, rarely in mammals (Fig. 616). ....
....Genus *Cryptocotyle* Lühe, 1899

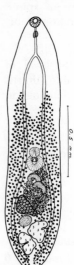

Key to species in Skrjabin (1964).
Life cycle: *C. lingua*—
Following oviposition, several days of incubation in running seawater are required for development of the miracidium. Pleurolophocercous cercariae develop in rediae in the marine snail, *Littorina littorea* and encyst in the skin and subcutaneous connective tissue of cunners. The development of black pigment in the cyst capsule results in "black spot" disease. The adult flukes develop in a variety of aquatic piscivorous birds as well as in dog, cat and rat (Stunkard, 1930).

Fig. 616. *Cryptocotyle lingua.*

8b. Body rectangular or pyriform; parasites of carnivorous mammals (one testis in *E. monorchis*) (Fig. 617, 618). ....
....Genus *Euryhelmis* Poche, 1926

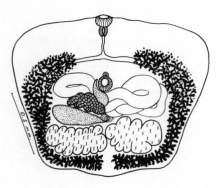

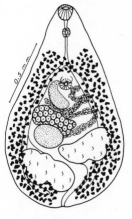

Fig. 617. *Euryhelmis squamula.*

Fig. 618. *Euryhelmis pacifica.*

Life cycle: *E. monorchis—*
Pleurolophocercous cercariae develop in rediae in the freshwater operculate snail, *Pomatiopsis lapidaria* and encyst in the skin and subcutaneous connective tissue of tadpoles and frogs of the Genus *Rana*. The natural definitive host is the mink. Experimental infections were established in cat and rat, the flukes attaining sexual maturity in about one week (Ameel, 1938).

Anderson and Pratt (1965) investigated the life cycle of *E. squamula*. Pleurolophocercous cercariae develop in rediae in *Bythinella hemphilli*. The cercariae encyst under the skin of frogs of the Genera *Rana* and *Ascaphus* and also in the newt, *Triturus cristatus*. Experimental infections were established in cat and hamster. Natural infections with the adult fluke have been reported from the raccoon and mink in North America.

9a. Ventral sucker sublateral. 10
9b. Ventral sucker median. 11
10a. Vitelline follicles restricted to hindbody; testes oblique; oral sucker subterminal, mouth ventral; esophagus twice length of pharynx (Fig. 619). ....
....Genus *Metagonimus* Katsurada, 1913

Although this genus is not represented in North America, it is included because of the importance of *M. yokogawai* as a parasite of human beings in the Far East. Embryonated eggs from feces of human beings are eaten by the snail, *Semisulcospira libertina*, in which the miracidia hatch and metamorphose to a sporocyst. Pleurolophocercous cercariae develop in daughter rediae and encyst under the skin of many species of freshwater fishes. The adult fluke develops in the small intestine of cat, dog, pig and human beings when infected fishes are eaten.

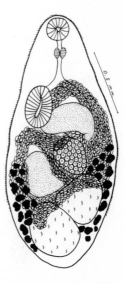

Fig. 619. *Metagonimus yokogawai.*

10b. Vitelline follicles in fore- and hindbody; testes opposite; oral sucker terminal, mouth anterior; esophagus very short or absent (Fig. 620). ....Genus *Metagonimoides* Price, 1931

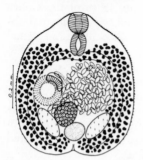

Fig. 620. *Metagonimoides oregonense.*

Life cycle: *M. oregonensis—*

Miracidia develop within 23 days after eggs are laid. Pleurolophocercous cercariae develop in rediae in freshwater operculate snails of several species of *Goniobasis*. Subsequently the cycle can follow two possible courses. Cercariae can either remain in the redia and develop to infective metacercariae or they can leave the redia and the snail and encyst in frogs. Experimental infections were established in hamsters but the natural definitive host is the raccoon (Ingles, 1935; Burns and Pratt, 1953; Lang and Gleason, 1967).

11a. Gonotyl spiny, sublateral, envelops genital pore; vitelline follicles restricted to hindbody (Fig. 621). ....
....Genus *Heterophyes* Cobbold, 1886

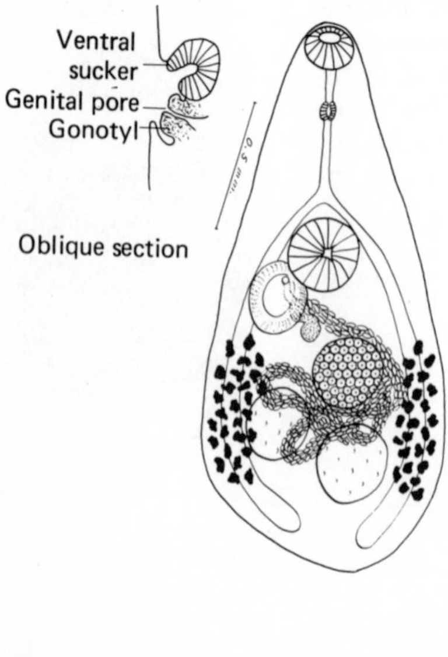

Ventral
sucker
Genital pore
Gonotyl

Oblique section

Species of this genus are not represented in North America but the genus is included because of the importance of *H. heterophyes* as a parasite of human beings in the Far and Near East. The life cycle is similar to that of *Metagonimus yokogawai*. The host snails are *Pirenella conica* and *Tympanotomus microptera* which in-

Fig. 621. *Heterophyes heterophyes.*

gest the embryonated eggs. The cercariae encyst in several species of fishes. The adult stage develops in the small intestine of cat, dog and human beings.

11b. Genital sucker absent. 12

12a. Vitelline follicles distributed in fore- and hindbody; testes opposite; in intestine of marine mammals (Fig. 622). ....
....Genus *Pricetrema* Ciurea, 1933

12b. Vitelline follicles restricted to hindbody. 13

13a. Body elongate or fusiform; ventro-genital sac contains a bulbous gonotyl; ventral sucker surrounds opening into ventro-genital sac; esophagus very short or absent; primarily intestinal parasites of birds (Fig. 623). ....
....Genus *Galactosomum* Looss, 1899

Key to species in Skrjabin (1964).

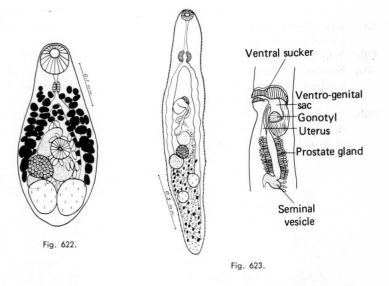

Fig. 622.

Fig. 623.

Fig. 622. *Pricetrema zalophi.* Fig. 623. *Galactosomum humbargari.* (Redrawn from Park, 1936.)

13b. Body pyriform; ventral sucker and ventro-genital sac not as described above; esophagus long. 14

14a. Vitelline follicles restricted to area around ovary and testes; seminal vesicle at least bipartite; ventro-genital sac contains U-shaped sclerite and ventral sucker (Fig. 624). ....
....Genus *Parastictodora* Martin, 1950

U-shaped
sclerite

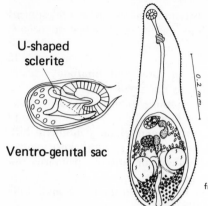

Ventro-genital sac

Fig. 624. *Parastictodora hancocki.* (Redrawn from Martin, 1950c.)

Life cycle: *P. hancocki—*
Parapleurolophocercous cercariae (Fig. 43) develop in rediae in the marine snail, *Cerithidea californica.* Metacercariae were found in the California killifish, *Fundulus parvipinnis* and in the mudsucker, *Gillichthys mirabilis.* Sexually mature flukes develop in chicks. The natural definitive host is unknown (Martin, 1950c).

14b. **Vitelline follicles distributed throughout most of hindbody; seminal vesicle not bipartite; ventro-genital sac without U-shaped sclerite (Fig. 625).** ....
....Genus *Apophallus* Lühe, 1909

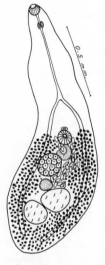

Fig. 625. *Apophallus brevis.*

Key to species in Price (1931) and in Morozov and Skrjabin (1952).
Life cycle: *A. venustus—*
Embryonated eggs in the feces of the host are eaten by the operculate snail, *Goniobasis livescens.* The miracidia hatch in the snail and pleurolophocercous cercariae eventually develop in daughter rediae. After leaving the snail, the cercariae penetrate several species of freshwater fishes and encyst in the muscles and skin. Suitable definitive hosts such as dog, cat, raccoon and great blue heron acquire the parasite by eating infected fishes (Cameron, 1937).
Miller (1941, 1946) investigated the life cycle of *A. brevis* which is similar to that of the above species except that the host snail is *Amnicola limosa* and the metacercariae occur under the scales of speckled trout, *Salvelinus fontinalis.* The presence of metacercariae in the skin causes "black spot" disease which is due to the development of black pigment in the connective

tissue capsules that the host produces around the cysts. The adult fluke develops in the loon, *Gavia immer* and the gull, *Larus dela-warensis*. Experimental infections were established in pigeons and kittens.

FAMILY CRYPTOGONIMIDAE Ciurea, 1933

Body small, oval, fusiform or elongate; pigmented eyespots present in some genera; oral sucker larger than ventral sucker, surrounded by a circle of large spines in some genera; ceca usually long; ventro-genital sac present, containing ventral sucker, genital pore and a gonotyl; testes two, usually opposite rarely oblique (nine in *Siphodera*); cirrus sac absent; ovary oval, lobed or follicular, anterior to testes or between testes; terminus of male and female reproductive ducts fused to form hermaphroditic duct which opens into ventro-genital sac; uterus usually extends posterior to testes; excretory vesicle V- or Y-shaped, arms extending forward to level of pharynx; parasites of fishes.

KEY TO GENERA

1a. **Oral sucker with a circle of large spines.** 2
1b. **Oral sucker without a circle of spines.** 4
2a. **Ovary in the form of a transverse band of follicles; vitelline follicles lateral to ovary and testes; intestinal parasites of freshwater fishes (Fig. 626).** ....
.....................Genus *Neochasmus* Van Cleave and Mueller, 1932
2b. **Ovary lobed.** 3
3a. **Parasites of freshwater fishes; ovary a transverse lobed mass; vitelline follicles lateral, between level of ovary and seminal vesicle (Fig. 627).** ....
...........................Genus *Allacanthochasmus* Van Cleave, 1922

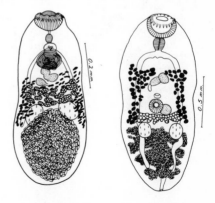

Fig. 626. *Neochasmus umbellus.* (Redrawn from Van Cleave and Mueller, 1932.)   Fig. 627.   *Allacanthochasmus varius.* (Redrawn from Van Cleave, 1922.)

Fig. 626.   Fig. 627.

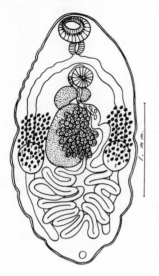

3b. **Parasites of marine fishes; ovary a spherical lobed mass; vitelline follicles lateral to ovary (Fig. 628).** .....
.... Genus *Paracryptogonimus* Yamaguti, 1934

Fig. 628. *Paracryptogonimus americanus.*

4a. **Nine testes, arranged in two longitudinal rows (5 and 4); parasites of marine fishes (Fig. 629).** ....
....Genus *Siphodera* Linton, **1910**

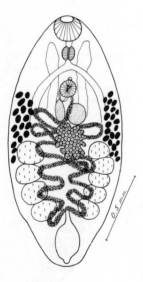

Life cycle: *S. vinaledwardsii*—
Pleurolophocercous cercariae develop in rediae in the marine snail, *Bittium alternatum.* The cercariae encyst in the fins and body wall of the summer flounder, *Paralichthys dentatus.* The adult fluke develops in the intestine of the toadfish, *Opsanus tau,* and the pigfish, *Orthopristis chrysopterus* (Cable and Hunninen, 1941, 1942b).

Fig. 629. *Siphodera vinaledwardsii.*

4b. **Two testes.** 5

5a. Testes elongate, located at posterior end of body; ventral sucker to right or left of median line; parasites in swim bladder and ovaries of catfish (Fig. 630). ....
....Genus *Acetodextra* Pearse, 1924

The genus contains one species, *A. ameiuri.* Gravid specimens tend to disintegrate, leaving only a mass of embryonated eggs. Due to the unusual habitat of the parasite, there has been some speculation regarding the method by which eggs escape from the body of the host. Those in the swim bladder are thought to escape by way of the pneumatic duct. Eggs in the ovaries leave with the eggs at spawning time. The life cycle is unknown (Perkins, 1950; Coil, 1954).

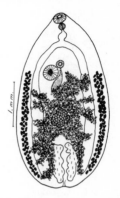

Fig. 630. *Acetodextra ameiuri.*

5b. Testes some distance from posterior end of body; ventral sucker median; intestinal parasites of marine and freshwater fishes. 6
6a. Intestinal ceca long, extending nearly to posterior end of body. 7
6b. Intestinal ceca short, extending only to midbody region. 8
7a. Body broadly oval; testes opposite or nearly so; gonotyl absent (Fig. 631). ....Genus *Metadena* Linton, 1910
Key to species in Skrjabin (1964).
7b. Body elongate; testes tandem or nearly so; seven to 11 gonotyls present, anterior to ventral sucker (Fig. 632). ....
....Genus *Multigonotylus* Premvati, 1967

Fig. 631. *Metadena crassulata.*
Fig. 632. *Multigonotylus micropteri.*

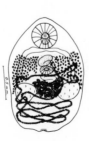

Fig. 631.

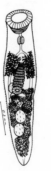

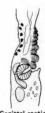

Sagittal section

Fig. 632.

8a. Vitelline follicles in lateral clusters along each side of eso-phagus; oral sucker large, terminal (Fig. 633). ....
.............................Genus *Caecincola* Marshall and Gilbert, 1905

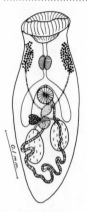

Fig. 633. *Caecincola parvulus.* (Redrawn from Marshall and Gilbert, 1905.)

Life cycle: *C. parvulus*—
Embryonated eggs are eaten by the fresh-water operculate snail, *Amnicola histrica*, in which pleurolophocercous cercariae develop in rediae. They leave the redia before they are fully developed and complete their development in the tissues of the snail. The cercariae encyst in the skin and fins of several species of centrarchid and cyprinid fishes. Metacercariae are infective for the definitive host after three weeks. The adult fluke develops in the pyloric ceca and in-testine of large-mouth bass, *Huro salmoides* and small-mouth bass, *Micropterus dolomieu* (see Lundahl, 1941).

8b. Vitelline follicles in lateral rows along intestinal ceca; body elongate or fusiform; pigmented eyespots present. 9
9a. Body elongate with transverse rows of scale-like spines; two ventral suckers in ventro-genital sac, one posterior to the other; hermaphroditic duct and genital pore between the ven-tral suckers (Fig. 634). ....Genus *Cryptogonimus* Osborn, 1903
9b. Body fusiform, nonspinous; one ventral sucker; genital pore anterior to ventral sucker; testes opposite; ovary lobed, median (Fig. 635). ....Genus *Centrovarium* Stafford, 1904

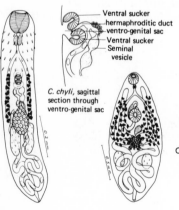

Ventral sucker
hermaphroditic duct
ventro-genital sac
Ventral sucker
Seminal vesicle

C. chyli, sagittal section through ventro-genital sac

Fig. 634. *Cryptogonimus chyli.* Fig. 635. *Centrovarium lobotes.*

Fig. 634.   Fig. 635.

SUPERFAMILY HEMIUROIDEA Faust, 1929

Miracidia spinous, without cilia, with one pair of flame cells; cercariae of cystophorous type, excretory system of stenostomate type with the main ducts fused dorsal to pharynx, develop in rediae; metacercariae in hemocoel of copepods; three hosts involved in life cycle; parasites in digestive tract of fishes and amphibians. The families Syncoeliidae, Accacoeliidae and Didymozoidae are placed in this superfamily temporarily until something is learned of their life cycles.

FAMILY HEMIURIDAE Lühe, 1901

Body elongate, fusiform or oval; cuticle nonspinous but may be provided with transverse cuticular plications, rows of scales or marginal serrations; in some genera the body is divided into a soma and an ecsoma or tail; suckers well developed; ceca long, frequently dilated near bifurcation; testes opposite, tandem or oblique; cirrus sac absent (present in Genus *Intuscirrus*?); terminus of male and female reproductive ducts fused to form hermaphroditic duct (= genital sinus) which is enclosed in a sinus sac (= false cirrus sac); seminal vesicle and prostate gland free in parenchyma; genital pore median, ventral to pharynx or intestinal bifurcation; ovary usually posterior to testes; vitelline glands tubular or in the form of two lobed or ovoid masses, or a rosette of digitiform tubes; uterus with descending and ascending limbs; eggs abundant, provided with polar filaments in some genera; excretory vesicle Y-shaped, with arms elongate and usually united dorsal to pharynx; parasites in the stomach of fishes, rarely in the pharynx and Eustachian tubes of amphibians.

In the few life cycles that are known, cystophorous cercariae develop in rediae in snails. The cercariae are thought to be eaten by copepods in the hemocoel of which metacercariae develop without encysting.

KEY TO GENERA

1a. Ecsoma (= tail) present (Fig. 637). 2
1b. Ecsoma absent (Fig. 649, 650). 14
2a. Vitelline glands tubular (Fig. 637). 3
2b. Vitelline glands in the form of two oval or lobed masses, or a rosette of digitiform tubes (Figs. 641, 651). 7
3a. Cuticle without transverse cuticular plications; body margins smooth. 4
3b. Cuticle with either transverse cuticular plications (Fig. 648) or rows of scales (Fig. 644). 5

4a. Ecsoma longer than soma; body very long (2 cm. or more)
(Fig. 636). ....Genus *Stomachicola* Yamaguti, 1934
4b. Ecsoma shorter than soma; body not unusually elongate (Fig.
637). ....Genus *Tubulovesicula* Yamaguti, 1934

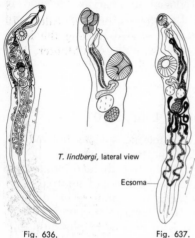

T. lindbergi, lateral view

Ecsoma

Fig. 636. *Stomachicola magnus.* (Redrawn from Manter, 1931.) Fig. 637. *Tubulovesicula lindbergi.*

Fig. 636.   Fig. 637.

5a. Seminal vesicle a thin-walled sac; prostate cells confined to
distal portion of prostatic duct (Fig. 638). ....
....Genus *Parectenurus* Manter, 1947
5b. Seminal vesicle bi- or tripartite. 6
6a. Prostate cells distributed along full length of prostate duct;
seminal vesicle tripartite; arms of excretory vesicle not united
dorsal to pharynx (Fig. 639). ....Genus *Dinurus* Looss, 1907

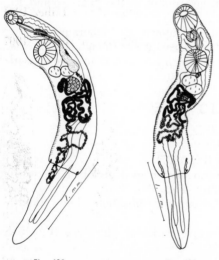

Fig. 638. *Parectenurus americanus.*
Fig. 639. *Dinurus scombri.*

Fig. 638.   Fig. 639.

6b. Prostate cells confined to distal portion of prostate duct; seminal vesicle bi- or tripartite; arms of excretory vesicle united dorsal to pharynx (Fig. 640). ....Genus *Ectenurus* Looss, 1907

7a. Body without transverse cuticular plications or rows of scales. 8

7b. Body with transverse cuticular plications or rows of scales....10

8a. Seminal vesicle bilobed, a narrow duct connecting the lobes (Fig. 641). ....Genus *Dissosaccus* Manter, 1947

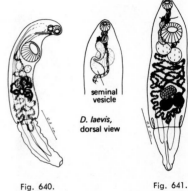

Fig. 640. *Ectenurus virgulus.* Fig. 641. *Dissosaccus laevis.*

seminal vesicle

D. laevis, dorsal view

Fig. 640.   Fig. 641.

8b. Seminal vesicle not bilobed as described above. 9

9a. Preacetabular pit present (Fig. 642). ....
....Genus *Lecithochirium* Lühe, 1901

9b. Preacetabular pit absent (Fig. 643). ....
....Genus *Sterrhurus* Looss, 1907

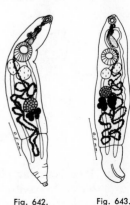

Fig. 642. *Lecithochirium microstomum.* Fig. 643. *Sterrhurus musculus.*

Fig. 642.   Fig. 643.

10a. Body having transverse rows of scales (Figs. 644, 645). 11
10b. Body having transverse cuticular plications. 12
11a. Seminal vesicle bipartite, thin-walled; vitelline glands con-
     sisting of two lobed masses; body scales numerous, arranged
     in close transverse rows (Fig. 644). ....
     ....Genus *Dinosoma* Manter, 1934
     Key to species in Skrjabin (1964).
11b. Seminal vesicle ovoid, thick-walled; vitelline glands con-
     sisting of two oval masses; body scales sparse (Fig. 645). ....
     ....Genus *Anahemiurus* Manter, 1947

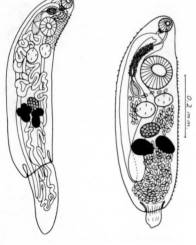

Fig. 644. *Dinosoma rubrum.* (Redrawn from Manter, 1934b.) Fig. 645. *Anahemiurus microcercus.* (Redrawn from Manter, 1947.)

Fig. 644.   Fig. 645.

12a. Preacetabular pit present; seminal vesicle bipartite and dorsal
     or anterior to ventral sucker; vitelline glands consisting of
     two lobed masses in midbody region (Fig. 646). ....
     ....Genus *Brachyphallus* Odhner, 1905

Preacetabular
pit

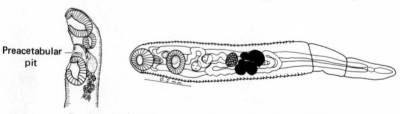

Fig. 646. *Brachyphallus crenatus.* (Redrawn from Lloyd, 1938.)

12b. Preacetabular pit absent; seminal vesicle some distance pos-
     terior to ventral sucker; vitelline glands consisting of two
     oval or indented masses in posterior third of body. 13

13a. Seminal vesicle bipartite, the anterior part thick-walled in
     some species (Fig. 647). ....Genus *Hemiurus* Rudolphi, 1809
13b. Seminal vesicle ovoid, thick-walled (Fig. 648). ....
     ....Genus *Parahemiurus* Vaz and Pereira, 1930

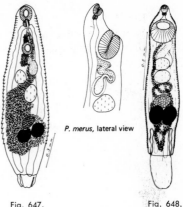

Fig. 647. *Hemiurus levinseni.* Fig. 648.
Parahemiurus merus.

P. merus, lateral view

Fig. 647.   Fig. 648.

14a. Seminal vesicle extending some distance posterior to ventral
     sucker. 15
14b. Seminal vesicle anterior or dorsal to ventral sucker. 18
15a. Vitelline glands in the form of two oval masses (Fig. 649).
     ....Genus *Opisthadena* Linton, 1910
15b. Vitelline glands consisting of a compact cluster of seven or
     more digitiform tubes. 16
16a. Ovary and vitelline glands pretesticular (Fig. 650). ....
     ....Genus *Macradenina* Manter, 1947

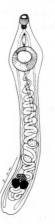

Fig. 649. *Opisthadena dimidia.* Fig. 650.
Macradenina acanthuri. (Redrawn from Manter, 1947.)

Fig. 649.   Fig. 650.

16b. Ovary and vitelline glands posttesticular. 17

17a. Body fusiform; vitelline glands consisting of seven digitiform tubes; ovary lobed (Fig. 651). ....
....**Genus** *Lecithaster* **Lühe, 1901**

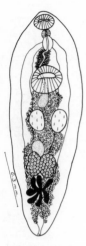

Life cycle: *L. confusus*—
Cystophorous cercariae develop in rediae in the marine snail, *Odostoma trifida*. The cercariae are eaten by the marine copepod, *Acarta tonsa*, in which metacercariae develop in the hemocoel without encysting. The adult fluke develops in the stickleback, *Apeltes quadracus* and the killifish, *Fundulus heteroclitus* and *F. majalis* (see Hunninen and Cable, 1943b).

Fig. 651. *Lecithaster salmonis.*

17b. Body elongate; vitelline glands in the form of 12 or more digitiform follicles; ovary not lobed (Fig. 652). ....
....**Genus** *Macradena* **Linton, 1910**

18a. Vitelline glands anterior to testes. 19

18b. Vitelline glands posterior to testes. 20

19a. Uterus spirally coiled; eggs with monopolar filaments (Fig. 653). ....**Genus** *Hemipera* **Nicoll, 1912**

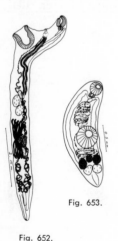

Fig. 652. *Macradena perfecta.* Fig. 653. *Hemipera nicolli.*

Fig. 653.

Fig. 652.

19b. Uterus looping, not spirally coiled; eggs without polar filaments (Fig. 654). ....Genus *Gonocerca* Manter, 1925

20a. Vitelline glands in posterior end of body; folds of uterus not extending posterior to glands. 21

20b. Vitelline glands separated from posterior end of body by some folds of uterus. 24

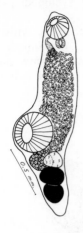

Fig. 654. *Gonocerca phycidis.*

21a. Vitelline glands in the form of two clusters of four or five large follicles each; eggs with unipolar filament; parasites in pharynx and Eustachian tubes of frogs (Fig. 655). ....
....Genus *Halipegus* Looss, 1899

Life cycle: *H. eccentricus—*
    Embryonated eggs from the feces of the frog are eaten by freshwater snails of the Genera *Physa* and *Helisoma*. Spinous, nonciliated miracidia hatch in the snail digestive tract, penetrate the intestinal wall, then metamorphose to a sporocyst which produces a generation of rediae. The latter produce cystophorous cercariae (Fig. 21) which, upon leaving the snail, are eaten by copepods of the Genera *Cyclops* and *Mesocyclops*. Metacercariae develop in the hemocoel of the copepods without encysting. Infected copepods are ingested by tadpoles in which developing stages of the parasite occur in the cardiac region of the stomach until the tadpole metamorphoses, after which the parasites migrate to the pharynx and Eustachian tubes where they mature. About three months is required for development to sexual maturity in the frog (Thomas, 1939).

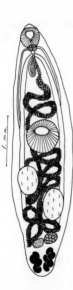

Fig. 655. *Halipegus occidualis.*

21b. Vitelline glands consist of two ovoid or spherical masses......22
22a. Eggs have unipolar filament; prostate gland weakly developed; parasites in stomach of snakes (Fig. 656). ....
....**Genus** *Vitellotrema* **Guberlet, 1928**
22b. Eggs without polar filament; prostate gland globose, well developed, parasites of fishes or frogs. 23
23a. Stomach parasites of marine fishes; ventral sucker in posterior half of body (Fig. 657). ....
....**Genus** *Gonocercella* **Manter, 1940**

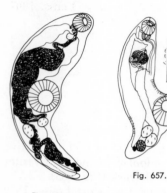

Fig. 656. *Vitellotrema fusipora.* (Redrawn from Guberlet, 1928.) Fig. 657. *Gonocercella trachinoti.*

Fig. 657.

Fig. 656.

23b. Stomach parasites of frogs and trout; ventral sucker in anterior half of body (Fig. 658). ....
...........................**Genus** *Deropegus* **McCauley and Pratt, 1961**

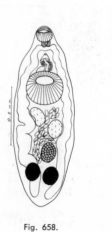

Fig. 658. *Deropegus aspina.*
Fig. 659. *Hysterolecitha rosea.*

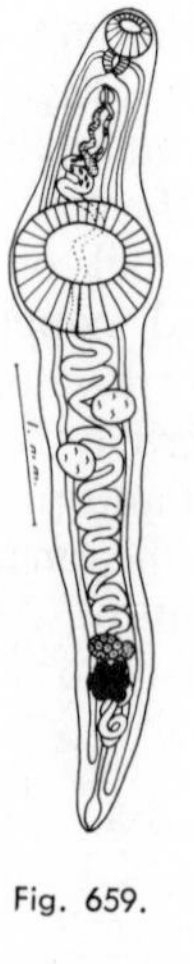

Fig. 658.   Fig. 659.

24a. Vitelline gland in the form of one cluster of seven club-shaped or rounded follicles. 25
24b. Vitelline gland in the form of two rounded or indented masses. 27
25a. Seminal vesicle tubular; prostate glands weakly developed or absent (Fig. 659). ....Genus *Hysterolecitha* Linton, 1910
25b. Seminal vesicle ovoid; prostate glands well developed. 26
26a. Vitelline gland a cluster of seven clubshaped follicles (Fig. 660). ....Genus *Lecithophyllum* Odhner, 1905
26b. Vitelline gland a cluster of seven rounded follicles (Fig. 661). ....Genus *Aponurus* Looss, 1907

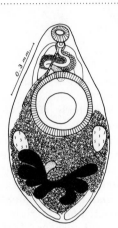

Fig. 660. *Lecithophyllum piriforme.*
(Redrawn from Linton, 1910.)

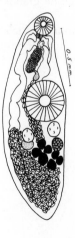

Fig. 661. *Aponurus intermedius.* (Redrawn from Manter, 1934b.)

27a. Testes oblique. 28
27b. Testes opposite. 29
28a. Sinus sac (= false cirrus sac) and hermaphroditic duct present (Fig. 662). ....Genus *Genolinea* Manter, 1925
28b. Cirrus and cirrus sac present; hermaphroditic duct absent (Fig. 663); parasite of marine sculpins. ....
....Genus *Intuscirrus* Acena, 1947

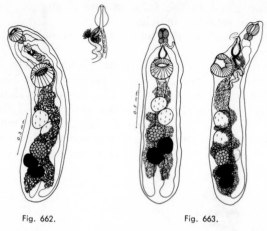

Fig. 662.   Fig. 663.

Fig. 662. *Genolinea laticauda.* Fig. 663. *Intuscirrus aspicotti.*

29a. Ventral sucker in anterior fourth of body (Fig. 664); parasite of moray eels. ....Genus *Dictysarca* Linton, 1910
29b. Ventral sucker in middle or posterior to middle of body.....30
30a. Seminal vesicle sac-shaped; prostate glands well developed;
vitelline glands compact, one on each side of ovary (Fig. 665).
....Genus *Derogenes* Lühe, 1900
30b. Seminal vesicle tubular; prostate gland inconspicuous, weakly
developed; vitelline glands compact, both to right of ovary
(Fig. 666). ....Genus *Leurodera* Linton, 1910

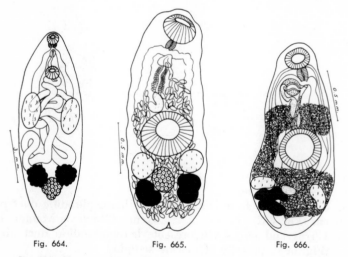

Fig. 664.   Fig. 665.   Fig. 666.

Fig. 664. *Dictysarca virens.* Fig. 665. *Derogenes crassus.* Fig. 666. *Leurodera decora.* (Redrawn from Linton, 1910.)

FAMILY ACCACOELIIDAE Looss, 1912

Body elongate, cylindrical, nonspinous; ventral sucker pedunculate; accessory suckers sometimes present; intestinal ceca with a pair of anterior diverticula, posterior end of ceca fused with excretory vesicle; testes two, tandem, in anterior half of body; ovary posttesticular; cirrus sac present (?); seminal vesicle long, convoluted, free in parenchyma; hermaphroditic duct sometimes present; genital pore median, anterior to peduncle; vitelline glands filamentous; uterus with long descending and ascending limbs; excretory vesicle Y- or V-shaped; intestinal parasites of ocean sunfish.

KEY TO GENERA

1a. Several accessory suckers on antero-dorsal surface of body and on peduncle of ventral sucker (Fig. 667). ....
....Genus *Odhnerium* Yamaguti, 1934
1b. Accessory suckers absent. 2
2a. Vitelline glands not extending anterior to peduncle; anterior cecal diverticula unbranched (Fig. 668). ....
....Genus *Accacladium* Odhner, 1928
2b. Vitelline glands extend anterior to peduncle; anterior cecal diverticula branched (Fig. 669). ....
....Genus *Accacladocoelium* Odhner, 1928

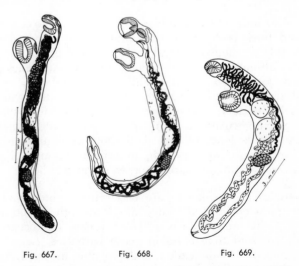

Fig. 667.   Fig. 668.   Fig. 669.

Fig. 667. *Odhnerium calyptrocotyle.* (Redrawn from Lloyd, 1938.)
Fig. 668. *Accacladium nematulum.* Fig. 669. *Accacladocoelium macrocotyle.*

FAMILY SYNCOELIIDAE Dollfus, 1923

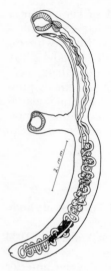

Body elongate, cylindrical, arched ventrally; ventral sucker at end of a long peduncle; intestinal ceca long, fused at posterior end to form cyclocoel; 16 to 20 testes; cirrus sac absent; seminal vesicle long, free in parenchyma; ovary single or follicular, posterior to testes; genital ducts fused to form hermaphroditic duct (= genital sinus); vitelline follicles few (5 to 7), posterior to ovary; uterus long, in numerous folds along the ceca; main excretory ducts extending far forward and united dorsal to pharynx; parasites in mouth and pharynx of marine fishes.

Only the Genus *Syncoelium* Looss, 1899 occurs in North America (Fig. 670). *S. filiferum* is a parasite of humpback salmon, *Onchorhynchus gorbuscha,* and blueback salmon,

Fig. 670. *Syncoelium filiferum.*

O. nerka in the Pacific Northwest.

FAMILY DIDYMOZOIDAE Poche, 1907

Body very long and thread-like or subdivided into a narrow anterior and thick posterior portion; oral sucker present but sometimes weakly developed; ventral sucker present or absent; pharynx present or absent; intestinal ceca long, narrow, sometimes partially atrophied; testes, ovary and vitelline glands tubular; ovary and vitelline glands posterior to testes; one or two testes; seminal vesicle usually present; uterus long, looped, extending throughout body; eggs operculate, contain spinous nonciliated miracidium; excretory vesicle long, tubular with short arms anteriorly; parasites in fins, mouth, muscles, skin, mucous membranes of pharynx, or in visceral organs of marine and freshwater fishes.

Trematodes in this family are either hermaphroditic or gonochoristic (separate sexes). They are frequently found encysted in pairs. Cable and Nahhas (1962a) report the occurrence of larval didymozoid trematodes in goose barnacles, *Lepas* sp. The spinous, nonciliated miracidium and probable use of a crustacean as second intermediate host indicate relationship with the Family Hemiuridae.

KEY TO GENERA

1a. Body subdivided into narrow anterior and thick posterior portions; ventral sucker absent; hermaphroditic; parasites in the mouth, pharynx, esophagus, stomach or coelom of marine fishes (Fig. 671). ....Genus *Didymocystis* Ariola, 1902

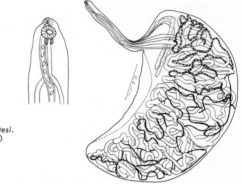

Fig. 671. *Didymocystis coatesi.*
(Redrawn from Nigrelli, 1939.)

1b. Body long, filiform or ribbon-like throughout. 2
2a. Sexes separate (gonochoristic), the sexual dimorphism not pronounced; testes parallel, extending through most of body; parasites in mouth and pharynx of marine fishes. ....
....Genus *Gonapodasmius* Ishii, 1935
2b. Hermaphroditic. 3
3a. Body ribbon-like; one testis; pharynx absent; parasites in mucous membrane of pharynx of marine fishes. ....
.............................Genus *Atalostrophion* G. A. MacCallum, 1915

3b. Body filiform, cylindrical; two testes; pharynx present; embedded in tissues of marine and freshwater fishes (Fig. 672). ......
.... **Genus** *Nematobothrium*
van Beneden, 1858

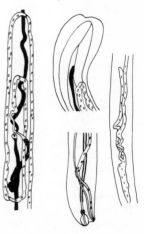

Fig. 672. *Nematobothrium texomensis.* (Redrawn from Self, Peters, and Davis, 1963.)

REFERENCES

BYCHOWSKY, B. E., 1957. Monogenetic Trematodes, Their Systematics and Phylogeny. Akad. Nauk. S.S.S.R. 509 pp. (Translated from the Russian) A.I.B.S. Wash. D.C.

DAWES, B., 1946. The Trematodes, with Special Reference to British and Other European Forms. 644 pp. Cambridge University Press.

SKRJABIN, K. I., 1947-1962. Trematodes of Animals and Man. 20 vols. Moscow, Russia.

─────, 1964. Keys to the Trematodes of Animals and Man. Translated from the Russian) 351 pp. University of Illinois Press, Urbana.

YAMAGUTI, S., 1958. Systema Helminthum: The Digenetic Trematodes of Vertebrates. Vol. 1, Pts. 1 and 2. Interscience Publishers, New York.

─────, 1963. Systema Helminthum: Monogenea and Aspidocotylea. Vol. 4. Interscience Publishers, New York.

PERIODICALS

ABDEL-AZIM, M., 1936. Ann. Trop. Med. Parasit. 30:351-356.

ADAMS, J. E. and W. E. MARTIN, 1963. Tr. Am. Micr. Soc. 82:1-6.

ALICATA, J. E., 1962. J. Parasit. 48:47-54.

ALLISON, L. N., 1943. Tr. Am. Micr. Soc. 62:127-168.

ALVEY, C. H., 1936. Parasitology 28:229-253.

AMEEL, D. J., 1934. Am. J. Hyg. 19:279-317.

─────, 1937. J. Parasit. 23:218-220.

─────, 1938. J. Parasit. 24:219-224.

─────, 1944. J. Parasit. 30:257-263.

ANDERSON, D. J. and R. M. CABLE, 1950. J. Parasit. 36:395-410.

ANDERSON, G. A. and I. PRATT, 1965. J. Parasit. 51:13-15.

ANDERSON, G. A., G. W. MARTIN and I. PRATT, 1966. J. Parasit. 52:704-706.

ANDERSON, G. A., S. C. SCHELL and I. PRATT, 1965. J. Parasit. 51:579-582.

ANDERSON, M. G., and F. M. ANDERSON, 1963. J. Parasit. 49:275-280.

─────, 1967. J. Parasit. 53:31-37.

ANGEL, L. M., 1954. Tr. Roy. Soc. S. Austral. 77:164-174.

ARAI, H. P., 1954. J. Parasit. 40:356-359.

BEAVER, P. C., 1929. J. Parasit. 16:13-23.

─────, 1937. Ill. Biol. Monog. 15(1):96 pp.

─────, 1939a. J. Parasit. 25:269-276.

─────, 1939b. J. Parasit. 25:383-393.

─────, 1941a. J. Parasit. 27:35-44.

─────, 1941b. J. Parasit. 27:347-355.

─────, 1943. J. Parasit. 29:65-70.

BENNETT, H. J., 1935. J. Parasit. 21:83-90.

─────, and A. G. HUMES, 1939. J. Parasit. 25:223-231.

BONHAM, K. and J. E. GUBERLET, 1938. Am. Midl. Nat. 20:590-602.
BRACKETT, S., 1942. J. Parasit. 28:25-42.
BURNS, W. C., 1961a. J. Parasit. 47:933-938.
————, 1961b. J. Parasit. 47:927-932.
BURNS, W. C. and I. PRATT, 1953. J. Parasit. 39:60-69.
BUTTNER, A., 1951. Ann. Parasit. 26:138-189.
BYRD, E. E., 1935. Tr. Am. Micr. Soc. 54:196-225.
————, 1937. Proc. U. S. Nat. Mus. 84(3010):183-199.
————, 1939. J. Tenn. Acad. Sci. 14:116-161.
———— and J. F. DENTON, 1938. J. Parasit. 24:379-401.
———— and J. F. DENTON, 1950. Am. Midl. Nat. 43:32-57.
————, and W. P. MAPLES, 1963. Zschr. Parasitenk. 22:521-536.
———— and R. J. REIBER, 1942. J. Parasit. 28:51-73.
CABALLERO, Y C. E., 1952. Rev. Med. Vet. Parasit., Caracas. 11:1-231.
CABLE, R. M., 1939. Proc. Indiana Acad. Sci. 48:201.
————, 1953. J. Parasit. 39:408-421.
————, 1954a. Biol. Bull. 106:15-20.
————, 1954b. J. Parasit. 40:71-76.
————, 1954c. J. Parasit. 40:202-208.
————, 1956. Parasitology 46:1-13.
————, 1962. J. Parasit. 48:419-422.
CABLE, R. M. and A. V. HUNNINEN, 1940. Biol. Bull. 78:136-157.
————, 1941. Biol. Bull. 81:279.
————, 1942a. Biol. Bull. 82:292-312.
————, 1942b. J. Parasit. 28:407-422.
CABLE, R. M. and F. M. NAHHAS, 1962a. J. Parasit. 48:34.
————, 1962b. J. Parasit. 48:536-538.
CAMERON, T. W. M., 1937. Can. J. Res. Sect. D. 15:38-51.
————, 1944. Can. J. Res. Sect. D. 22:6-16.
————, 1945. Can J. Comp. Med. 9:245-254; 283-286; 302-311.
CARNEY, W. P., 1967. Can. J. Zool. 45:131-134.
CHANDLER, A. C., 1932. Proc. U. S. Nat. Mus. 81(Art. 16):1-15.
————, 1942. Tr. Am. Micr. Soc. 61:156-167.
CHANDLER, A. C. and R. RAUSCH, 1947. Tr. Am. Micr. Soc. 66:283-292.
CHENG, T. C., 1957. J. Parasit. 43:60-65.
————, 1961. J. Parasit. 47:469-477.
CHING, H. L., 1960. Proc. Helm. Soc. Wash. 27:53-62.
————, 1961. Proc. Helm. Soc. Wash. 28:130-138.
CHU, G. W. T. C. and C. E. CUTRESS, 1954. J. Parasit. 40:515-524.
CHUBRIK, G. K., 1952. Zoologicheski Zhurnal 31:653-658 [in Russian].
COIL, W. H., 1954. J. Parasit. 40:101.
CORT, W. W. and S. T. BROOKS, 1928. Tr. Am. Micr. Soc. 47:179-221.
CORT, W. W., S. BRACKETT and L. J. OLIVIER, 1944. J. Parasit. 30:309-321.
CRANDALL, R. B., 1960. J. Parasit. 46:289-307.
CRAWFORD, W. W., 1937. J. Parasit. 23:389-399.
————, 1938. J. Parasit. 24:35-44.
————, 1940. J. Parasit. 26 (Sect. 2):38.
DAWES, B., 1942. Parasitology 34:266-277.
DEBLOCK, S. and C. COMBES, 1965. Bull. Soc. Zool. France 90:101-117.

DeGiusti, D. L., 1962. J. Parasit. 48(Sect. 2):22.
DeMartini, J. D. and I. Pratt, 1964. J. Parasit. 50:101-105.
Denton, J. F., 1941. J. Parasit. 27(Sect. 2):13-14.
—————, 1944. J. Parasit. 30:277-286.
—————, 1945. J. Parasit. 31:131-141.
—————, 1962. J. Parasit. 48(Sect. 2):22.
Dery, D. W., 1958. J. Parasit. 44:110-112.
Dickerman, E. E., 1934. Tr. Am. Micr. Soc. 53:8-21.
—————, 1945. Tr. Am. Micr. Soc. 64:138-144.
—————, 1948. J. Parasit. 34:164.
—————, 1954. J. Parasit. 40:311-315.
Dobrovolny, C. G., 1939a. Tr. Am. Micr. Soc. 58:121-155.
—————, 1939b. J. Parasit. 25:461-470.
Dollfus, R. Ph., 1937. Ann. Parasit. 15:57-73; 164-176; 259-281.
—————, 1958. Ann. Parasit. 33:305-395.
Dollfus, R. Ph., J. Callot and C. Desportes, 1935. Ann. Parasit. 13:12-20.
Dubois, G., 1938. Mem. Soc. Neuchâtel. Sci. nat. 6:1-535.
—————, 1955. Bull. Soc. Neuchâtel. Sci. nat. 78:53-65.
—————, 1968. Mem. Soc. Neuchâtel. Sci. nat. 10:260 pp.
Edwards, S. R. and F. M. Nahhas, 1968. Calif. Fish and Game 54:247-256.
Erickson, D. G. and F. G. Wallace, 1959. J. Parasit. 45:310-322.
Etges, F. J., 1953. J. Parasit. 39:643-662.
Feldman, S. I., 1941. J. Parasit. 27:525-533.
Fischthal, J. H. and L. N. Allison, 1941. J. Parasit. 27:517-524.
—————, 1942. Tr. Am. Micr. Soc. 61:53-56.
Frankland, H. M. T., 1955. Parasitology 45:313-351.
Gallien, L., 1932. C. R. Acad. Sci., Paris 194:1852-1854; 195:77-79.
—————, 1933. C. R. Acad. Sci., Paris 196:426-428.
Goodchild, C. G., 1943. Biol. Bull. 84:59-86.
—————, 1948. J. Parasit. 34:407-427.
Goodchild, C. G. and D. E. Kirk, 1960. J. Parasit. 46:219-229.
Goto, S., 1895. J. Coll. Sci. Imp. Univ., Japan 8:1-273.
Groves, R. E., 1945. Tr. Am. Micr. Soc. 64:112-132.
Guberlet, J. E., 1928. J. Helm. 6:205-218.
Guberlet, J. E., 1936. Am. Midl. Nat. 17:954-964.
Hall, J. E., 1959. J. Parasit. 45:327-336.
—————, 1960. Am. Midl. Nat. 63:226-245.
Hand, C. and M. Voge, 1952. J. Parasit. 38:57-58.
Hanson, M. L., 1950. Proc. Helm Soc. Wash. 17:74-89.
Hargis, W. J. Jr., 1955a. Quar. J. Fla. Acad. Sci. 18:33-47.
—————, 1955b. Tr. Am. Micr. Soc. 74:203-225.
Harshey, K. R., 1937. Proc. Indian Acad. Sci. 5:64-75.
—————, 1939. J. Tenn. Acad. Sci. 14:332-340; 421-437.
Herber, E. C., 1938. J. Parasit. 24:549.
—————, 1939. J. Parasit. 25:189-195.
—————, 1942. J. Parasit. 28:179-196.
Hoffman, G. L., 1955. Proc. Iowa Acad. Sci. 62:638-639.
—————, 1956. J. Parasit. 42:435-444.

————, 1958a. Exp. Parasit. 7:23-50.

————, 1958b. J. Parasit. 44:416-421.

HOFFMAN, G. L. and C. E. DUNBAR, 1963. J. Parasit. 49:737-744.

HOLL, F. J., 1928. J. Elisha Mitchell Scient. Soc. 43:181-183.

HOPKINS, S. H., 1931. J. Parasit. 18:79-91.

————, 1933. Tr. Am. Micr. Soc. 52:147-149.

————, 1934a. Ill. Biol. Monog. 13(2):1-80.

————, 1934b. Science n. s. 79:385-386.

————, 1937. J. Parasit. 23:94-97.

————, 1941. J. Parasit. 27:395-407.

HORSFALL, M. W., 1933. Science n. s. 78:175-176.

————, 1934. Tr. Am. Micr. Soc. 53:311-347.

————, 1935. Proc. Helm. Soc. Wash. 2:78-79.

HSÜ, D. Y. M., 1937. Tr. Am. Micr. Soc. 56:478-504.

HUGGHINS, E. J., 1954. Tr. Am. Micr. Soc. 73:1-15; 221-236.

HUGHES, R. C. and P. G. BERKHOUT, 1929. Pap. Mich. Acad. Sci., Arts, Letters 10:483-488.

HUNNINEN, A. V. and R. M. CABLE, 1941. Biol. Bull. 80:415-428.

————, 1943a. Tr. Am. Micr. Soc. 62:57-68.

————, 1943b. J. Parasit. 29:71-79.

————, 1934. J. Parasit. 20:325.

INGLES, L. G., 1933. Univ. Calif. Publ. Zool. 39:163-178.

————, 1935. Tr. Am. Micr. Soc. 54:19-21.

IZIUMOVA, N. A., 1956. Parasit. Sborn. Zool. Inst. Akad. Nauk. S. S. S. R. 16:229-243.

————, 1959. Parasit. Sborn. Zool. Inst. Akad. Nauk. S. S. S. R. 18:295-303.

JAHN, T. L. and L. R. KUHN, 1932. Biol. Bull. 62:89-111.

JAMES, B. L., 1964. Parasitology 54:1-41.

JOHNSTON, T. H. and L. M. ANGEL, 1951. Tr. Roy. Soc. S. Austral. 74: 66-78.

JORDAN, H. E., 1963. Dissertation Abstracts 23:4472-4473.

JORDAN, H. E. and E. E. BYRD, 1967. Tr. Am. Micr. Soc. 86:67.

KAGAN, I. G., 1951. Tr. Am. Micr. Soc. 70:281-318.

————, 1952a. Tr. Am. Micr. Soc. 71:20-44.

————, 1952b. Am. Midl. Nat. 48:257-301.

————, 1953. J. Inf. Dis. 93:200-206.

KATHERINER, L., 1904. Zool. Jahrb. Suppl. 7 Festschr. 70 Geburtst. A. Weismann 7:519-550.

KEARN, G. C., 1963. Parasitology 53:253-263.

KELLY, H. M., 1926. Proc. Iowa Acad. Sci. 33:339.

KINGSTON, N., 1965. Can. J. Zool. 43:745-764.

KNIGHT, R. A. and I. PRATT, 1955. J. Parasit. 41:248-255.

KNISKERN, V. B., 1952. Tr. Am. Micr. Soc. 71:317-340.

KRULL, W. H., 1931. Tr. Am. Micr. Soc. 50:215-277.

————, 1933. J. Parasit. 20:109.

————, 1934a. J. Wash. Acad. Sci. 24:483-485.

————, 1934b. Proc. Helm. Soc. Wash. 1:5.

————, 1934c. Tr. Am. Micr. Soc. 53:408-415.

————, 1934d. J. Parasit. 20:326-327.

————, 1935a. Tr. Am. Micr. Soc. 54:118-134.

————, 1935b. Parasitology 27:93-100.

————, 1935c. Proc. Helm. Soc. Wash. 2:77.

————, 1935d. Pap. Mich. Acad. Sci., Arts, Letters 20:697-710.

————, 1936. Proc. Helm. Soc. Wash. 3:56-58.

————, 1937. Proc. Helm. Soc. Wash. 4:75-78.

KRULL, W. H. and C. MAPES, 1952. Cornell Vet. 42:253-285; 339-351; 464-489; 603-604.

————, 1953. Cornell Vet. 43:199-202; 389-410.

KRULL, W. H. and H. F. PRICE, 1932. Occ. Pap. Mus. Zool. U. Mich. 237:1-38.

KULWIEC, Z., 1929. Arch. Hydrobiol. Rybact. 4:277-281.

LANG, B. Z., 1968. J. Parasit. 54:945-949.

LANG, B. Z. and L. N. GLEASON, 1967. J. Parasit. 53:93.

LA RUE, G. R., 1957. Exp. Parasit. 6:306-349.

LAUTENSCHLAGER, E. W. and T. C. CHENG, 1958. Tr. Am. Micr. Soc. 77:451-454.

LEE, H. F., 1962. J. Parasit. 48:728-739.

LEIGH, W. H., 1946. Am. Midl. Nat. 35:460-483.

————, 1954. J. Parasit. 40(Sect. 2):45.

————, 1958. J. Parasit. 44:379-387.

LEIGH, W. H. and R. B. HOLLIMAN, 1956. J. Parasit. 42:400-407.

LEUCKART, R., 1882. Arch. Naturgesch. 48:80-119.

LEZOTTE, L. A. JR., 1954. J. Parasit. 40:148-162.

LINTON, E., 1910. Carn. Inst. Wash. Publ. 133:11-98.

————, 1928. Proc. U. S. Nat. Mus. 73 (Art. 1):1-36.

————, 1940. Proc. U. S. Nat. Mus. 88(3078):1-172.

LITTLE, P. A., 1930. Parasitology 22:399-413.

LLOYD, L. C., 1938. J. Parasit. 24:103-133.

LUHMAN, M., 1935. J. Parasit. 21:274-276.

LUNDAHL, W. S., 1941. Tr. Am. Micr. Soc. 60:461-484.

LYNCH, J. E., 1933. Quar. J. Micr. Sci. n. s. 76:13-33.

MACCALLUM, G. A., 1913. Zbl. Bakt. Abt. 1. Orig. 68:335-337.

————, 1917. Zoopathologica 1:43-75.

McCOY, O. R., 1927. J. Parasit. 14:127-128.

————, 1929. Parasitology 21:220-225.

————, 1930. J. Parasit. 17:1-13.

McINTOSH, A., 1932. J. Parasit. 19:32-53.

————, 1934a. Parasitology 26:463-467.

————, 1934b. Proc. Helm. Soc. Wash. 1:2-4.

————, 1935. J. Parasit. 21:53-55.

————, 1937. Proc. Helm. Soc. Wash. 4:21-23.

McLEOD, J. A., 1937. J. Parasit. 23:456-466.

————, 1940. Can. J. Res. Sect. D. 18:1-28.

McLEOD, J. A. and G. E. LITTLE, 1942. Can. J. Res. Sect. D. 20:170-181.

McMULLEN, D. B., 1934. J. Parasit. 20:248-250.

————, 1935a. J. Parasit. 21:52-53.

————, 1935b. J. Parasit. 21:369-380.

————, 1936. J. Parasit. 22:295-298.

————, 1937. J. Parasit. 23:235-243.

McMULLEN, D. B. and P. C. BEAVER, 1945. Am. J. Hyg. 42:128-154.
MACY, R. W., 1931. J. Parasit. 18:28-33.
————, 1933. Tr. Am. Micr. Soc. 52:247-254.
————, 1934. Univ. Minn. Agr. Exp. Sta. Tech. Bull. #98:71 pp.
————, 1939. J. Parasit. 25:281.
————, 1940a. J. Parasit. 26:279-286.
————, 1940b. Proc. Minn. Acad. Sci. 8:39-41.
————, 1960a. J. Parasit. 46:662.
————, 1960b. J. Parasit. 46:337-345.
————, 1964. J. Parasit. 50:564-568.
MACY, R. W. and W. D. BELL, 1968. J. Parasit. 54:761-764.
———— and J. R. FORD, 1964. J. Parasit. 50:93.
———— and D. J. MOORE, 1954. J. Parasit. 40:328-335.
———— and ————, 1958. Tr. Am. Micr. Soc. 77:396-403.
MAGATH, T. B., 1918. J. Parasit. 4:58-69.
MALDONADO, J. F., 1945. J. Parasit. 31:306-314.
MANTER, H. W., 1925. J. Parasit. 12:11-18.
————, 1931. Parasitology 23:396-411.
————, 1934a. Carn. Inst. Wash. Pap. Tortugas Lab. 28:167-180.
————, 1934b. Carn. Inst. Wash. Pap. Tortugas Lab. 28:257-345.
————, 1940a. Rep. Allan Hancock Pacific Exped. 2(14):325-497.
————, 1940b. Carn. Inst. Wash. Pap. Tortugas Lab. 33:1-19.
————, 1942. Tr. Am. Micr. Soc. 61:349-360.
————, 1944. J. Wash. Acad. Sci. 34:86-89.
————, 1947. Am. Midl. Nat. 38:257-416.
————, 1949. Am. Midl. Nat. 41:432-435.
————, 1954. Tr. Roy. Soc. N. Zealand 82:475-568.
MANTER, H. W. and H. J. VanCLEAVE, 1951. Proc. U. S. Nat. Mus. 101(3279):315-340.
MAPES, C. R., 1951. Cornell Vet. 41:382-432.
MAPES, C. R. and W. H. KRULL, 1951. Cornell Vet. 41:433-444.
MARGOLIS, L. and G. C. PIKE, 1955. J. Fish Res. Bd. Canada 12:97-120.
MARKELL, E. K., 1953. J. Parasit. 39:45-51.
MARSHALL, W. S. and N. C. GILBERT, 1905. Zool. Jahrb. Syst. 22:477-488.
MARTIN, W. E., 1938. Biol. Bull. 75:463-474.
————, 1939a. Biol. Bull. 77:65-73.
————, 1939b. J. Parasit. 25(Sect. 2):18.
————, 1940. Biol. Bull. 79:131-144.
————, 1950a. J. Parasit. 36:552-558.
————, 1950b. Tr. Am. Micr. Soc. 69:194-209.
————, 1950c. J. Parasit. 36:360-370.
————, 1951. J. Parasit. 37:297-300.
————, 1956. Tr. Am. Micr. Soc. 75:117-128.
————, 1964. Tr. Am. Micr. Soc. 83:270-272.
MARTIN, W. E. and J. E. ADAMS, 1961. J. Parasit. 47:777-782.
———— and J. W. BAMBERGER, 1952. J. Parasit. 38:105-110.
MATHIAS, P., 1925. Bull. Biol. France et Belgique 59:1-123.
MEADE, T. G. and I. PRATT, 1965. J. Parasit. 51:575-578.
MENZIES, R. J., 1946. J. Parasit. 32:428-430.

MILLER, J. H., 1954. J. Parasit. 40:255-270.
MILLER, M. J., 1940. Can. J. Res. Sect. D. 18:333-335; 423-434.
————, 1941. J. Parasit. 27(Sect. 2):12.
————, 1946. Can. J. Res. Sect. D. 24:27-29.
MIZELLE, J. D. and V. BLATZ, 1941. Am. Midl. Nat. 26:105-109.
————, and SR. M. A. DONAHUE, 1944. Am. Midl. Nat. 31:600-624.
MOROZOV, F. N. in K. I. SKRJABIN, 1952. Trematodes of Animals and Man 6:153-615.
MUELLER, J. F., 1934. Roosevelt Wild Life Annals 3:335-373.
————, 1936. Tr. Am. Micr. Soc. 55:55-72; 457-464.
————, 1938. Am. Midl. Nat. 19:220-235.
MURRELL, K. D., 1963. J. Parasit. 49:116.
————, 1965. J. Parasit. 51:600-604.
MYER, D. G., 1960. J. Parasit. 46:819-832.
NAJARIAN, H. H., 1953. Science n. s. 117:564-565.
————, 1954. J. Morph. 94:165-197.
————, 1961. J. Parasit. 47:625-634.
NAJIM, A. T., 1950. J. Parasit. 36(Sect. 2):19.
NICKERSON, W. S., 1902. Zool. Jahrb. Syst. 15:597-624.
NIGRELLI, R. F., 1939. Tr. Am. Micr. Soc. 58:170-178.
NOBLE, A. E. and J. T. PARK, 1937. Tr. Am. Micr. Soc. 56:344-347.
NORRIS, G. R. 1945. Doctoral Dissert. Ohio State Univ. No. 65:527-528.
OCHI, S., 1930. Okayama Igakkai Zasshi 42:388-402.
ODHNER, T., 1902 Zbl. Bakt. Abt. 1. Orig. 31:58-69; 152-162.
OGATA, T., 1934. Sci. Rep. Tokyo Bunrika Daigaku 2(B):45-53.
OLIVIER, L. J., 1940. J. Parasit. 26:447-477.
OLSEN, O. W., 1937a. Tr. Am. Micr. Soc. 56:311-339.
————, 1937b. J. Parasit. 23:13-28.
————, 1940. Zoologica 25:323-328.
OSBORN, H. L., 1903. J. Morph. 18:1-44.
————, 1905. Zool. Jahrb. Anat. 21:201-242.
OWEN, H. M., 1946. J. Parasit. 32:553-562.
PALOMBI, A., 1930. Publ. Staz. Zool., Napoli 10:111-149.
————, 1931. Boll. Zool. Torino 2:165-171.
————, 1934a. Publ. Staz. Zool., Napoli 13:438-478.
————, 1934b. Publ. Staz. Zool., Napoli 14:51-94.
————, 1937. Riv. Parassit. Roma 1:1-12.
————, 1949. Arch. Zool. Torino 34:203-408.
PAPERNA, I., 1963. Bamidgeh, Bull. Fish Culture Israel 15:8-28.
PARK, J. T., 1936. Tr. Am. Micr. Soc. 55:360-365.
PATTEN, J. A., 1952. J. Parasit. 38:165-182.
PAUL, A. A., 1938. J. Parasit. 24:489-510.
PEARSE, A. S., 1949. Proc. U. S. Nat. Mus. 100(3255):25-38.
PEARSON, J. C., 1956. Can. J. Zool. 34:295-387.
————, 1959. J. Parasit. 45:155-174.
————, 1961. Parasitology 51:133-172.
PENNER, L. R. and B. FRIED, 1963. J. Parasit. 49:974-977.
PERKINS, K. W., 1950. J. Parasit. 36(Sect. 2):27.
PETERS, L. E. JR., 1955. J. Parasit. 41(Sect. 2):36.
————, 1961. Am. Midl. Nat. 65:436-445.

PRATT, H. S., 1914. Arch. Parasitologie 16:411-427.
PREVOT, G., 1966. Ann. Parasit. 41:233-242.
PRICE, E. W., 1929. Proc. U. S. Nat. Mus. 75(Art. 18):1-39.
————, 1931. Proc. U. S. Nat. Mus. 79(Art. 17):1-6.
————, 1932. Proc. U. S. Nat. Mus. 81(Art. 13):1-68.
————, 1934. Proc. Helm. Soc. Wash. 1:1-2.
————, 1936a. Proc. Helm. Soc. Wash. 3:31-32.
————, 1936b. Proc. Helm. Soc. Wash. 3:32-34.
————, 1937. J. Wash. Acad. Sci. 27:114-130; 146-164.
————, 1938a. Proc. Helm. Soc. Wash. 5:48-49.
————, 1938b. J. Wash. Acad. Sci. 28:109-126; 183-198.
————, 1939a. J. Wash. Acad. Sci. 29:63-92.
————, 1939b. Proc. Helm. Soc. Wash. 6:80-92.
————, 1942. Proc. Helm. Soc. Wash. 9:39-56.
————, 1943a. J. Wash. Acad. Sci. 33:44-54.
————, 1943b. Proc. Helm. Soc. Wash. 10:10-15.
————, 1961a. Proc. Helm. Soc. Wash. 28:4-9.
————, 1961b. Proc. Biol. Soc. Wash. 74:127-156.
————, 1962a. Proc. Helm. Soc. Wash. 29:1-18.
————, 1962b. J. Parasit. 48:402-418.
PRICE, H. F., 1931. Am. J. Hyg. 13:685-727.
RALPH, P. H., 1938. Tr. Am. Micr. Soc. 57:376-382.
RANKIN, J. S. JR. 1939a. Am. Midl. Nat. 21:476-488.
————, 1939b. Tr. Am. Micr. Soc. 58:431-447.
————, 1940. Biol. Bull. 79:439-451.
————, 1944. Tr. Am. Micr. Soc. 63:30-43.
REMLEY, L. W., 1942. Tr. Am. Micr. Soc. 61:141-155.
REYNOLDS, B. D., 1938. Parasitology 30:320-323.
ROBINSON, H. W., 1952. J. Parasit. 38:368.
RODGERS, L. O., 1941. J. Parasit. 27:153-157.
————, and R. E. KUNTZ, 1940. Wasmann Collector 4:37-40.
ROWAN, W. B., 1955. Tr. Am. Micr. Soc. 74:1-21.
SCHELL, S. C., 1962. Tr. Am. Micr. Soc. 81:137-146.
————, 1965. J. Parasit. 51:587-593.
————, 1967a. J. Parasit. 53:569-576.
————, 1967b. J. Parasit. 53:1000-1004.
SCHEURING, L., 1922. Zool. Jahrb. Anat. 44:265-310.
SCHILLER, E. L., 1959. Tr. Am. Micr. Soc. 78:65-76.
SCHROEDER, R. E. and W. H. LEIGH, 1965. J. Parasit. 51:594-599.
SEITNER, P. G., 1951. J. Parasit. 37:223-244.
SELF, J. T., L. E. PETERS and C. E. DAVIS, 1963. J. Parasit. 49:731-736.
SHIBUE, H., 1951. Jap. Med. J. 4:315-324.
SILLMAN, E. I., 1953. J. Parasit. 39(Sect. 2):21.
————, 1962. Tr. Am. Micr. Soc. 81:43-65.
SINITZIN, D. F., 1931. Zschr. Parasitenk. 3:786-835.
SMITH, R. J., 1967. J. Parasit. 53:287-291.
————, 1968. J. Parasit. 54:283-285.
SOGANDARES-BERNAL, F. and R. D. LUMSDEN, 1963. J. Parasit. 49:264-274.
SPROSTEN, N. G., 1946. Tr. Zool. Soc. London 25:185-600.

STANG, J. C. and R. M. CABLE, 1966. Am. Midl. Nat. 75:404-415.
STUNKARD, H. W., 1928. Ann. Parasit. 6:303-320.
————, 1930. J. Morph. Physiol. 50:143-191.
————, 1934. Bull. Soc. Zool. France 59:447-466.
————, 1935. J. Parasit. 21:359-364.
————, 1936. J. Parasit. 22:354-374.
————, 1938a. Biol. Bull. 75:145-164.
————, 1938b. Biol. Bull. 75:308-334.
————, 1940. J. Parasit. 26(Sect. 2): 33-34.
————, 1943. Biol. Bull. 85:227-237.
————, 1958. J. Parasit. 44:225-230.
————, 1959. Biol. Bull. 117:562-581.
————, 1961. Biol. Bull. 120:221-237.
————, 1964a. Biol. Bull. 126:163-173.
————, 1964b. Biol. Bull. 126:467-489.
STUNKARD, H. W. and R. M. CABLE, 1932. Biol. Bull. 62:328-338.
———— and M. C. HINCHCLIFFE, 1951. Anat. Rec. 111:529-530.
———— and ————, 1952. J. Parasit. 38:248-265.
————, C. H. WILLEY and Y. RABINOWITZ, 1941. Tr. Am. Micr. Soc. 60:485-497.
SZIDAT, L. 1931. Zschr. Parasitenk. 3:160-172.
————, 1937. Zschr. Parasitenk. 9:529-542.
————, 1939. Zschr. Parasitenk. 11:239-283.
————, 1962. Zschr. Parasitenk. 22:196-213.
TALBOT, S. B., 1933. Parasitology 25:518-545.
TENNENT, D. H., 1906. Quar. J. Micr. Sci. n. s. 49:635-690.
THOMAS, A. P. W., 1883. Quar. J. Micr. Sci. n. s. 23:99-133.
THOMAS, L. J., 1939. J. Parasit. 25:207-221.
TRAVASSOS, L., 1944. Monog. Inst. Oswaldo Cruz 2:357 pp.
TRIPATHI, Y. R., 1957. Indian J. Helm. 7:5-22.
————, 1959. Indian J. Helm. 9:1-149.
ULMER, M. J., 1951. Tr. Am. Micr. Soc. 70:189-238; 319-347.
————, 1952. Anat. Rec. 113:613-614.
————, 1960. J. Parasit. 46:813-814.
VANCLEAVE, H. J., 1922. Proc. U. S. Nat. Mus. 61(Art. 9):1-8.
———— and J. F. MUELLER, 1932. Roosevelt Wild Life Annals 3:5-71.
———— and ————, 1934. Roosevelt Wild Life Annals 3:161-334.
VAN HAITSMA, J. P., 1931. Pap. Mich. Acad. Sci., Arts, Letters 13:447-516.
VENARD, C. E., 1941. J. Tenn. Acad. Sci. 16:379-383.
VERNBERG, W. B., 1952. J. Parasit. 38:327-340.
VILLELLA, J. B., 1953a. J. Parasit. 39(Sect. 2):20.
————, 1953b. J. Parasit. 39(Sect. 2):21.
————, 1954. J. Parasit. 40:470-472.
WALKER, J. H., 1937. Proc. Soc. Exp. Biol. Med. 37:245-248.
————, 1939. Tr. Am. Micr. Soc. 58:404-430.
WALL, L. D., 1951. Tr. Am. Micr. Soc. 70:173-184.
WALLACE, F. G., 1935. J. Parasit. 21:143-164.
————, 1940. J. Parasit. 26(Sect. 2):37.
———— and L. R. PENNER, 1939. J. Parasit. 25:437-440.

WALLACE, H. E., 1941. Tr. Am. Micr. Soc. 60:309-326.
WARD, H. B. and S. H. HOPKINS, 1931. J. Parasit. 18:69-78.
WEST, A. F., 1961. Am. Midl. Nat. 66:363-383.
WETZEL, R., 1930. Proc. U. S. Nat. Mus. 78(Art. 3):1-4.
WHARTON, G. W., 1940. J. Parasit. 26:497-518.
WILLEY, C. H., 1930. Anat. Rec. 47:364.
————, 1936. J. Parasit. 22:68-75.
————, 1941. Zoologica 26:65-88.
WILLIAMS, C. O., 1942. J. Parasit. 28:467-475.
WILLIAMS, R. R., 1960. Ohio J. Sci. 60:323-326.
WISNIEWSKI, W. L., 1958. Acta Parasit. Polon. 6:289-307.
WOLFGANG, R. W., 1955. Can. J. Zool. 33:113-128.
WOODHEAD, A. E., 1929. Tr. Am. Micr. Soc. 48:256-275.
————, 1930. Tr. Am. Micr. Soc. 49:1-17.
WOOTTON, D. M., 1957. Biol. Bull. 113;302-315.
WUNDER, W., 1926. Biol. Zbl. 46:748-755.
————, 1929. Zschr. Fischerei Neudamn Berlin 27:511-545.
YAMAGUTI, S., 1937. J. Parasit. 23:431-432.
————, 1938. Jap. J. Zool. 7:609-611.
YOUNG, R. T., 1953. J. Wash. Acad. Sci. 43:88-93.
ZELLER, E., 1872. Zschr. Wiss. Zool. 22:1-28.
————, 1876. Zschr. Wiss. Zool. 27:238-274.

INDEX AND PICTURED GLOSSARY

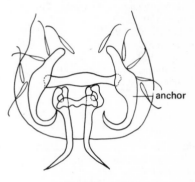

Fig. 673. Anchor

343

B

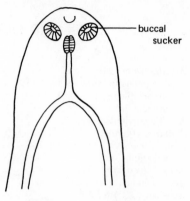

Fig. 674.　Buccal sucker

C

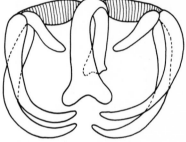

Fig. 675. Clamp

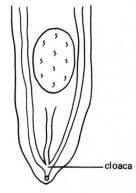

Fig. 676. Cloaca

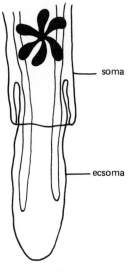

Fig. 677. Ecsoma

F

G

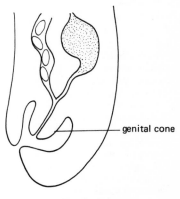

Fig. 678. Genital cone

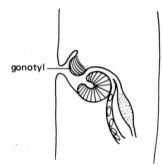

gonotyl

Fig. 679. Gonotyl

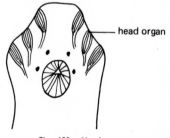

head organ

Fig. 680. Head organ

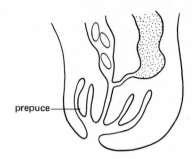

Fig. 681. Prepuce

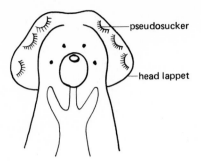

Fig. 682. Pseudosucker

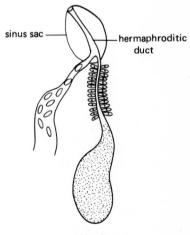

Fig. 683. Sinus sac

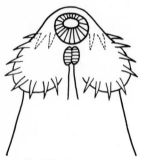

Fig. 684. Spiny collar

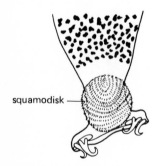

squamodisk

Fig. 685. Squamodisk